Storytelling, Narrative,
and the Thematic Apperception Test

CLINICAL PSYCHOLOGY
A Guilford Series

STORYTELLING, NARRATIVE, AND
THE THEMATIC APPERCEPTION TEST
Phebe Cramer

Forthcoming

ASSESSMENT OF UNCONSCIOUS PROCESSING
Joel Weinberger

STORYTELLING, NARRATIVE, AND THE THEMATIC APPERCEPTION TEST

PHEBE CRAMER

THE GUILFORD PRESS
New York   London

© 1996 The Guilford Press
A Division of Guilford Publications, Inc.
72 Spring Street, New York, NY 10012

Printed in the United States of America

This book is printed on acid-free paper.

Last digit is print number: 9 8 7 6 5 4 3 2 1

Library of Congress Cataloging-in-Publication Data
Cramer, Phebe.
   Storytelling, narrative, and the thematic aperception test / Phebe Cramer.
      p. cm. — (Assessment of personality and psychopathology)
   Includes biographical references and index.
   ISBN 1-57230-094-9
   1. Thematic Apperception Test. I. Title. II Series.
RC473.T48C73   1996
616.89′075—dc20   96-5520
                                              CIP

Preface

Storytelling occurs all over the world, at every age of life. Stories may refer to historical events, be fantastic, purposely deceptive, or educational. They entertain, instruct, amuse, and comfort. Characteristically, they convey some intention, some explanation, some theme that adds to our understanding of life.

The increasing interest in the narrative form of thought recognizes the importance of stories for understanding human nature. Our personal history consists not only of biographical "facts." Rather, it is the way in which these facts are strung together, the context in which they are placed, and the intermingling of cause and effect that gives a unique construction to each individual life. In this sense, each life is a constructed story, not reducible to historical fact.

From this vantage point, stories provide abundant material for studying the human psyche. They allow us to enter into the complex patterns, textures, tangents, and byways that constitute each individual. This book discusses some of these patterns and offers systematic approaches for their exploration.

One of the greater pleasures I experience as a college professor is the surprise and amazement that students express when they discover themselves in their own stories written for the Thematic Apperception Test (TAT). Typically, they enter my class in Personality Assessment with a preformed opinion regarding the TAT. This opinion is one of skepticism or outright disbelief that such an "unscientific" procedure could provide any important information. In one of the first exercises of the class, I ask the students to write out several TAT stories. Despite their skepticism, most students take this assignment seriously and make an effort to create a variety of stories. Some time later, in a different context, I ask them to write a brief autobiography. When this has been completed, I ask them to compare the story protocols with the autobiography and to note any consistent or recurring themes in the two documents. Most students are astonished to discover how self-revealing they have been in their original stories. Their experience is something like, "I can't believe I said that and didn't know I was saying it!" For many of them, this is a significant, mind-expanding moment, lifting the veil of "objectivity" that has impeded their vision for some time.

Attitudes toward the validity of the TAT are shifting in the academic research front, as well. In a review of more than 100 published research articles on the TAT (Spangler, 1992), the predictive validity of the TAT-based measure of achievement motivation was compared with that of questionnaire methods. Using the technique of meta-analysis to summarize the results of these studies, findings obtained from more than 15,000 subjects were analyzed. This very thorough study showed that, on average, the TAT measure of achievement motivation was successful in predicting various outcome measures, and that the predictive validity of the TAT measure was stronger than that based on questionnaire methods. Especially important were the findings that the TAT was most successful in predicting outcome when this involved long-term behavioral trends, such as career success, while self-report questionnaires were more successful in predicting short-term choice behavior. The thoroughness and sophistication of this recent analysis should put to rest earlier criticisms regarding the predictive value of the TAT-based measure (e.g., Entwisle, 1972).

The invitation to write this book, and to present new ideas and approaches to the understanding of storytelling, came from Sidney J. Blatt, friend and colleague, and Seymour Weingarten, Editor-in-Chief of the Guilford Press. I thank them for providing this opportunity. I am also indebted to Richard Q. Ford and Anne de Gersdorff for providing materials discussed in Section III of the book. Earlier discussions with Robert May enhanced my understanding of his approach to the exploration of gender identity. Susan Engel was especially helpful with discussions of the narrative approach to psychological understanding. My thanks also to the reference librarians of the Sawyer Library at Williams College for unfailing assistance in locating materials, information, and references. Finally, I thank my daughters, Mara and Julia, with whom I have shared many stories.

Contents

Section I
ORIGINS OF THE THEMATIC APPERCEPTION TEST

One	Introduction	3
Two	The TAT	9

Section II
INTERPRETATION OF THE TAT

Three	Narrative and Storytelling	21
Four	Context and Storytelling	36
Five	The TAT and the Life Story Narrative	50
Six	Gender Identity: An Interpretive Perspective	70
Seven	Defense Mechanisms: Another Intepretive Perspective	84

Section III
STUDIES OF CLINICAL PATIENTS

Eight	The Storyteller's Narrative	103
Nine	The Anaclitic/Introjective Perspective: Two Personality Organizations	130
Ten	The Intepreter's Perspective: TAT and Psychopathology	153

Section IV
CHANGING NARRATIVES:
STUDIES OF NORMAL DEVELOPMENT

Eleven   Developmental Differences in TAT Stories: 179
              Children and Adolescents
Twelve   Developmental Differences in Adult TAT Stories   210

Section V
RESEARCH ISSUES WITH THE TAT

Thirteen   General Issues in TAT Research   233
Fourteen   Questions of Reliability and Validity   250
Fifteen   The TAT in Personality Research Today   270
Sixteen   The TAT in Clinical Research Studies: 295
               Further Examples
Seventeen Conclusion   319

               Notes   323
               References   341
               Index   363

Storytelling, Narrative,
and the Thematic Apperception Test

• SECTION I •

ORIGINS
OF THE THEMATIC
APPERCEPTION TEST

• ONE •

Introduction

Storytelling has a long tradition in human history. The famous epic poems—the *Iliad* and the *Odyssey* from the ninth century B.C., the *Aeneid* (20 B.C.), the East Indian *Mahabharata* and *Ramayana* (fourth century A.D.) and the Norse Sagas from the 13th century A.D., in company with the Bible's 39 Old Testament books (13th–first century B.C.) and 27 New Testament books (first century A.D.), have been the significant means by which man told "his-story," recording for posterity the oral legends that had been recounted for many years to willing listeners. In this way, history was known within one generation and was communicated from one generation to the next. That there were embellishments and modifications, exaggerations, and omissions from what may have been the "factual" events is largely irrelevant. The story, as it was presented, was the storyteller's way to introduce a truth about the cultural identity of those who heard the story—a psychological truth, a moral truth, and an intellectual truth. The culture and character of the Greeks, who listened to Homer's stories, were portrayed for them in the representation of the world described in the *Iliad* and the *Odyssey*. The *Aeneid* provided a glorification of their culture to the Romans, thus serving a nationalistic purpose. The Indian epic poems, including the *Bhagavadgita*, were a rich source book of Hindu life, legend, and thought, while the Norse sagas kept alive the persons and events that shaped the Northern world. The Bible continues to inform the lives of millions of people today. As noted in the current century by Henry Murray, the father of storytelling in contemporary psychology, "The soul of a people is mirrored in their legends" (1938, p. 728).

Recently, psychology has taken a new interest in stories, or narratives. It has been suggested that storytelling is used to construct *meaning* in our lives (see, e.g., Howard, 1991). The particular meaning one gives to an experience will be shaped by the story one uses to explain its occurrence. Those who employ a scientific story may well find a different meaning

3

from those who invoke a religious or a historical story. From this perspective, *culture* may be conceptualized in terms of a group of individuals who share common stories to interpret and provide meaning to their lives. In this context, education becomes a process of initiating young people into the dominant stories of their culture. These stories make an important contribution to establishing the identity of a culture (Howard, 1991).

On the individual level as well, identity is related to storytelling. It has been suggested that identity may be conceptualized as a life story which the individual constructs for him- or herself, consciously or unconsciously (McAdams, 1988a). The construction of the individual's story will be influenced by the dominant stories of the culture, but which of these stories are chosen (e.g., scientific or religious), and which roles in the stories are identified with, will contribute to the ultimate uniqueness of each individual's life story. Both existing stories and stories newly constructed provide meaning to life. It is by living in and through the chosen and the constructed story that life becomes meaningful.

Children, too, find out about the world through stories.[1] Whether it is the amusing antics of Curious George or the immersion into the imaginative world of Narnia,[2] dimensions of psychological reality are revealed to those who are yet too young to make their own discoveries through action in the real world. And how early society uses stories to inculcate the stereotypical myths in children: Cinderella, whose dreary, abused, and self-sacrificing life is rewarded by the appearance of Prince Charming; Tom Sawyer, who escapes the respectable world of adults to live free, but ultimately returns because his conscience will not allow an innocent man to be wrongly punished; Huckleberry Finn, who has no place in the respectable adult world but learns about the value of all human life, including that of a runaway slave; Mary Poppins, who embodies the mysterious secrets and magical powers of the as yet incomprehensible adult world; and even Winnie the Pooh and friends, who present to the child universally recognizable human character types in animal form. These, and many others, are the stories that have created the schema in children's minds about the human condition.

Today, there is another storyteller who shapes reality for children, with stories in which people are bashed, sliced, tortured, and blown up but rise again, as did the Phoenix, only somewhat the worse for having been so brutalized. These are stories in which cars travel at incredible rates of speed, leave the ground to soar over rivers, navigate mountain roads on two wheels, and crash into tractor-trailers, only to have the occupants emerge unscathed and walk away. Such is the reality of stories today, as told by the television set, videocassettes, and the movies absorbed by hundreds of thousands of children.[3] These stories also present a schema for children in which the world is understood to be a place where

the occurrence of unbridled aggression and violence without consequence is the norm. The disastrous enactment of these schemas in real
life by some children is a tragic demonstration of the importance of
stories in the child's development.[4]

As much as being a recipient of stories, we are also storytellers. We
tell each other stories about what happened in the past, what happened
today, and what we hope might happen in the future. Sometimes, we tell
the same story again, an occurrence that often increases as we get older.
Sometimes the details of the story change, and even the characters may
vary from one telling to the next. But the stories continue, one generation
to the next.

Each story is one person's explanation of his or her psychological
reality. Although individual realities often overlap to a considerable extent,
each story is also personally unique. Nowhere is this better and more
beautifully illustrated than in the enticing dramas of Lawrence Durrell's
Alexandria Quartet, or in the shocking, blatant discrepancies among the
storytellers of Kurosawa's film *Rashomon*. In life, the story of each person—
the story that he or she tells—is unique; it is like no one else's story.

If this is true—that each story is a unique, individual expression—it is
not surprising that some psychologists look to the narrative as a prime
and singular source of information about the individual who has created
the tale. In the themes, but also in the nuances, the subtleties, and the
omissions, the life schema carried about by that individual is manifest. In
describing what has happened, or what may happen, each individual will
formulate a story guided by a schema that is harbored within. To hear or
to read these stories is to be given a glimpse into the unique nature of a
person's psyche.

Psychotherapists are among those who listen to stories carefully,
concerned not so much for their veridicality with what "really happened"
but rather listening for the core theme that marks the stories as variants
on an underlying narrative—a personal representation of the individual's
experience and understanding of what life is about.[5]

Of course, there are those people who cannot, or will not tell stories.
Of those who refuse, it is probably safe to say that they have some inkling
that storytelling is self-revealing, and, for some reason, they do not wish
to expose themselves. When faced with a request to tell a story, they may
refuse altogether, or, more commonly, they may tell another person's
story—that is, they may respond with a stereotyped plot that has been
gleaned from the popular media or from a book they have read. The
telling of someone else's story informs us of something important—
namely, the defensiveness of the individual around self-revelation—but we
are kept at bay from discovering the particular life narrative of this person.
Not all people will tell us their story.

Of those who will, some will tell short stories, some will tell long stories, some will provide only the barest outline, while others will smother the structure in voluminous details and many side pathways. Some stories are characterized by multithematic complexity, whereas others are almost repetitively single-minded, as if to say, "See, this is what it is about!" in case we, the naive listener, might miss the point. Although it is said that a picture is worth a thousand words, it is probably also true that it takes a thousand words, at least, to present the schematic picture of life—the narrative—that each individual carries within.

This book is about a particular kind of storytelling. Known as the Thematic Apperception Test (TAT), and used by psychologists for nearly 60 years, the stories told by thousands and thousands of individuals about a small set of black-and-white pictures have formed the basis of intensive study by psychologists who believe that stories will reveal aspects of human nature that may otherwise remain unknown and silent. This systematic approach to storytelling has provided a method to investigate those original, highly personal themes that constitute the unique personality of each individual. The stories of the TAT are life's stories.

To understand the TAT, its own story should be known. This book attempts to tell that story. The history and development of the test are discussed in Chapter 2.

A story is a narrative, and the interest of social scientists in narrative as a means for representing experience has grown rapidly during recent years. The second section of the book explores the implications of the story as narrative. Although the term "narrative" may be used in different ways—for example, narrative may refer to the product or to the process involved in creating the product—it seems clear that TAT stories belong more to the realm of narrative thought than to positivist operationalism.

In the broadest sense, narrative may be considered a mode of communication used to represent experience. A description of this mode of thought, including its significance for the meaning of reality and truth, is discussed in Chapter 3. The idea that narrative must always be understood in context is further discussed in Chapter 4, and examples of the influence of context on storytelling are provided. The remaining three chapters in this section raise the issue of the interdependence of the storyteller's narrative and the story interpreter's narrative in the process of explicating TAT stories. In Chapter 5, the stories of college students are considered in terms of the individual story lines portrayed. The personal significance of these story lines is seen as they are related to similar narrative representations in the students' autobiographical sketches. In Chapter 6, an approach to interpretation of TAT stories, which is itself based on a narrative account of experience, is described. Here, the interpreter's narrative perspective—which is concerned with gender identity—is superimposed on the storyteller's narrative. From this interaction, or "dialogue," between the storyteller's and interpreter's narratives, a new perspective on the meaning of the story is created. This interpretive perspective is then applied to the stories of the college students discussed in the previous chapter, illustrating how an interpreter's narrative may enhance the meaning to be found in stories told. Research studies supporting the assumptions of this narrative approach are discussed at the end of the chapter.

The last chapter in this section presents another interpretive perspective—one that focuses on the use of defense mechanisms in the process of storytelling. The rationale behind this perspective is explained, research evidence is provided, and, again, the approach is applied to the stories of the college students, showing the rich potential of narrative stories for yielding multidimensional descriptions of personality.

The third section of the book is devoted to discussions of the use of the TAT with clinical patients. Chapter 8 provides a detailed discussion of two individuals, one female, one male, who are patients in a small, psychoanalytically oriented hospital. Clinical information from the therapists and from case conferences is presented along with the TAT stories these patients told at the time of admission to the hospital and after some months of treatment. Here, the patients' own story lines, and the change in their themes over time are discussed. In addition, the interpretive perspectives of gender identity and defense mechanisms are used to enhance our understanding of these patients and the changes that occur after a period of treatment.

Chapter 9 is also devoted to the study of clinical patients. Four individuals from the same psychiatric hospital were selected to illustrate how a particular form of personality organization is manifest in TAT stories. Two of these patients (one female, one male) show an anaclitic personality organization; two others (one female, one male) show an introjective personality organization.[6] The ways in which these different personality organizations are revealed in the narrative stories of these patients are illustrated. Again, the interpretive perspectives of gender identity and defense mechanisms are used to enhance the meaning derived from the stories.

Chapter 10 again focuses on different interpretive perspectives that are used to assess psychopathology in TAT stories. Themes that are frequently found in the stories of the borderline personality disorder and the narcissistic personality disorder are discussed and illustrations are provided. A new method for assessing borderline pathology, based on the developmental level of object representations in the TAT stories, is explicated and illustrated.

The fourth section of the book is devoted to a description of the ways in which narratives change with age. Chapter 11 discusses the use of the TAT with children and provides examples of stories from children of different ages, as well as demonstrations of how the same children's stories change as the children develop. Research information based on the TAT that shows the developmental changes that occur in gender identity, defense mechanisms, object relations, achievement motivation, and emotional stance is discussed. Chapter 12 focuses on developmental studies of older people, illustrating how adult narratives also change with age.

The fifth and final section of the book concentrates on the use of the TAT for research studies. As is true for all research, the well-crafted study is more likely to yield meaningful results; to accomplish such results, the researcher should be aware of factors that may confound or disrupt the study. Chapter 13 considers a few of these factors, such as the choice of TAT pictures and the influence of the length of stories told. Chapter 14 raises the issues of reliability and validity. Here, new approaches to these psychometric issues appropriate to narrative material are discussed. Chapter 15 discusses research using carefully developed coding schemes to assess the strength of motives and other personality dispositions, as revealed in TAT stories. Finally, Chapter 16 reviews a number of clinical research studies that have used the TAT to investigate both physical and psychological aspects of health and pathology.

Several reviews of the use of psychological tests by practicing clinicians indicate that the TAT continues to be one of the most widely used methods for clinical assessment. A search of published research abstracts[7] reveals that more than 1,000 studies using the TAT have been published between 1970 and 1995. This book includes many of these references, as well as a number of significant earlier publications. Clearly, the TAT continues to be an important instrument for clinicians and researchers. I hope that the new systematic approaches to interpretation and new understanding about the appropriate psychometric approaches for narrative material that are discussed in this book will enhance this valuable method for the study of the human psyche.

In telling this story about storytelling, one cannot but be impressed with the enormous number of stories that have been collected in research studies of individuals over the years. Some of these stories have been preserved and made available to other researchers[8]; others linger in old filing cabinets or displaced cardboard boxes. Unlike reams of numbers on data sheets, these stories contain revelations awaiting discovery; one hopes they will be preserved for future study.

TWO

The TAT

HISTORY

Prior to Morgan and Murray

Before the development of the TAT, there were several precedents in the academic literature for the use of storytelling as a means for understanding personality (Tomkins, 1947). Just after the turn of the century, two papers appeared which described the use of storytelling about a set of pictures as a technique for determining personality and developmental differences in boys and girls (Brittain, 1907; Libby, 1908). However, this approach remained in obscurity until 1932, when a psychiatrist working at a busy clinic made use of a standard set of eight pictures to carry out the assessment of juvenile delinquents with whom he did not have time to establish the rapport needed for successful interviewing (Schwartz, 1932).

Development of the TAT

Three years later, a paper describing the TAT was presented by Morgan and Murray (1935). Arising from a psychoanalytic context, the test was conceived of as a shortcut method to discovering the hidden fantasies of patients. The rationale for the test was based on two "facts": First, according to Morgan and Murray, when a person "attempts to interpret a complex social situation he is apt to tell as much about himself as he is about the phenomenon on which attention is focused"; and second, "a great deal of written fiction is the conscious or unconscious expression of the author's experiences or fantasies" (Morgan & Murray, 1935, p. 289). The mechanism that accounts for these two facts, said the authors, is projection, which is facilitated by the TAT procedure. "At such times the person is off his guard, since he believes that he is merely explaining objective occurrences" (p. 289). Also, the test instructions do not focus attention directly on the subject but, rather, stress an interest in the more abstract process of "creative imagination."

These two factors were perhaps made even more prominent in this first version of the TAT by certain differences in the instructions for that test, as compared to later versions. In the first presentation of the TAT, subjects were told that the TAT picture was to be used as the illustration (e.g., in a magazine or book) for the story the subject told,[1] thus putting greater emphasis on the role of the external stimulus in determining the subjects' responses. Also, in addition to describing the procedure as a test of creative imagination, the instructions for the first version told subjects that the TAT was a test of "literary imagination," thus stressing intellectual or esthetic factors somewhat removed from the subject's more personal concerns.

In developing the TAT, Morgan and Murray began with several hundred pictures which they presented to a number of subjects for storytelling. From this larger set, they selected 20 that elicited good stories. The main features of this final set of pictures were, first, that each picture should suggest a critical situation that might serve as a "trellis" to support the development of "every root fantasy" (Morgan & Murray, 1935, p. 290) and, second, that there be at least one character in the picture with whom the subject could identify. For this latter reason, separate pictures were needed for men and women, boys and girls, children, young adults, and elderly persons.

In an attempt to validate the assumption that stories told about the TAT would be a shortcut to discovering significant unconscious material, Morgan and Murray carried out a research study with 50 men ages 20 to 30. The stimulus pictures were administered individually.[2] After the storytelling was complete, the subjects were queried about the source of their fantasy material. From these inquiries, it appeared that the story material came from four sources: books and movies (i.e., the media); actual events in the lives of friends or family; personal experiences, either objective or subjective, in the subject's life; and the subject's conscious and unconscious fantasies. The last two categories served to validate the authors' assumption that TAT stories would provide personally meaning-ful material about the storyteller. The first two categories, although apparently derived from nonpersonal experiences—that is, apparently about persons other than the self—were also felt to have personal signifi-cance insofar as the subject selectively remembers, or chooses to report on, certain stories and events while ignoring others; those that are selected by the subject to report on are assumed to be personally meaningful.

Morgan and Murray stated that every single subject projected his or her own experiences or preoccupations onto the stories, and that some of the stories were obvious autobiographies. However, the authors felt it was not the possibility of eliciting autobiographical information that made the TAT important; that purpose is better served by direct questioning. Rather, they believed that the value of the TAT lay in its usefulness as a method to discover unconscious fantasies. Although the stories are given as conscious fantasies, "Like dreams, they must be interpreted if one is to arrive at the unconscious trends which determine them" (Morgan & Murray, 1935, p. 293).

As an aid in this interpretation, a conceptual scheme for classifying fantasies was outlined. The dynamic structure or plot of the fantasy was designated a *thema*, which consisted of three aspects (although not all aspects need be expressed in any one thema). The three important features were described as the driving motivational force in the subject, referred to as *need*; the objects (or group of objects) toward which or away from which the force is directed, referred to as the environmental *press*; and the *outcome* of the interaction of need and press, expressed in terms of a subjective feeling (e.g., satisfaction or dissatisfaction).

In their paper, Morgan and Murray presented two case studies, providing autobiographical material, TAT stories, and examples of their analyses of the thema in the stories. On the basis of these and other test results, they concluded that the TAT was a valid method for discovering personally relevant dynamic material a subject would not directly expose, as well as fantasies of which a subject may be entirely unconscious.

Explorations in Personality

Three years later, Murray's book *Explorations in Personality* was published (Murray, 1938). This work was a landmark in psychology, presenting both Murray's theory of personality and a model for personality assessment. Both were to influence the direction of the study of personality for years to come. The first half of the book, devoted to Murray's theory, provided detailed definitions, descriptions, and illustrations of 29 "needs" and 20 environmental "press" situations, each of the latter containing a number of subcategories. The other half of the book presented the 25 assessment procedures used at the Harvard Psychological Clinic to study a group of 28 Harvard students, young men chosen from the fields of arts and sciences by the Harvard Employment Office and paid for their time to participate in the assessment study.

A discussion of the TAT appears in three places in the second half of the book. As part of the first assessment procedure experienced by each student—a roundtable conference with several staff members—three pictures which were not part of the standard set of 20 were presented.[3]

This procedure, administered at first by Christiana Morgan and subsequently by Erik Homburger (Erikson), used the standard TAT instructions for storytelling. The subject's responses to these pictures were used to determine whether any subjects should be removed from the study; in fact, no subjects were removed.

The next discussion of the TAT in the book occurs when it is described as the 18th procedure used in the assessment battery. This description, written by Morgan and Murray, was largely based on the 1935 article (Murray, 1938, p. 530, footnote). However, a new case study is included, with autobiography and TAT stories, along with an analysis of the thema, needs, and press for each story. Three of the TAT pictures used are reproduced. These pictures are quite similar to their counterparts in the final published version of the test, but they are not identical, indicating that the pictures were redrawn after this assessment study.

The use of the TAT is illustrated for a third time in the extensive case study of Earnst (Murray, 1938, chapter 7). The section of this chapter that deals with the TAT was written by Christiana Morgan. Although many of the TAT stories are not given, the predominant thema, needs, and press are identified and discussed. The relationship between these TAT thema and those thema discerned from the autobiographical material makes clear again, as did the 1935 paper, that the theoretical model of thema = need + press → outcome might be applied equally well to life history information as to TAT stories.

As mentioned previously, this book provided the model for personality assessment that was to be used by psychologists in their selection of military personnel[4] and for the conduct of research studies[5] in years to come. Murray (1938, p. 705) felt that the development of the assessment method was the book's greatest contribution. Among the procedures used, Murray concluded that those designed to evoke imagery and fantasy (e.g., the TAT) produced the most significant data.

Toward the end of the book, Murray commented on the need for verification of some of the exciting hypotheses regarding personality dynamics that emerged from the analyses of TAT data. He stated that he looked forward to the development of the TAT into a standardized procedure for "the systematic investigation of covert mental processes" (p. 729). With regard to the question of verification (validity), Murray referred readers to his 1937 article, in which "several techniques of verification" (1938, p. 729) were tried out, after the completion of the assessment study.

In this later paper (Murray, 1937), three methods are mentioned which had actually been used in an attempt to validate TAT findings. The first method relies on "matching" the TAT protocols with results obtained from other tests or with biographical data obtained from the storytellers.

Murray reports that such matching was done successfully for 10 subjects. A second suggested method is to use the TAT to guess the occurrence of certain childhood experiences and then to determine the accuracy of this guess through an interview with the subject. A third method was to use the TAT results to make predictions about future behavior. For this purpose, the TAT stories of 15 Harvard subjects were used to predict their relative hypnotizability. The rank-order correlation between predicted hypnotizability and actual hypnotizability, which was established later, was quite good (rho = .72).

THE THEMATIC APPERCEPTION TEST

Following these publications on the TAT, the final version of the test, with an accompanying manual describing administration and scoring procedures, was published in 1943 by the Harvard University Press.

The Stimulus Cards

Prior to this published form, there had been three earlier versions of the stimulus pictures (Rapaport, Gill, & Schafer, 1946). The original set of pictures, used by Morgan and Murray, were apparently never available for general use outside the Harvard Psychological Clinic. A second set of pictures was produced at the Clinic and made available for general professional use.[6] These TAT cards, in a smaller-format photographed edition, included 10 pictures of males and females, 10 of males only, and 10 of females only. The third version of the TAT was a revised, big-format photographed edition produced by the Harvard Psychological Clinic. The fourth and final version was the Harvard University Press printed edition.[7]

The Harvard University Press edition of the TAT has been in use for nearly 50 years. It consists of 31 standard cards, one of which is blank. The remaining 30 cards are designated for use as follows: seven for boys and men, seven for girls and women, one each for boys alone, men alone, girls alone, women alone, boys and girls, and men and women. The remaining 10 cards are to be used by all individuals. Thus, a complete TAT would consist of 20 stimulus pictures for any one individual. In clinical practice, it is rare to administer all 20 cards; the use of 10 or less pictures is more common. A description of each of the 31 cards, along with an excellent discussion of the typical themes elicited, has been provided by Bellak (1975), Holt (1978), and Rapaport et al. (1946), among others. Other important aspects of the pictures, such as their form, complexity, and bizarreness, have been discussed by Henry (1956).

Method of Administration

The standard procedure for administering the TAT is presented in Murray's (1943) manual. After seating the subject in a chair, the examiner provides the following instructions:

> This is a test of imagination, one form of intelligence. I am going to show you some pictures, one at a time; and your task will be to make up as dramatic a story as you can for each. Tell what has led up to the event shown in the picture, describe what is happening at the moment, what the characters are feeling and thinking; and then give the outcome. Speak your thoughts as they come to your mind. Do you understand? Since you have fifty minutes for ten pictures, you can devote about five minutes to each story. Here is the first picture. (Murray, 1943, p. 3)

Murray's (1943) instructions suggest that each TAT card should be responded to for about 5 minutes, although many examiners do not adhere strictly to this interval, relying instead on the subject to indicate when his or her response is complete. A related issue is the length of time the stimulus picture should be presented to the storyteller, and whether the picture should remain in view throughout the storytelling or be removed after a stated interval. At a later date, Murray suggested that the picture should remain in view for only 10 seconds (see Bellak, 1975, p. 41); a study by Stang, Campus, and Wallach (1975) found that the rated pleasantness of 27 TAT pictures decreased in a linear fashion from a 10-second to a 60-second exposure duration.

When the subject has completed telling the story, if any parts of the original instructions have not been responded to, the examiner may ask the subject for the relevant information (e.g., "And how was the little boy feeling?"; "Then how does the story end?"). This kind of inquiry is generally done immediately after the story is told. Some examiners may make an additional inquiry after all the stories have been told, asking, for example, which picture/story the subject liked the best or least, and why, or inquiring about personal associations to the pictures/stories—as Morgan and Murray did in their original 1935 paper.[8]

For research purposes, the TAT is often administered to a group of subjects, all of whom write their stories at the same time. Atkinson (1958) has provided a standard format for group administration of the TAT.

The Projective Hypothesis

As described by Morgan and Murray (1935), the crux of the test lies in the assumption that subjects will project onto the stories their own needs, motives, expectancies, and anxieties—that they will interpret ambiguous pictures of social situations in terms of their own experiences and unconscious fantasies. In this process, projection is used as a mechanism of thought organization in which the private world of the individual is projected onto the external reality (see Rapaport, 1951, p. 388). Using this mechanism, the subject is largely unaware of the revelation of personally significant material through its attribution to the characters in the picture/story. How is it that this personal material circumvents normal inhibition or censorship? That is, what is it about the TAT that facilitates the use of projection?

As suggested by Morgan and Murray, there are two important aspects of the test situation that might encourage the use of projection. First, the attentional focus in the test is on the stimulus pictures—something outside the subject, provided by the examiner, for which the subject is not responsible. Someone else drew these pictures, someone else is presenting them, someone else is asking for a story to be told about pictures, and so on. This exterior focus encourages a tendency to externalize, which in turn facilitates the use of projection.

Second, the instructions to the subject tend to divert attention from the subject's personal concerns (needs, wishes, fears, anxieties, etc.). Instead, the more abstract realm of creative imagination is stressed. Unless subjects happen to have a conflict around this aspect of themselves, the focus on a somewhat esoteric domain should lessen anxiety about personal involvement in the task. But even if storytellers are threatened by the idea of being creative, or having creativity evaluated, they are no less likely to be unaware of the personal revelation aspect of their stories. In any case, the subjects' stories are fulfilling the external request for demonstrating creative imagination; they are not generally perceived as being about the subject's own self.

PREVIOUS BOOKS ON THE TAT

There have been several long books, or significant sections of books, previously written about the TAT. The first of these was published about 10 years after Morgan and Murray's 1935 paper, and most of the others appeared over the following 10 years. In addition to describing the test itself and the process of test administration, each of these works provides a rationale or scheme for interpreting the stories. Although all these works assumed a psychodynamic orientation toward the understanding of personality, some were more eclectic in this regard (e.g., Tomkins, 1947; Henry, 1956; Shneidman, 1951), and others were more firmly rooted in psychoanalytic theory (e.g., Bellak, 1954, 1975; Holt, 1951, 1978;

Rapaport et al., 1946; Rosenwald, 1968). Stein's (1955) approach was closely tied to Murray's original conceptions of needs, press, and cathexes as these are expressed in TAT stories. Shneidman's (1951) book was unique in that each of the 15 chapters was written by a different psychologist, describing his or her personal approach to interpreting the same TAT protocol. Tomkins's (1947) book stands apart from the others in the expression of greater concern for research possibilities with the TAT and the attendant problems of reliability and validity; Murstein (1963) provided a sourcebook for theory and research. The work of Rapaport et al. (1946, 1968) provided extensive discussions of the use of the TAT for the diagnosis of various psychopathological conditions. Several of these approaches were summarized by Wyatt (1947), who described a further method of analysis. A recent work (Smith, 1992) has described the methods of content analysis currently used in TAT research, as well as various theoretical issues associated with the interpretation of the TAT.

CLINICIANS' USE OF THE TAT

To conclude this section, it is interesting to consider how frequently the TAT is used by practicing clinical psychologists. Several surveys have inquired about the tests most frequently used in clinical settings. For example, in 1982, questionnaires were sent to 458 psychologists practicing in five different types of psychiatric institutions (Lubin, Larsen, & Matarazzo, 1984; Lubin, Larsen, Matarazzo, & Seever, 1985). The respondents were asked to indicate the frequency of use of 30 psychological tests, chosen because they had been ranked in a 1969 survey as those most frequently used (Lubin, Wallis, & Paine, 1971). With a 48% response rate from those contacted, the TAT was ranked fifth out of the 30 tests (preceded by the Wechsler Adult Intelligence Scale [WAIS], the Minnesota Multiphasic Personality Inventory [MMPI], the Bender Gestalt Visual Motor test, and the Rorschach), based on the number of times the test was mentioned as being used. This finding was generally consistent with that of surveys taken in 1969, 1959, and 1946 (Lubin et al., 1971; Sundberg, 1961), all of which found the TAT to be among the top five tests used by clinicians.[9]

A second survey, in 1984, queried 400 members of the Society for Personality Assessment, with a 51% return (Piotrowski, Sherry, & Keller, 1985). Respondents were given the names of 18 popular psychological tests, as determined from previous surveys, and were asked to indicate on a 5-point scale the frequency with which they used each test. Based on total mentions of usage, the TAT was found to rank fourth, following the

Wechsler scales, Rorschach, and MMPI. In a follow-up study 4 years later, a survey was made of test usage in 900 outpatient mental health centers (Piotrowski & Keller, 1989), with a 46% usable return. Again, based on total mentions of usage, the TAT was found to rank sixth.

Another survey (Archer, Maruish, Imhof, & Piotrowski, 1991) examined test usage with adolescent clients. From 600 requests, 165 respondents provided usable data. The TAT was included among the 10 most frequently used instruments, with the WAIS, the Rorschach, and the MMPI being the most popular tests.

A further study of 107 psychologists working in 36 juvenile forensic psychological clinics (Haynes & Peltier, 1985) asked how often the TAT was included as part of the complete psychological evaluation of male adolescent delinquents. The distribution of responses was "U-shaped"; 32% of the psychologists reported using the TAT in less than 10% of their evaluations, while another 33% reported using it in more than 90% of their evaluations, yielding an overall mean usage of 51%. The most frequent reasons given for *not* using the TAT were time constraints (43%), client level of intelligence (18%), and limited verbal interaction capacities (12%).

From these surveys, one may conclude that the TAT is, in fact, frequently used by clinicians in a number of psychiatric settings. In fact, Obrzut and Boliek (1986) conclude from surveys that thematic techniques have become increasingly valuable in clinical assessment. The consistently high rate of usage of the TAT over a nearly 25-year period despite a rather negative attitude on the part of the clinical faculty at some universities toward the value of projective techniques, as pointed out by Lubin et al. (1984), is striking.[10] Apparently, that negative attitude is not very influential in determining test usage because several projective techniques (TAT, Rorschach, House–Tree–Person, and Draw-a-Person) still ranked among the top 10 in frequency of use in 1991. Moreover, there seems to be agreement across clinicians working in different settings as to which are the most useful cards from which to obtain information helpful in diagnostic and psychodynamic formulations of the patient.[11]

SUMMARY

The contribution of the early books on the TAT to a sensitive and insightful use of the test by large numbers of clinicians cannot be overstated. Those students who were reared in this tradition have learned the importance of the TAT for determining character structure, ego functioning, and interpersonal dynamics. Although less central for psychodiagnosis than, say, the Rorschach, the TAT continues to be a prime assessment approach for the practicing clinician. Yet, it is significant that a number of these early advocates of the TAT refer to the absence of a systematic scoring scheme to delineate the findings. For some, this was a tangential concern, one for researchers to worry about; for clinical use, the single most important factor in determining success with the TAT was the capacity of the interpreter and his or her "thorough understanding of dynamic psychology" (Holt, 1951, p. 210). For others, a scoring system was a more pressing concern, and attempts were made to establish some kind of coding scheme (e.g., Bellak, 1954; Shneidman, 1951; Tomkins, 1947). These systems, however, were sometimes highly complex and cumbersome, with even their proponents acknowledging that an illustration of the scoring scheme "may well discourage the reader from even attempting to score the TAT" (Tomkins, 1947, p. 41).

With regard to the issue of scoring, it might be fairly said that those authors who attempted to set up a scheme that would capture the psychological processes involved in storytelling ended up with a complex, unwieldy approach that discouraged its use, whereas those who took a more "objective" approach ended up with checklists that had lost the flavor and psychological significance of the stories. Thus, although there was some research being conducted with the TAT during this period,[12] it was hampered considerably by the lack of a systematic approach to objectifying the TAT data. Nevertheless, among clinicians the TAT has continued to be one of the most frequently used procedures.

• SECTION II •

INTERPRETATION OF THE TAT

THREE

Narrative
and Storytelling

NARRATIVE CONSTRUCTIONS

For the past several years, there has been a discussion among psychologists regarding the nature of two different modes of thought, and some disagreement as to which of these is more likely to provide insight into human lives. One of these, the logicoscientific mode, has dominated American psychology since the advent of behaviorism. Now, as the behaviorist paradigm for psychological inquiry wanes, new models emerge. One of these is based on the narrative mode of thought, which only recently has made inroads into academic psychology. Interestingly, although narrative is about stories and storytelling, this perspective has not been brought to bear directly on work with the TAT.[1] Closely tied to this discussion about modes of thought are larger philosophical questions about the nature of reality and the nature of truth. In turn, these questions lead to further differences between the two modes in conceptions of causality and in the nature of verification.

Two Modes of Thought

Behaviorism fits firmly into the mode of thought referred to as logicoscientific, paradigmatic, or propositional—a mode following, intellectually, from logical positivism. In its extreme form—"if you can't see it, it doesn't exist"—unseeables, such as "drives," were accounted for by operational definitions, using such observables as "number of hours of food deprivation" or "number of bar presses to obtain food" as the objective, countable events that became the meaning of "hunger drive." Yet, it was always assumed that these events referred to ("meant") something underlying,

21

something within the organism, probably within the brain, that *was* drive. And here, as Gergen (in Spence, 1982, p. 292) has pointed out, lies a problem rarely considered by psychologists operating in the behaviorist, positivist mode—namely, that *meaning* can not be verified or falsified. In the case of "drive," although bar presses or hours elapsed are observable, the theoretical *meaning* of those observables—in this case, drive—cannot be proven to be true or false. There is no observable referent of the meaning; it depends on the observer's system of interpretation. This becomes clear when we adopt an alternative frame of interpretation for the same set of observables; bar pressing may now be interpreted to indicate anxiety, or even boredom. But these alternative meanings, as with drive, can be proven neither true nor false. They, too, are the result of an interpretation. There is no observable referent that is clearly, uniquely, and indisputably "hunger drive," "anxiety," or "boredom." Thus, even within the logicoscientific mode of functioning, psychologists are dependent on interpretive context for assigning psychological meaning to observable behavior. We will return to the importance of context and interpretation later.

The goal of the logicoscientific mode of thought is to establish abstract, universal truth conditions—truth that is independent of context. This goal is pursued by using procedures for formal and empirical proof, along with logical arguments and hypotheses that can be tested against observables. The prototype of the goal is seen in highly abstract, formal mathematical systems in which ever more abstract categories are developed and then related to one another to form a system that represents reality. Implicit in this mode of thought is the belief that there *is* one immutable reality, waiting to be discovered.

Influenced by 19th-century science, Sigmund Freud attempted to follow the paradigmatic mode of thought. Freud's recurring metaphor for his work was as an archaeologist who was delving into the past in order to uncover the historical truth[2] of the patient's life (see Freud, 1937/1959; Schafer, 1992; Spence, 1982). As is characteristic of this mode of thought, Freud assumed that past events continued to exist in the patient's memory, unchanged and immutable. By uncovering these "facts," this "truth," he believed that understanding and then cure would ensue. In fact, Freud believed that attempts to reconstruct the psychological past were facilitated in a way that the archaeologist's excavations were not, because he found that past psychological events were repeated by the patient in the present, both inside and outside the therapeutic situation. Although the current manifestations of the past might be modified or distorted, it was assumed that the original event remained buried in memory, unchanged. By focusing on reconstructing the immutable past, Freud hoped to avoid criticism that his method was based on suggestion or subjectivity, as well as to counteract disbelief in the material that he discovered (Spence, 1982).

The idea that psychological or other investigation should be aimed at discovering the "aboriginal world"—the original, given, unsullied reality (Bruner, 1986, p. 37)—has been called into question by Bruner (1986), Sarbin (1986), Spence (1982), and Schafer (1992), among others. They have noted that throughout the history of man an alternate mode of thought has been present and has been used repeatedly to explain, enlighten, instruct, and inspire human actions. This mode—narrative thinking, or storytelling—is intended to convince or persuade another of its true-to-life representation of experience. Central to narrative thinking is a concern for human intentions and actions and for the vicissitudes and consequences of these (Bruner, 1986). Further, narratives focus on people and on the causes of their actions and on subjective experience (Vitz, 1990). Through the use of concrete and interpersonal situations, narrative thought presents the particulars of experience in time and place—that is, particulars in a context—in contrast to paradigmatic thought, which is concerned with propositions demonstrating logical or scientific universals separated from any emotional or specific context (Vitz, 1990). Rather than searching for universal abstractions, narrative thought aims at putting the more general human condition into the particulars of experience (Hermans, Kempen, & van Loon, 1992).

Reality and Truth

Narrative *reality* also differs from paradigmatic reality. Whereas the latter is defined as historical truth—the "aboriginal reality" mentioned above—narrative reality is a description that aims at verisimilitude (Bruner, 1986; Vitz, 1990) and that recognizes a variety of perspectives that may be brought to bear on rendering an experience comprehensible (Bruner, 1986). Thus each mode of thought has a different method for ordering experience and construing reality. The contrast here is between a conception of reality as single, fixed, and forever and reality as relative and context based, known through multiple perspectives. As Bruner (1986) has written:

> The moment that one abandons the idea that "the world" is there once and for all immutably, and substitutes for it the idea that what we take as the world is itself no more nor less than a stipulation couched in a symbol system, then the shape of the discipline alters radically. And we are, at last, in a position to deal with the myriad forms that reality can take—including the realities created by story, as well as those created by science. (p. 105)

These differences in the nature of historical and narrative reality have implications for procedures of "proof" or verification.

> With science, we ask finally for some verification (or some proof against falsification). In the domain of narrative and explication of human action, we ask instead that, upon reflection, the account correspond to some perspective we can imagine or "feel" as right. The one, science, is oriented outward to an external world; the other, inward toward a perspective and a point of view toward the world. They are, in effect, two forms of an illusion of reality—very different forms. (Bruner, 1986, pp. 51–52)

Narrative truth, focused inward, depends on interpretation and especially on the interpretation of human intentionality. These interpretations can be judged for their rightness, but not in terms of their correspondence to "an aboriginal 'real' world out there" (Bruner, 1986, pp. 158–159). Rather, narrative truth depends on how well the interpretation captures an experience, and the degree to which it embodies features of continuity, closure, and the pieces "fitting together."[3]

The importance of interpretation for narrative truth is part of a larger concern regarding the role of construction in determining reality. If reality is based on personal constructions, it is important to realize that these constructions are formulated in part in terms of what others have thought before us. Our current view of reality depends on previous constructions. Further, as we develop, both as individuals and as a society, our construction of reality does and will change, a point made so clearly by the work of Piaget and cultural anthropologists. "We do not operate on some sort of aboriginal reality independent of our own minds or the minds of those who precede or accompany us" (Bruner, 1986, p. 96). In the narrative mode of thought, reality is constructed, not found.

Interestingly, Freud toward the end of his career moved from an insistence on the archaeological model and the search for historical truth toward a position in which he suggested that the "truth" may be unobtainable, and that the therapist may need to fill in the gaps, to "construct" the truth. With this important change in his point of view, he moved from stressing the role of "interpretation" in the work of the analyst to the conception of "construction."

> "Construction" is by far the more appropriate description. "Interpretation" applies to something that one does to some single element of the material, such as an association or a parapraxis. But it is a "construction" when one lays before the subject of the analysis a piece of his early history that he has forgotten, in some such way as [to construct a narrative]. (Freud, 1937/1959, p. 363)

It is clear in Freud's writing on this issue, however, that he still believed that the historical fact existed, unaltered, immutable; although not always recoverable, the analyst could surmise or construct the missing data. Now, the curative agent became not the return of the repressed but a conviction of the truth of the constructed narrative.

> The path that starts from the analyst's construction ought to end in the patient's recollection, but it does not always lead so far. Quite often we do not succeed in bringing the patient to recollect what has been repressed. Instead of that, if the analysis is carried out correctly, we produce in him an assured conviction of the truth of the construction which achieves the same therapeutic result as a recaptured memory. (Freud, 1937/1959, p. 368)

Verification

This shift from the goal of uncovering hidden memories to a focus on creating a meaningful and believable construction raises the problem of verification. Working in the "historical truth" model, there is but one truth. But when reality is constructed, the way is open for multiple interpretations, or constructions, for the same set of data. Here we face the problem that in trying to understand or interpret the psychological nature of the individual, we are dealing not only with the narrative construction of that individual but also with the narrative construction brought to the situation by the interpreter. And although there may be but one single narrative, or set of narratives, characteristic of the individual under study, there is the possibility of as many interpretative narratives as there are interpreters. Thus one of the main difficulties with the narrative mode of thought is, that if reality is constructed, how does one decide which construction is "true."

This dilemma has been well described by Steele (1986):

> Hermeneutics, which is the art or science of interpretation, has since its inception been concerned with the interpretation of text and contexts. . . . While positivism has always maintained the existence of the fact as a near sacrosanct unit of information unadulterated by human interests and secured by objectivity, hermeneutics does not seek a grounding in fact. It maintains that a fact is a construction, a part of a whole. The fact both gives to and takes meaning from the context of explanation in which it is situated. (p. 259)

Thus the meaning of a text, or, in a larger sense, the interpretation of a life, will inevitably depend on the interplay between the storyteller's narrative and the interpreter's construction—that is, on the interpersonal context in which meaning is constructed.

NARRATIVE INTERPRETATION INVOLVES A DIALOGUE

To conceive of narrative interpretation as dialogue, in which the narrative of the storyteller is informed by the narrative of the interpreter and vice versa, is to again make clear how there can be no single absolute interpretation of a storyteller's narrative.

Faced with this situation of multiple interpretative narratives, which cannot be validated by reference to past historical fact, how does one choose among the alternatives? Different solutions to this question have been proposed by different theorists. Steele (1986), based on the philosopher Karl Popper's writings, proposes that narratives be evaluated not in terms of whether they are true but rather in terms of whether they are false. Just as science proceeds by refuting the null hypothesis, so the value of narratives should be determined by the "falsification criterion." If the narrative disagrees or conflicts with observations, one can decide that it is false. These observations may include the narrative itself, which may be determined to be false by noting such distortions as omission of relevant data, inconsistencies, or tailoring of accounts to disguise inconsistencies.

Spence (1982) proposes a different solution to the question of how to choose among possible narratives, at least as this applies to interpretation in the psychoanalytic setting. Rather than focusing on the historical truth or falsity of the narrative, an interpretation might instead be considered an artistic production. For, says Spence, "the historical truth of the interpretation is not necessarily relevant to its clinical impact (read aesthetic experience)" (p. 269). Artistic truth is not necessarily connected with historical truth but does have its own standards as to adequacy and goodness, as does a "good narrative" (Bruner, 1986). "The artistic model is one alternative to the archaeological approach. We no longer search for historical accuracy but consider the interpretation in terms of its aesthetic appeal" (p. 270).

Alternatively, Spence suggests that narratives (interpretations) might be considered pragmatic statements—that is, statements that have the purpose of inducing oneself or others to believe something is true even though it is not known and could not possibly be known whether the statements are true, as when a politician says, "I am going to win the election next week."

Perhaps most critical to this question of how to choose among narratives is the position that interpretations "are to be primarily considered as means to future effects and not the result of past causes" (Spence, 1982, p. 274). That is, the value of an interpretation will be found in the effect it produces.

Our search for verification of the interpretation should be "forward looking," rather than searching in the past for substantiating historical fact. As Freud noted, if an interpretation is incorrect, it results in the therapeutic dialogue coming to a halt; "if nothing further develops, we may conclude that we have made a mistake" (Freud, 1937/1959, p. 363). On the other hand, an interpretation that is followed by the emergence of new material has produced an event that serves as an indirect confirmation of the adequacy of the interpretation.

In sum, the clinical stories with which we work, that is, the narratives of patients—their life history, fantasies, dreams, or TAT stories—do not correspond to historical fact. Whatever the earlier life experiences were, the material has since been transformed into a psychological narrative. Each narrative thus constructed serves as a context for the transformation of further experience into narrative form, creating what Schafer has termed "story lines" (Schafer, 1992, p. 35) through which individuals represent themselves.[4]

At the same time, we who interpret patients' narratives do so by means of our own narratives, our own story lines.

The application of these narratives provides the context through which the patient's narrative is understood. This "dialogue" between two narratives will, in successful therapeutic relationships, bring about a change in both the patient's and the therapist's narrative. Some story lines will serve as structures to which material may be assimilated; at the same time, emergence of new material may require accommodation and change in existing story lines.

> No single designation of an action may be presented as final, definitive, exclusive, or conclusive. Narrative priority may be given to a particular description of an action only after carefully spelling out a context of aims, conventions, circumstances, and practices, or at least when there is ample reason to assume that the listener or reader knows this context very well. The description to be given of an action depends on the kind of account one wants to give of it. No action can be presented intelligibly or usefully if it is not in the context of an implicit or explicit narrative. The narrative context helps readers understand the description being employed at the same time as the description contributes to the further development and persuasiveness of the narrative account. (Schafer, 1992, p. 45)

NARRATIVE AND THE TAT

What are the implications of narrative theory for working with the TAT? First, and most obvious, is the need to recognize that with the TAT, we are working with narrative material. To do this successfully requires the listener to have a "narrative sensitivity," a certain way of listening to the story.

Narrative Sensitivity

This sensitivity, or narrative set, has been discussed by Wyatt (1986) as a "basic orientation, a way of listening and organizing" (p. 201). It includes an awareness that stories refer to something more than, or different from, the surface content, something that may not be consciously available to the storyteller, or that he or she may not have intended to reveal. The listener should be sensitive to implicit as well as explicit meanings in the material. Gertrude Stein notwithstanding, a story about a rose may be about more than a rose.

In addition, stories are understood to reflect process—the transformation of experience into story lines—rather than being references to discrete historical events. Because there is a need to order and integrate experience, there is a tendency for the storyteller to "work over" the same thematic material, to repeat story lines, to express the same story line in multiple variations (see Edelson, 1993). Narrative sensitivity includes an alertness to this repetition. There is, in addition, a belief on the part of the listener that, owing perhaps to the storyteller's need for unity and consistency, it will be possible to recognize the underlying story lines as they are revealed in the narrative.

In short, narrative sensitivity, as it applies to working with the TAT, involves going beyond the material given—beyond the surface arrangement of words, phrases, pauses, starts, and stops—to find story lines that are repeated in various forms and with different content but are used to express the storyteller's unique way of organizing experience. Sensitivity to these recurring patterns is essential in working with the TAT.

Meaning as Constructed

Narrative theory also tells us that TAT stories should not be approached as windows into the historical past, or as X rays revealing some critical event or engram in the unconscious. Stories do not reflect historical truth; they provide a version of the underlying narrative, and they represent the storyteller's reworking of experience into patterns, or story lines, that serve to make experience comprehensible and meaningful. The storyteller thereby constructs his or her world, and this construction is used both to explain new experiences and to direct effort at coping with these experiences. It is for these latter reasons that the discovery of the story lines in the storyteller's constructions is important, not because they may or may not reveal historical truth.

Further, the meaning of a TAT story is not to be found in "observables," for, as discussed earlier, there are no observable referents of meaning. Its meaning lies in the connections and patterns of experience that are both revealed and discovered in the story. We, the listeners, construct this meaning through interpretation.

Context

Narrative theory continually stresses the importance of context, a factor that cannot be overlooked when working with the TAT. Story interpretation should occur within the framework of all the relevant contextual factors. The most obvious of these is the TAT picture, which serves as the immediate stimulus for story production. Different pictures pull for different story lines (see Chapter 13). The context also includes the situational features of the testing situation—the reason for testing, the place, the examiner, and so on—as well as the intrapsychic reaction of the storyteller to these features. Beyond this is the personal context of the storyteller: health, ethnicity, age, gender, business/educational background, intelligence, and so on. "Blind analysis" of TAT stories (i.e., analysis without knowledge of the contextual factors and their effects) is inevitably of limited value.

The importance of context for the interpretation of TAT stories also has implications regarding the level of analysis that may be considered meaningful. Not only is the story to be understood as set in a physical and psychological context; the words that comprise the story themselves occur in a linguistic context. The meaning of an isolated phrase, or a single word, often cannot be interpreted without knowing the context in which it occurs.

Consider the meaning of the phrase "The boy stood up" when occurring in several different "simple" linguistic contexts. "The boy stood up" arouses a certain image, or meaning, in our mind. If, however, we change the linguistic context by adding two words, "The boy stood up the girl," a completely new interpretation of "stood up" is made. This change in interpretation can not be fully explained by noting that a grammatical object—the girl—has been added to the sentence, as is apparent in the further sentence, "The boy stood up the hill," which produces yet another meaning. Can this difference in interpretation be dealt with by noting that the first object is human whereas the second is inanimate? The failure of such a mechanical scheme is seen in the further change of meaning when another human object is added to the stem, as in, "The boy stood up to the teacher." Can the new word, "to," be independently described in such a way as to explain the changed interpretation of "stood up"? Or, consider the following two versions, both of which are highly similar, grammatically yet clearly lead to different interpretations: "The boy stood up against all odds," and "The boy stood up against the wall."

We have, in this illustration, provided six different interpretations of the phrase "stood up," each of which is revealed only through the context in which "stood up" is embedded. Even the meaning of individual words is highly susceptible to context, as demonstrated convincingly in experimental studies of semantic priming[5] and humor based on punning.

It may seem quite unnecessary to stress the point that the interpretation of narrative material is dependent on context, but I have done so in order to demonstrate that the interpreter's narrative, or perspective, should be one that does not destroy context. The linguistic context—the ordering and sequencing of elements—is essential for understanding narratives. And context, we have noted, extends beyond the linguistic matrix. Context includes the intentions, aims, and wishes of the storyteller, as well as the situation in which the story is told. "Deprived of the actual context, the explicator of such a text must supply his own, and the resulting interpretation may shed less light on the . . . [storyteller] than on the hopes and fears of the explicator" (Spence, 1982, pp. 285–286).

Context thus includes the narrative of the interpreter. Narrative theory alerts us to the point that both the story interpreter and the storyteller bring their own narratives to the task of story comprehension. In this way, the interpretation of TAT stories involves a dialogue, between the story lines of the storyteller and the perspective of the story interpreter. Clearly, the perspective, or system of explication, that the interpreter applies to the TAT story will construct meaning for that story; the meaning of a story is intimately linked with the system of interpretation. It is equally clear that there are as many ways in which a story may be interpreted as there are interpretive narratives. Should this be cause for distress? On the contrary, the possibility of multiple interpretations indicates the richness of narrative material.

Multiple Perspectives

We do not live out our lives with a single story line. The complexities of human nature are expressed in a multitude of patterns, some intermingling, some kept isolated. It is this very complex state of affairs that is expressed through narrative. Disentangling that complexity in narratives *requires multiple perspectives.*

In thinking about the TAT, it is thus useful to keep in mind that the story*teller*'s narrative is expressed via multiple story lines. The story *interpreter*, depending on his or her purpose, may "listen with a third ear"—that is, with free-floating attention but without firm preconceptions—in an attempt to recognize those story lines that are idiosyncratic to the storyteller. In fact, this is probably never fully possible, for every interpreter begins with at least a few basic categories of experience that will shape the listening process. It is then really a matter of the degree to which the interpreter's narrative is intermingled with the storyteller's narrative in arriving at the meaning of a TAT story. On the one hand, the interpreter may focus entirely on the narrator's story lines as they emerge and are found to be repeated in the stories told. The interpreter is not committed to finding any particular pattern, any particular story line, but is oriented to discovering story lines as these occur in the stories. Repetition of similar story lines in narrative data will call attention to their importance for the narrator. In this case, the interpretation of the stories will largely be based on the storyteller's narrative and minimally on that of the interpreter. This is the preferred approach when using the TAT for purposes of clinical case study.

At the other end of the continuum, the interpreter may consciously apply the story lines from his or her own narrative as a way of organizing the material. Here, the interpreter will look into the stories for patterns or descriptions of experience that coincide with the narrative constructed by the interpreter. One example of this, discussed in Chapter 6, is Robert May's narrative of deprivation and enhancement. It is May's contention that stories may be characterized by one of two narrative forms, distinguished by the pattern, or trajectory, of events. In one form, the story begins on a high note: Actions are successful, affect is positive, self-concept is elevated. Then, as in many dramatic constructions, there is a turning point, after which things go downhill: Actions fail, affect is negative, and self-concept drops. This is the "enhancement followed by deprivation" story. The second narrative pattern described by May is characterized by the reverse trajectory: The story begins with episodes of failure, sadness, and disappointment, but, after a critical turning point, there is success, happiness, and fulfillment. Using carefully constructed categories to characterize the occurrence of these patterns in TAT stories, May and others have found the first narrative to be characteristic of the stories of men, whereas the second pattern occurs more frequently in the stories of women. As we will see in Chapter 6, these two narratives may also be found in the historical myths and folk tales of the world.

Other approaches to story interpretation, such as the coding schemes developed to assess various motivational dispositions (see Chapter 15), although not strictly narrative in their design, share some features with narratives. Perhaps the best known among these is the coding scheme for the "need for achievement." To assess the presence of this motivation as revealed through stories, the interpreter applies a set of disparate categories to the story. Aspects of the story that fit these categories are scored, yielding an overall numerical score that indicates the strength of achievement motivation in the story and, by inference, in the storyteller.

Although this method does not meet all the criteria for narrative—for example, the motivation score is not dependent on the order in which the categories occur, and the scoring of a category is not influenced by the context in which it occurs—still, the overall approach to assessing motivation in this way does make certain narrative assumptions. First, before any category may be scored, the interpreter must consider the story as a whole, to determine the major theme of the entire story. This decision cannot be made without considering the interrelationship of the story components and the way in which they are organized to result in some intended point of view or outcome that can only be understood in the context of knowledge about the earlier parts of the story. Only if, after this consideration, the story is determined to have a central thematic line focused on the motive in question (i.e., only if this is a narrative primarily about that motive) may the coding interpretation proceed.

Second, the coding systems developed for the various motivational dispositions are all based on a common hypothesized underlying pattern of experience—that is, on a narrative. This narrative prototype characterizes human motivation as consisting of a sequence of events that begins with the arousal of a motive or need. The narrative continues with the arousal being closely followed by some anticipation of success or failure in attaining the goal that would satisfy the need. The sequence continues with the individual engaging in some activity that is instrumental to attaining or not attaining the goal. The context in which this activity occurs is important, for there may be an obstacle to attaining the goal, due either to some block in the external world or to some problem within the person. The narrative sequence ends with positive affect if the goal is attained or negative affect if it is not. This abstract form of the motivational narrative has been translated into various versions, depending on the particular motive under consideration—for example, achievement. These versions are made explicit, so that it is possible to determine the degree to which any TAT story coincides with any motive version (i.e., to determine the degree to which the storyteller's narrative is explained by the interpreter's motivational scoring scheme).

Whether, then, the story interpreter uses an approach that is fully or only partially a narrative approach, it is the interplay between the interpreter's and the storyteller's narrative that creates a dialogue. On the one hand, the storyteller's narrative is used to substantiate the story interpreter's narrative, which, in turn, may or may not be modified by this encounter. On the other hand, the interpreter's narrative provides meaning to the storyteller's narrative. To really understand stories, there is thus an ever-shifting point of reference. The narrative of the storyteller influences and determines the narrative of the interpreter, which, so modified, is used in turn to understand the story. This continual shifting in point of reference and revising of story lines is the narrative dialogue. How this process is used to establish interpretive schemes for the TAT is further discussed in the chapters that follow.

Does this mean that every interpretive scheme for stories is narrative? Clearly not. Mechanical attempts to interpret stories by counting the frequency with which certain words or word types occur are clearly not narrative approaches. Such word counts destroy the form of the story (the pattern, the sequence) and ignore context and intention as though irrelevant for comprehension. Likewise, scoring schemes that rely on checklists to characterize what the storyteller did and did not say overlook the important qualities that make one story different from another—different not because of using different words but because the words are arranged in different ways to convey different meanings. Word counts and checklists cannot convey these narrative differences. Borrowing an axiom from Gestalt psychology, a narrative is more than the sum of its parts.[6]

Intention

In considering the nature of the narrative dialogue, we made mention of the interpreter's *intention*. Intention, like context, is an integral part of narrative. Just as the interpretive narrative will be determined by the intention of the interpreter (e.g., case study vs. motivation research), so the TAT story itself must also be understood as expressing psychological intentions, and as reflecting how human interaction is based on those intentions. Listening with narrative sensitivity involves recognizing the importance of intentions—their origin, their nature, their effects—for understanding the story. Intentions are among those unobservable connections that lie between facts and that explain the facts. TAT stories without intentions are not really stories at all but rather are best described as picture descriptions.

In this connection, it may be helpful to keep in mind Bruner's (1986) description of the essential features of a story. Stories, Bruner (1986) has suggested, involve two "landscapes" simultaneously present. The "landscape of action" (p. 14) includes an agent, an intention or goal, a situation, an instrument, and something that may be referred to as a "story grammar" (p. 14). The "landscape of consciousness" (p. 14) consists of "what those involved in the action know, think, or feel, or do not know, think, or feel" (p. 14). These two components of stories, while present simultaneously, are distinct: "It is the difference between Oedipus sharing Jocasta's bed before and after he learns from the messenger that she is his mother" (Bruner, 1986, p. 14).

Thus, in addition to noting the "action" of the story, the intentions and the perpetrators and obstructors of those intentions, we will simultaneously pay attention to the consciousness or lack of consciousness surrounding those intentions.

Verification

Finally, narrative theory contributes to our thinking about approaches to verifying TAT interpretations. Narrative theory points out that there is no way for working backward, from effect to cause. With the TAT, we may believe that the story is "caused" by the storyteller's narrative, his or her representation of experience, but we cannot prove this, for example, by going back inside the individual and extracting an independently existing narrative for comparison. Rather, narrative theory indicates that the value of an interpretation is to be determined in terms of its effect. The question becomes: What does this interpretation of a story help us to understand that another one does not? Rather than searching for evidence from the past that might validate our interpretation of the TAT, we may instead look to the future to see whether the interpretation will illuminate other aspects of the storyteller's life that are currently cloudy or unknown, or, alternatively, whether future information will show the interpretation to be false. The criterion for a "good" interpretation then becomes whether it will produce new meanings, clarify current puzzles, or demonstrate new relationships as yet unknown. The question then is, What do we now understand about what may happen in the future that we did not understand before? And, what can we now predict about this person that we could not predict before? Verification always lies ahead, not behind.

SUMMARY

This chapter has described the difference between narrative thought and logicoscientific thought. We have seen that narrative reality, truth, and verification are not based on historical fact but rather depend on verisimilitude. Narrative truth and the meaning of stories will be found in forward-looking connections to other aspects of the storyteller's life rather than in attempts to demonstrate historical truth.

This chapter has also expressed the view that the TAT *is* a narrative and *expresses* a narrative. For this reason, the interpreter requires narrative sensitivity—a belief in implicit meanings and underlying story lines. From this viewpoint, the TAT story represents a construction of reality, not a reconstruction. Whereas the narrator creates meaning through the construction of story lines, the listener creates meaning through interpretation, which is itself a construction. In this way, narrative interpretation involves a dialogue between the narrator and the interpreter.

Narrative constructions are also influenced by context and reflect intentions. Although the narrator may or may not be aware of these, the interpreter must be. Further, due to the richness of narrative stories, they may be interpreted from multiple perspectives, each as "true" as the other. In the chapters that follow, we consider several of these perspectives for interpreting TAT stories.

• FOUR •

Context and Storytelling

S torytelling as a means for communicating profound insight into human nature has been with us for a long time. But, as indicated in the previous chapter, it is only recently that psychology has recognized this form of communication as valid and as an alternative to the logicodeductive method borrowed from other scientific disciplines. Narrative thinking involves imagination and the description of concrete, human situations that appear to be true. It is a way of rendering a reality that recognizes human motivation, subjective experience, and the importance of time and place for understanding what is being communicated. In contrast to propositional thinking, which demonstrates logical or scientific universals that transcend the particular and are context independent, narrative thinking is tied to emotions, intentions, and most especially to the particular context in which these occur (Bruner, 1986; Hermans et al., 1992; Vitz, 1990).

CONCEPTS OF NARRATIVE

Although there is considerable agreement that narrative is an important concept in understanding individual lives, there is less consensus about the nature of this concept. Narrative has been variously referred to as a root metaphor for interpreting a life (Sarbin, 1986), as a story told by a person to describe the self, or, alternatively, as a model for determining action (Sarbin, 1986) as influenced by level of ego development (McAdams, 1988a) and as the overt expression of underlying, unconscious "mandates" or "scripts" (Alexander, 1988; McAdams, 1988b; Tomkins, 1978). In these renditions of the concept, narrative is something that resides within the person who is "telling the story"; it is something that shapes, or *is*, the story being told. As we will see, however, narrative may also refer to the point of view, or perspective, of the person who is interpreting the story.

NARRATIVE IN PSYCHOANALYSIS:
MULTIPLE INTERPRETATIONS

The importance of narrative as an approach to understanding humankind has also become popular within the realm of psychotherapy and psychoanalysis.[1] The idea that the patient will repeatedly enact "his or her story" for the therapist to hear, and that it is this narrative rather than historical truth that is important, has been discussed by Edelson (1993), Luborsky (1984), Schafer (1992), and Spence (1982). However, in these writings, it is not only the patient's narrative that is recognized as important. Equally important is the narrative the therapist brings to the dialogue. It is the intermingling of these two narratives that creates a story of the patient's life.

Schafer (1992) expresses this most clearly:

> I do not regard the self as an entity found in nature and available for detached study by nonparticipant observers. Selves are told through dialogue, in words, images and enactments, and they are retold by observers whose narrative preferences and strategies express specific aims, values and competencies. (p. xvi)

This focus on the role of the interpreter brings additional meaning to the statement that narrative is context dependent: namely, the discovered narrative of the storyteller is dependent on the narrative preference of the discoverer. As Schafer (1992) notes about the therapist, whatever is "found" in the patient's story depends on what the observer is looking for. The *narrative of the observer*—in the case of the therapist, what is understood, on the basis of theory and experience, about the patient's past and current life, and about the nature of the therapeutic relationship—provides the context for interpreting the story. This context provides a new and different way to understand the patient's narrative.

The reinterpretation of a patient's life by therapists with different narratives has been strikingly demonstrated by several classical examples in the history of psychoanalytic interpretation. Each interpretation, or construction, provides a plausible explanation of the meaning of the narrative within the predominant theoretical context existing at the time the interpretation was constructed. But, as that context changed, a new interpretive narrative was brought to bear on the original narrative data, with a different outcome.

Classical examples of multiple interpretation in psychoanalysis have occurred when the same narrative data have been interpreted by two or more individuals, as in Freud's classic Schreber case. At least four different interpretations of this case have been offered: that of Schreber himself (Schreber, 1903), that of Freud (1911/1959), that of Keen (1970), and that of Schatzman (1973). The case of Little Hans was interpreted according to psychoanalytic theory by Freud (1909/1955), and again by Wolpe and Rachman (1960) using the narrative of behaviorism. Freud's own dream of Irma has also been subject to alternative interpretations. The first explication was presented by Freud (1900/1953) himself in *The Interpretation of Dreams*; the reinterpretation was by Erikson (1954, 1968). Freud's original analysis of the dream was constructed using the narrative he had created as a theory to explicate hysteria and, subsequently, dreams and the process of dreaming—a narrative stressing unconscious inner conflict, defense, and wish fulfillment. Erikson's reinterpretation, however, is through the narrative of "identity," with the same data now being interpreted as illustrations of identity confusion, negative identity, and identity restoration.

Equally interesting are occasions in which one interpreter changes his or her own narrative, allowing for a comparison of the "before and after" interpretations of the same data. Such is the case in Kohut's (1979, 1984) two analyses of Mr. Z. Here, the same analyst treated the same patient on two different occasions using two different psychoanalytic narratives. The first analysis was based on the classical psychoanalytic model; the second occurred within the framework of psychoanalytic self psychology. The interpretations offered to the patient (i.e., the narratives constructed) were quite different on the two occasions. Nevertheless, each analysis, judged within its own time–space context, was deemed success-ful, in the sense of producing symptom remission.

This shifting of interpretive narratives can also take place within a single individual. Schafer (1992, p. 10), for example, discusses a patient whose perception of herself in the mirror, although physically unchanged, was experienced by the patient as having changed as her "self-narrative" changed. Previously, she perceived (interpreted) herself as being ugly. However, as a result of therapy, her personal self-narrative no longer included the need to protect herself from intimate encounters; as a consequence, she no longer had the need to interpret herself as ugly. Then, as the narrative applied to the same image changed, so did the perception, which was no longer ugly.

Spence (1982) also described a case in which a single patient used alternative narratives to explain the same data. In this case, the historical data consisted of the patient's refusing, as an adolescent boy, to wear eyeglasses, although he was nearsighted. This fact was interpreted by the patient in terms of four different successive narratives. Initially, the explanatory narrative centered around the adolescent wish not to be different, not to stand out from his or her peers. This narrative then shifted to recalling a concern that glasses would make him appear feminine or girlish. A third narrative explanation then emerged, centering around a belief that wearing glasses might actually weaken his eyes, so that by avoiding glasses he was in fact strengthening his vision. The final narrative included the wish that he might strengthen his eyes so that he could enlist in the Air Force and become a hero (Spence, 1982, pp. 290-292).

In these examples, we may ask, which narrative is true? Is Erikson's interpretation of Freud's dream any more true than Freud's own construction? Is there greater verity to Kohut's second analysis of Mr. Z, as compared to the first? As Spence (1982) points out, each story has a piece of the truth, but explanatory narratives cannot be verified by appealing to facts. Narrative explanations deal with meaning and with the connections between facts, and these cannot be observed. As discussed earlier, there are no directly observable referents for meaning. In the case of the developing nearsighted adolescent boy, each of the explanatory narratives had existed in the past, but they were inside his head, changing into new variants over time, and were never fully in awareness. They guided his behavior and his feelings about himself, but they left no visible record, no trace in the past, that could be validated. Yet clearly these changing narratives have a reality—an important meaning—for understanding this man's adolescent development.

INTERPRETIVE CONTEXT: PERSPECTIVES

The idea that in the stories people tell, we may find the themes that are central to their lives, reflective of their life history, and indicative of the way in which they construct reality is not new and was previously referred to as the projective hypothesis (see Rapaport, 1951). Indeed, Murray (1937) went to some lengths to demonstrate how the themes discernible in TAT stories reflect the basic personality patterns and associated life history of the individual. He illustrated this at some length in his discussion of "Earnst" (Murray, 1937), who was one of a group of closely studied Harvard students. But Murray, too, had his "narrative" which consisted of needs, press, and the combination of these into "thema," which were then used to understand the individual's life.[2]

More recently, Tomkins (1978) and Alexander (1988) used the notion of "scripts" as guiding rules for detecting individual patterns in such narrative material as autobiographies or TAT stories. Identifying these scripts, however, is based on certain rules for determining what in the material is important and what is not. These identifiers and the rules for developing scripts become the observer's narrative through which the storyteller's narrative is interpreted. Thus, in every case of narrative interpretation, it is clear that not only are story*tellers* influenced by their narratives but also that story interpreters are influenced by theirs. That is, the narrative of the interpreter provides a context, or a perspective, through which the story is interpreted.

In addition to the thema and script narratives, there have been other interpretive approaches used with the TAT. Clinicians often approach TAT stories as being reflections of the "life history" of the individual—that is, that the storyteller will relate personal narrative patterns and "thematic lines" (McAdams, 1988a). Some researchers have adopted motivational perspectives, investigating the needs for achievement, power, affiliation, and intimacy (e.g, Boyatzis, 1973; McClelland, Atkinson, Clark, & Lowell, 1953; McAdams, 1980; Winter, 1973). Others have used a narrative derived from sexual physiology and cultural experience to investigate sexual identity (May, 1980). Still others have adopted perspectives based on concepts from clinical psychology, focusing, for example, on defense mechanisms (Cramer, 1987, 1991a) and object relations (Westen, 1991a). Some of these interpretive perspectives have been discussed at length elsewhere (see Smith, 1992; McAdams, 1988a; Winter, 1973); others are examined in later chapters of this book.

It is clear from this brief discussion that even though the narrative of the story being interpreted may remain constant, when the narrative of the story interpreter changes, the resulting psychological meaning of the story will change. It is equally clear that there is no one meaning for a single narrative; there are as many meanings as there are interpretive narratives. For the sake of clarity, in the following discussion, I use the term "narrative" to refer to the storyteller's contribution, and the term "perspective" to refer to that of the interpreter.

Does this mean that story interpretation is hopelessly subjective, and that, as such, there is nothing substantial to be gleaned from storytelling procedures? If by "subjective" we mean that what we see is largely determined by what we are looking for, then story interpretation is clearly subjective. However, this need not reduce story interpretation to the realm of highly personalized, idiosyncratic speculations. Determination of reliability—in the sense of the same result over time, or the same result produced by an independent observer—is readily obtained by applying the same, clearly defined perspective to the story on another occasion or

by another observer.[3] Determination of validity, of psychological meaningfulness, will depend on the degree to which any interpretation fits into
a larger context of theoretically related psychological variables and on the
degree to which observations that previously appeared disparate can now
be subsumed under this interpretation. In other words, the validity of
story interpretation will depend on its goodness of fit within the broader
context of the person's psychological life.

THE CHOICE OF INTERPRETIVE PERSPECTIVE

It is clear that the perspective brought by the interpreter to the TAT story
will determine the way in which the story is understood. The question
then becomes, Which perspective shall the interpreter adopt? And how
specifically defined will this perspective be? The chapters that follow
provide a variety of answers to these questions.

Some perspectives consider the life history of the storyteller as the
relevant interpretative scheme, as discussed in Chapter 5. Other perspectives are based on concepts defined with considerable specificity, such as
various motivational dispositions (e.g., need for achievement; see Chapter
15), mechanisms of defense (see Chapter 7), and sexual identity (see
Chapter 6). Still other perspectives are based on concepts broader than
a specific motive but less inclusive than a life history. Examples of these
broad abstractions include Rosenwald's (1968) narrative of "levels"[4] and
Holt's (1951) "story-as-dream" narrative, discussed below.

Yet other perspectives may focus on aspects of psychopathology and
personality organization, guided by clinical theory and intuition (see
Chapters 8, 9, and 10). The application of these more broad-ranging
concepts depends largely on the intuitive skills of the interpreter.

Chapters 5, 6, and 7 of this first section of the book are devoted to
several perspectives that have been found useful for TAT interpretation.
In each case, the rationale for these interpretive approaches is followed
by a demonstration of how they are used to interpret individual stories.
In addition, research studies based on larger groups of individuals that
support the validity of these perspectives are described.

TAT PICTURES AS CONTEXT

Thus far I have been focusing on the narrative of the storyteller and the
perspective of the story interpreter, overlooking the defining feature of
the TAT—the TAT cards themselves. This is yet another "context" to be

considered when interpreting a TAT story. Psychologically naive storytellers assume that the story told comes from the picture; that is, that the
entire narrative is determined by the picture rather than the storyteller.
This is often seen in TAT stories that begin with a comment such as
"*Obviously*, this is a picture of two people having an argument." That this
is not so obvious is clear when the next person looks at the same picture
and says, "These two people are deep in thought."

Of course, the pictures are *of something*, and this fact leads to what is
called "card pull." Different TAT cards pull for certain kinds of story
content; research studies of this issue are presented in Chapter 13. But
even here, the narrative of the storyteller will be an important factor in
determining how the content of the pictures is perceived. For example,
Card 17BM depicts a man clinging to a rope. A sizable percentage of
storytellers looking at this card will see a man climbing *up*, while another
large group will see the man climbing *down*. Does this matter? The answer
to this question depends on the perspective of the story interpreter. If the
interpreter is working with the deprivation–enhancement perspective for
assessing sexual identity (see Chapter 6), it will matter; if the interpreter
is focusing on intimacy motivation, it may not matter. Again, the same
TAT picture may be described as a rock climber clinging to the rope to
save his life, but in addition one storyteller may add the statement,
"However, he is not afraid," while another mentions the images of death
that rush through the climber's mind. Do these brief additions make a
difference? If the interpreter approaches the story with an interest in
defense mechanisms, the answer is yes; if the perspective is focusing on
achievement motivation, these two differences are not critical.

THE STORYTELLING CONTEXT: ISSUES

Before considering the specific perspectives for TAT interpretation, let
us take a moment to consider the storytelling context. The TAT involves
telling stories about a standard set of pictures—stories that convey information about the storyteller's experience, including historical, motivational, and defensive organizations, among others. But also, and important, the stories include the storyteller's ideas about the test and the test
situation, the reason for testing, and the motivation for taking part in it.
These interpersonal and situational dynamics provide the context for the
storytelling. As such, they will influence the stories told. This context,
including but not limited to the examiner's instructions, will set the
storytelling in motion.

How is the storyteller's experience of this context revealed? One
interpretive framework that is helpful here comes from psychoanalytic

dream theory (Freud, 1905/1962, 1908/1959; Holt, 1951; Edelson, 1993). Although dreams and stories are not identical processes, they share several features. Both are set in motion by an external stimulus; in the case of the dream, this is the "day residue"; in the case of the TAT, it is the stimulus picture. Just as many day residues are not seized upon to prompt a dream, not all stimulus pictures will connect, dynamically, with central motives or conflicts of the individual. But some will, and the arousal of psychologically meaningful needs, affects, or motives are then worked over, modified, disguised, or otherwise reformulated, either through the "dream work" or, for the TAT, through formulating a story that meets the request of the examiner. The end point of this process in the dream frequently involves some wish fulfillment. In the TAT story, there is an outcome associated with positive or negative affect. Owing to the external source of the original stimulus—the day residue or the TAT picture—the dreamer or storyteller is somewhat absolved from responsibility for the nature of the end product, and in this way some of the mechanisms of censorship are evaded.[5]

In interpreting a patient's dreams, clinicians often listen with an ear to locating representations of themselves in the dream. Thoughts, feelings, and attitudes of the patient about the therapist are discovered in this way. In a similar manner, attitudes, reactions, and feelings of the storyteller about the testing situation and the tester may appear in TAT stories, especially in the first story, and especially when the testing situation is an interpersonal one (e.g., a dialogue between tester and testee) as compared to a group testing situation in which the storyteller writes, rather than tells, his or her stories.

Illustration: Story as Comment on the Research Context

If we approach the TAT story from the perspective that it reflects the storyteller's experience of the testing situation and the tester, we will have a helpful interpretive tool, one that will guide our efforts to hear what the story is telling us. In the following illustrative stories, I take the point of view that the storyteller's perceptions of the examiner—his beliefs about the kind of person she is and why she is engaged in this enterprise—will influence and be revealed in the stories told.

The situational context for the storytelling in the following example was as follows: A 21-year-old male college student agreed to participate in a research study being carried out by a fellow student, but only after several phone calls from the female experimenter.[6] He arrived somewhat late, apologizing that he got held up. He was met at the door of the experimental room by a female professor, who led him into a darkened experimental room where he was asked to lie down on a cot, with the student experimenter sitting in a chair above and behind him. The experimenter then gave him the instructions for storytelling, but she made a mistake, saying, "Speak your louds [*sic*]—uh, your louds [*sic*] (*laughs*)—uh, your thoughts out loud," indicating her nervousness with this, her second pilot subject. At this point, she produced the first TAT card, which he took with his left hand, as he did each subsequent card.

Story 1

The subject then told the following story to TAT Card 6GF, which depicts a young woman seated, with an older man standing behind and above her.

> "This young lady is a reporter for a magazine and she's doing a story on a very wealthy corporate executive who has been accused of being involved in illegal activities and she's unable to get in touch with him in his office. He will not return her calls. So finally she comes right to his house and comes to the door and the maid lets her in and says, 'Well, why don't you wait for him in the study.' And so she goes in and sits down. It's a very darkened room and she's a little nervous but she's determined to get this story and to find out the truth about the guy. And suddenly—when you get to where the picture's at right now—he comes up behind her and startles her, saying something along the lines of, 'So you're the one who's been bothering me at my office.' And then he sits down. She asks him some questions which he gives nondescript answers to. She's unable to get her story there but she stands up in a huff and says, 'One way or another I'm going to get to the bottom of this.' "

In this story, there are a number of veiled references to the testing situation, to the examiner, and to the experience of the subject in that situation. However, the representation of this experience in the story shifts between the two characters, as described below.

To begin, the young woman in the picture is described as someone who, as a reporter, wants to get a story from the man—indeed, this is the task of the student experimenter. Like the male subject, the man described will not return her calls. In the opening part of the story, then, the young woman in the picture takes on attributes of the female experimenter, and the man represents aspects of the subject.

At this point in the story there is a shift in roles; the woman "comes to the door" and thus becomes the character who temporarily represents the experience of the storyteller as he entered the experimental room. This character is led into a darkened room by the maid, just as the subject was led into a darkened room by the female professor.

Then, there is a second shift, and the woman again represents the female experimenter in that "she's a little nervous," just as the experimenter was, but she is "determined to get this story," as was the experimenter. This is followed by a third shift, in which the man comes up behind the woman (in keeping with the objective reality of the picture) and startles her, whereas, in fact, the female experimenter sat behind the subject and may have surprised him with her request for creative storytelling.

A final shift occurs when the man sits down, the woman questions him and attempts to get a story, but he is resistant and refers back to the initial bother of the phone calls—again, a fairly direct description of the testing situation. The story ends with a sense that the woman's quest for a story has been temporarily blocked but that she will persevere and eventually be successful, just as occurred in the actual testing situation.

Using the interpretive perspective of "story as description of experience in testing situation," the text reads as a nearly verbatim account of what has actually transpired between the experimenter and the subject. Element by element, it is a "good fit."

But our interpretation is not complete. We may also focus on the story from the point of view of what it tells us about the attitude and feelings of the storyteller toward the woman examiner.

First, it is striking how any activity or assertive stance is attributed to the female character. In contrast, the male uses defensive maneuvers of avoidance or evasion. He avoids returning the reporter's calls and gives her nondescript answers when she appears. This passive–aggressive defensive stance then allows him to shift the blame to her—that she has been bothering him—rather than it is he who has been attempting to hide himself in order to prevent the discovery of some possibly illegal activities. With one exception, all the action in the story is attributed to the female, who is portrayed as assertive, intrusive, and irritable. That the issue of male–female relations and gender roles may be of more general importance for this man is hinted at in his characterization of the male figure in the TAT picture as a "very wealthy corporate executive," while the woman is a "young lady." This attitude regarding social status is also seen in the storyteller's addition to the story of a woman who is a "maid," one that comes entirely from the mind of the storyteller for there is no third person in the TAT picture.

Overall, then, the storyteller appears to experience the storytelling situation as one in which the intrusive female experimenter will, through her persistent assertion, discover in him some hidden, unacceptable aspect of himself which, if revealed, would put him in jeopardy. He attempts to defend himself against this through avoidance and the attribution of responsibility to the woman.

Story 2

Following the initial story just discussed, the subject told three more stories to different TAT pictures. After this, the experimenter, as part of a planned manipulation, told the male student that his stories were among the worst that she had ever heard. This comment drastically alters the interpersonal context in the testing situation. In the next story told, we might expect to find the effect of this markedly changed context.

Just after the sharp criticism, the experimenter handed the subject TAT Card 7BM, which depicts a young man in the foreground with an older man standing to the side and somewhat in back of the younger man. The subject told the following story:

"This is a story of a person overcoming a great impairment. This young man all his life from the time he was young wanted to be a concert pianist and wanted to play the piano professionally. And he practiced from the time he was four or five and worked at it 3 to 4 hours a day. The problem was that he came from a very poor family. In addition to the fact that he had to play the piano, that he wanted to play the piano, and wanted to work at it every day, he also had to work a job to help support his family. . . . So basically he worked in a construction mill and sawed lumber and those kind of things. So, about the time he was about 17, he was in an accident and his left hand was damaged so that he was unable, he lost the mobility and was unable to play the piano, and he was distraught. And then he met this other man that we see in the picture, this older man, who introduced him to compositions and pieces that had been written specifically for being played with one hand. . . . The young man became a fantastic piano player and as a result of really working at it and being able to use that one hand to play these fabulous pieces, he also was able to get the motivation to bring his left hand back into use. And although not fully, he was able to overcome this impairment and as a result of the fact that he had an impairment, he became actually quite a success story, not necessarily for his piano playing, obviously people who have two fully functioning hands could play better, but he played so well he was more, it's more a story of perseverance and uh, and as a result he was very successful."

The psychological effect of the experimenter's critical comments are almost immediately evident in this story, which incorporates her statement of incompetence in the opening reference to the "impairment" of the young man. This impairment has been brought about in the context of the young man having practiced hard in a creative pursuit and having tried hard to support his family.

From the perspective of "story as comment on the testing situation," the opening of this latter story may be interpreted as reflecting the storyteller's current experience. He had worked hard to carry out the experimenter's instructions to be creative and he had tried to support his fellow student in her work. But, as the story continues, in the process of supporting his family, his left hand was damaged through an accident. This is an unusual response to the picture, and it is heard, through the present perspective, as a result of the storyteller's experience in the testing situation. In his attempt to help his fellow student by accepting her pictures with his left hand, his creative capacity was damaged by her criticism.

Whether one wishes to interpret the story about the damaged left hand as being a symbolic representation of castration brought about by the female experimenter's criticism and as exemplifying the need for identification with a nurturing older man to restore the functioning of the damaged phallus, or whether one thinks of the impairment as representing a damaged self-esteem which is restored through such identification, the experience of the testing situation and the tester is clearly represented in the story.

Taking the two stories together, we see the storyteller's experience of the research context. The examiner is perceived as dangerous to his manhood and his self-esteem. The fear that she may be instrumental in exposing his inadequacies creates the need to utilize defensive strategies. These include passive opposition and diminishing her importance, and, where possible, identification with a supportive older male.

But here we have shifted to a new perspective, namely, that the mechanisms of defense that form part of an individual's adaptive repertoire will be expressed in the stories told. This subject is discussed further in Chapter 7.

Illustration: Story as Comment on the Clinical Context

For individuals who are patients in treatment—particularly if that treatment is intense, as may occur in a psychiatric hospital—the patient's experience of the clinical context is often expressed in the TAT stories. This may be seen in the following story from a young woman who was hospitalized at a treatment facility that offered intensive psychotherapy as well as a full range of other activities. The story was told about TAT Card 12M, which shows one man lying on a cot and a second man standing above him, with a raised arm.

> "The man is casting some kind of spell. That sounds a little peculiar but . . . in order to make her . . . speak freely to him without her being aware of it at all after it is done. She is a very reserved woman and

she never speaks to him of what she's thinking or hearing. She tries hard not to tell him anything and he is very curious about her. Guess that is it. [*hearing?*] Oh, I said, 'or feels.' "

It is not difficult to understand this story as reflecting the patient's experience both of the testing situation and of the therapy process. She, the patient, tries hard not to reveal anything about herself, while he, the clinician, is trying to find out about her. In addition, there is an element of suspicion—that he will take control and make her disclose information without her being aware of what is happening, and against her will. Interestingly, at the same time that the patient strives not to reveal anything about herself, her story alerts us to the possibility that she experiences auditory hallucinations, when she says "she never speaks to him of what she's thinking or *hearing*." However, when the clinician queries her at the end, she denies this possible revelation by stating that she said "*feels*," not "*hears*."

Two further examples illustrate how the experience of the treatment context may be expressed in the stories. The following two stories came from a male patient at the same psychiatric hospital. The first story was told about a picture from the original Harvard Psychological Clinic edition of the TAT (see Chapter 2). The picture shows two men drawn schematically; one is placed above the other, with arms extended toward the lower man's head.[7]

"Sort of makes me think of a psychiatrist and his patient, picking the patient's brain. . . . There are spirits floating on the air and a sea underneath them. I am having a hard time with this one. The one at the top is the spiritual one, picking the head of the one below, who is more of a physical one. The spiritual one at the top has an arm like a thunderbolt, symbolizing that it is more powerful."

After several more stories, the patient was given TAT Card 12M, and he told the following story:

"There is a man sleeping and he has been going through hell and this is like a spirit who has come to where he is sleeping in order to heal him. When he awakens, he is a much more together person—I wish that would happen to me."

Again, it is not difficult to hear these stories as reflecting the clinical context in which the patient finds himself. However, the experience of this man is rather different from that expressed by the first patient. The current patient describes a situation in which the clinician is the strong, powerful one who will extract the needed information without resistance from the patient. The clinician is also felt to be a healer, someone who will make the patient feel better, and someone whose help is desired. The relevance of this second story to the patient's own situation is made clear in his closing comment.

SUMMARY

In this chapter, we have continued to discuss the concept of narrative and its relevance for the interpretation of TAT stories. Whereas the narrative of the storyteller provides the basis for the story, the *interpretation* of the story will depend on the narrative or perspective of the story interpreter. In the first part of the chapter, examples from the psychoanalytic literature of the use of multiple perspectives to interpret classical case studies is reviewed, raising again the issue of truth for narrative material. The importance of interpretive context for understanding TAT stories and a variety of alternative perspectives for approaching story interpretation are considered.

The second part of the chapter expands on the importance of context in working with narrative material. Storytelling with the TAT occurs in the context of pictorial cues that function in interaction with the storyteller's personal narrative to produce a story. Beyond this, there is the larger situational context in which the storytelling occurs. The influence of this context—whether one of research study or of clinical assessment—on the narrative produced is illustrated in several example stories. Again, the "dialogue" nature of narrative is demonstrated in that the context influences the narrative produced, depending on the storyteller's experience of that context, that is, depending on the interaction of the storyteller's narrative with the context.

The remaining chapters in this section of the book discuss in detail three different narrative perspectives for the interpretation of TAT stories.

• FIVE •

The TAT and the Life Story Narrative

I n the broadest sense, TAT productions may be thought of as reflections of the storyteller's "life story." In the same way that novels, especially first novels, tend to be autobiographical, TAT stories often mirror the important life themes of the storyteller. This is seen in the concerns and conflicts of the central characters, in the way in which interpersonal relationships are represented, in the sequencing of central episodes or units of the story, and in the story outcome. In a sensitive reading of an individual's stories, the reader begins to "hear" the repeated themes and understands them to be the central patterns of the storyteller's personality—patterns that both organize the person's experience of the world and are organized by these experiences.

The assertion that the central themes of a narrator's TAT stories are indeed manifestations of his or her life story and not simply imaginative constructions without personal relevance is seen most clearly when, in addition to the stories themselves, we know something about the life history of the storyteller. In the four case studies presented in this chapter, the interrelationships between the TAT themes and autobiographical material are made clear.

COLLEGE STUDENTS: CASE STUDIES

To illustrate the point that the TAT reflects central themes from the life story of the storyteller, I asked students who were beginning the study of personality assessment to write several stories in response to TAT-like cards and then, several weeks later, in a different context, to write a brief autobiography selecting aspects of their lives that they considered impor-

50

tant. This information provides the opportunity to identify story themes that reflect life history themes.

Don

Autobiographical Material

The first case study comes from a college senior, the youngest son from an academic family. In his autobiography Don,[1] who is obviously bright, commented several times about his realization that he was smarter than his high school classmates, and that while they had to study, he did very well academically without much effort. Don went on to say that this pattern was disrupted only on his entrance into college, where his easy A's turned into C's and D's. In his second semester of college, he made an important personal connection with the baseball team and its coach, and his grades began to improve. Now in his senior year, he describes with pleasure his successful attempts to develop relationships with classmates.

A close reading of this student's autobiography indicates that it revolved around two main themes. The first theme concerns his older brother. Don describes in poignant detail his reactions to the occasional absences from the family of this brother—absences that would cause him considerable worry. This anxiety was augmented by the fact that he could not remember, at these times of absence, what his brother looked like.

> "I went crying to my mother because I couldn't remember what he looked like. Even after she showed me his school picture, I was unable to visualize him without looking at a picture to jar my memory. This minor trauma still bothers me, as it proved to be somewhat foreshadowing of later events." On a subsequent occasion, when his brother again left home, Don "became very scared of once again forgetting about him. The year was one filled with anxieties and worries over his absence."

Subsequently, he felt that these worries were premonitions of his brother's early death, caused by an accidental fall that occurred while the brother was away at college. His mother informed Don of the accident, and together they went to be with his brother, who never regained consciousness. His very great pain about this loss led to a thwarted suicide attempt (jumping from a ledge) and subsequently to a strong cynicism stemming from a feeling that no one cared for his departed brother. His cynicism was intensified by the murder of a good friend's older brother and by the accidental death of another friend. As she had for his brother's fatal accident, it was his mother who informed him of his friend's fate.

A second theme that ran through Don's autobiography was the

contrast between his parents' persistent opinion of him as being their "little angel" and his own rebellious and minor criminal activities. In addition to drinking, drugs, cutting classes, and gambling, he was involved in petty thievery and shoplifting, for which he was arrested. Don recounts, in three places in his autobiography, the escalation of these delinquent activities until he was "caught" by some authority. In each case, he describes as the outcome his parents being upset by the revelation of his misbehavior:

> "Then we got caught. My folks were pretty devastated by this whole thing, I think, and they knew for sure I wasn't their little angel."

TAT Story

Don's first projective story was written about a picture depicting two people sitting on a bench near a river; a large bridge spans the river.[2]

> "This is Mr. and Mrs. James Smith. Their son Bill committed suicide almost 7 years ago, by jumping off this bridge. This is the first time they have been able to come here and really think about their son. They are torn by emotions and memories of the happy times they spent with their son. Their one overriding fear is for their youngest son, Donald, who has turned very depressed and has trouble making friends since his older brother's suicide. The Smiths are extremely worried that Donald may also take his own life in a fit of deep depression. The thought of losing a second son in this way tears at their souls. Donald refuses professional help and seems angry with his mother often. Even in this hour of stress, as his parents attempt to finally accept their son's death, Donald is off playing baseball with his friends from college."

The autobiographical nature of this story is quite clear. It begins with the older son dying after a fall from a height, as did the storyteller's oldest brother. That this fall is turned into a suicide in the story suggests that the anxieties and worries the storyteller felt about his brother when they were separated continue to plague him and to create concern about the real reason or responsibility for the fatal fall. Also, these early worries and "forgettings" of his brother suggest that Don may have felt angry about his brother's absences, as well as conflicted over these angry feelings toward a brother who was so important to him. Further, the fact that his brother died when he was once again away from the family suggests that the death may have occurred in a psychological context of anger over his absence, with ensuing guilt not only over the anger but now over the possible consequences of that anger.

The story continues as the younger son becomes depressed and it is feared he will follow the older brother, as was the case with the storyteller. The reference to being "angry with his mother often" is not further explained in the story, and its referents in the autobiography are not as clear as those to the death and suicide attempt of the sons. However, because the autobiography makes a point of stating that it was his mother who informed Don of both his brother's fatal accident and also of his friend's fatal accident, it is possible that Don's anger about those occurrences has been associated with, or partially displaced onto, his mother as the bearer of bad tidings. After all, when he was younger, it was his mother who could make his brother reappear (by showing his picture) when Don was unable to visualize him. The uneasy foreshadowing aspect of this memory also hints at some unconscious sense of responsibility for his brother's fate.

Finally, the story concludes with the surviving son coping with his stress by becoming involved with baseball and with his college friends, again reflecting the life of the storyteller.

A second story from Don expresses the other theme of his autobiography—the contrast between his parents' view of him as the bright, shining angel and his delinquent behavior, which was hidden from them until it reached a level that could no longer be overlooked. The picture for this story portrayed a person standing near a large flask, one hand upraised. A sheet of paper, with some markings on it, is in the lower left-hand corner.

"Mark Parker is a lab scientist at MIT doing independent research on genetics and DNA. He is currently hot on the trail of an amazing breakthrough sure to win him a Nobel Prize in chemistry and get him world renown. As he progresses through the final stage of his work, he notices some odd readouts on his computer printout of data. Shocked by the revelation that his great discovery may, in fact, never materialize, he rushes over to his equipment and pulls out the one beaker of material which is producing the faulty data, crucial to his experiment. As Dr. Parker stares into the beaker, he thinks about his enormous time commitment to his work and the ridicule that will come from his peers if the experiment he has staked his reputation on fails. It would be very easy for Dr. Parker to remedy the situation and get rid of the evidence and present his other findings as proof of his theory, but that would break the ethical code of research science. As he stares blankly into the offending beaker, Dr. Parker thinks of fame, glory, money, success, shame, guilt and responsibility. As the beaker is crushed in the heat of the incinerator in the building's cellar, his only thought becomes 'I wonder if anyone will ever find out.' "

This story portrays the powerful conflict between the wish to maintain society's image of the hero as bright, shining, and successful ("fame, glory, money, success") and the moral dilemma that in order to maintain this image he must engage in dishonest, unethical behaviors ("shame, guilt, responsibility"). Significantly, his potentially great future was dashed by the shocking revelation that there is one faulty beaker in the environment on which he had staked his life's ideals. His concern around the destruction of this beaker is whether or not he will get caught. Again, the autobiographical theme emerges. Repeatedly, Don's parents' image of him as an angel is disrupted by his delinquent behavior. Repeatedly, this bright young man manages to get caught, thereby forcing his parents to attend to his conflict. In the story, the dilemma is brought about by one beaker that does not behave as it should. The storyteller is responsible for the destruction of that beaker, and the issue of getting caught is related to that act. It seems likely that this errant beaker and its ultimate destruction in some way symbolizes Don's departed brother. The description of staring into the beaker recalls Don's need to stare at a picture of his brother in order to visualize him when he is absent. The beaker being crushed in the cellar resonates with the result of his brother's fall. In this context, the question of being "caught" for misbehavior then takes on a significant new meaning: Namely, will others hold him responsible for the death of his brother? The existence of such unconscious guilt helps explain Don's retrospective uneasiness about his absent brother, as well as the need to be caught and punished.

In these two stories, the parallels with the life history of this young man are abundantly clear. It is important to remember that these stories were written during the first class meeting of the semester. Don had no idea how they would be used. Likewise, in writing the autobiography, there was no suggestion that this would be linked with the TAT stories. Nevertheless, the parallel themes in the two narratives are striking. However, the stories provide something more than a narrative recounting of the factual events of Don's life. In the stories, some of the emotion attached to the traumatic life events appears; this is not expressed or made clear in the autobiography.

DeeDee

Autobiographical Material

In contrast to Don, DeeDee (the preferred nickname, from childhood, of a female college senior) writes an autobiography in which there is very little discussion of significant events. Rather, the focus is on the nature of family relationships and the personalities of family members. DeeDee is the youngest of four sisters. She describes the four of them in similar positive terms. In fact, the perceived similarity among the four girls turns out to be a source of consternation for DeeDee.

> "One thing that has always bothered me is that of all my mom's thousands of pictures, there are *none* of me alone. I'm always flanked by my damn sisters."

Although the four sisters are described as currently getting along well, there was considerable conflict, jealousy, and arguing during adolescence.

DeeDee's relationship with her mother is described as generally sanguine, having had many positive features when she was younger. Currently, however, she perceives her mother as weaker and overly dependent on her husband and children and having a difficult time functioning on her own.

Considerable attention in the autobiography is devoted to her father, who DeeDee describes as "overbearing, suffocating, demanding, and tyrannical." However, she immediately qualifies this statement by saying that this is the way she, her sisters, and her mother felt about him when the girls were children. Now, she continues, her father has tried "to be nicer, and to establish close relationships with his daughters, who deep down he truly adores, but he blew it." DeeDee acknowledges considerable guilt over her inability to accept her father's current offers of closeness—"it's so hard to be nice to him"—that often occur in the context of his insensitive domination: "Cancel all plans, I'm coming up this weekend."

At her father's insistence, the family continually moved around the country during DeeDee's childhood. This moving around inevitably resulted in a repeated series of disrupted relationships for DeeDee, her sisters, and her mother. DeeDee cites these father-dominated moves as the most influential part of her childhood.

> "Probably the most influential part of my childhood was the fact that my dad was always picking us up and moving us to different parts of the United States. Just when my mom and we would make new friends and get adjusted, off we'd go again."

Her father also insisted she adopt a more "mature" name as she grew older. However, DeeDee resumed her childhood nickname when she left home to begin college. Strikingly, she focuses on the importance of her name in establishing her own identity, separate from her sisters and parents:

"Maybe my name means so much to me because it's the one thing I have that no one else can share with me or take away."

This concern about her own identity, as separate from the family's percepts of her, is well expressed in the concluding paragraph of her autobiography:

"Everyone says I'm gifted with intelligence and 'special,' but I think that's a load of crap. [I know] I've internalized my dad's ambition for me. . . . I like to think I am a strong, independent person who has a lot of good friends and qualities, but sometimes I feel unloved and lonely. I never have 'dates' like so-called 'normal' people, and have had pitifully few significant relationships. This upsets me, because the one thing I'm sure I really want in life is to get married and have children. . . . I'm a romantic at heart."

In this autobiography, it is possible, as in Don's, to identify two central themes. One theme focuses on the dominating, controlling nature of DeeDee's father, on the disruptions in relationships that he caused, and on her current unwillingness to forgive him for the pain he caused all the women in the family. The other recurring theme is a feeling of having been lost in the crowd of sisters, a strong wish to identify herself as separate and unique from them, and a continuing feeling of a split between her external self, seen as strong and independent, and an internal self that feels weak and unloved.

TAT Story

DeeDee's story was written about a picture showing one person in the foreground, with a beaker and sheet of paper to the side. The story included crossed-out words, which are indicated below.

"This is a [classical—word crossed out] composer of classical music from the 17th century. He is examining a gift presented to him mysteriously by an anonymous admirer of his music. She has been watching him for months and has fallen in love, but he does not know this or who she is. The note with the package merely said 'With [unloving—word crossed out] undying love and devotion, an ardent admirer.' The [note—word crossed out] mystery has intrigued him enough to drop the sheet music he has been working on, and now he stands contemplating the mysterious suitor.
    "Sarah is the daughter of a count and is obligated to marry a count chosen for her by her father. But she is not in love with the count, she finds him quite dull. Her secret passion is music, and

whenever she can she sneaks away from her ladies-in-waiting to hear Roberto's symphonies. She has fallen madly in love with him from afar, but does not know how to approach him, nor what would happen if she dared to break her engagement to the count. She feels hopeless, so she sent the note and gift but knows she can do no more. She must give up—that was her final act of love and now, done, she must heed to her family's wishes.

"Roberto will pursue this mysterious admirer with all his heart. He will hire several investigators to track her down. He has been lonely and looking for a wife with a love for music and for romance, and she is what he needs. [Eventually—word crossed out] But Sarah has moved off with her new husband and the two never meet."

This story may be understood as representing DeeDee's conflicted feelings about relationships with men. In the first part of the narrative, her longing for a romantic relationship is clearly described. However, the conflict around this possibility quickly breaks through when DeeDee makes a "slip." Presumably wishing to describe positive feelings of the woman for the man, she instead initially characterizes the feelings as "unloving." This "error" is crossed out, but the attempt to shift to the positive is not complete, for the choice of a substitute expression, "undying" is negative in both its components ("un" and "dying"). It is only through the juxtaposition of the two negatives that a positive sentiment can be expressed.

In the next paragraph, we are provided with a reason for the heroine's conflict. Her father has dictated that she marry someone else, a man who is just like him. Her conflict around not knowing how to approach her own "secret passion" stems from her fear around what would happen if she disobeyed her father. She feels helpless and hopeless to escape from this paternal domination.

In addition to this more obvious theme of father controlling daughter's life and relationships, there are also hints that the "classical composer" may embody DeeDee's representation of another aspect of her father, the one who "truly adores" her. From afar, she longs for some closeness with this man, with whom she identifies. However, his modus operandi is "to track her down," in the same overbearing, intrusive manner of her father. However, as with her father (due to the previous history of paternal tyranny) she cannot allow closeness—she can "do no more" to further the relationship; "she must give up" despite his efforts to reach her.

Two other details of this story resonate with some unique features of DeeDee's autobiography. The first is her need to differentiate her interests from those of the family, and to "sneak away from her ladies-in-waiting," a striking echo of being "always flanked by my damn sisters." The second is voiced in the outcome that the two main characters "never meet" because "Sarah has moved off" as a result of her father's domination. This seems a clear echo of "my dad was always picking us up and moving us to different parts of the United States. Just when we would make new friends . . . "

Again, it is clear that the narrative themes from the autobiography are also present in the TAT story. Also, as in the case of Don, DeeDee's story helps explicate the somewhat puzzling statement in her autobiography that although she consciously longs for a partner, marriage, and children, romantic relationships do not seem to develop. Through her story we become aware of internal conflicts about heterosexual relationships perhaps most succinctly characterized as "approach–avoidance" conflicts. The resulting helpless feeling in the story is tied to feelings of paternal domination as well as to the conflicted emotional connection to the father. The conjunction of these elements illuminates some of the factors that may contribute to DeeDee's lack of romance.

Marie

In the preceding two cases, I have considered the autobiographical material first and then noticed the corresponding narrative themes in the projective stories. In the next example, I proceed in the opposite direction, first considering the story and then the autobiography. The storyteller is a female college senior.

TAT Story

About the picture of a person standing near a beaker,[3] Marie wrote:

> "There is a person in the background, but the room is extremely dark so we, the observers, can only see his hand. There is also a man in the picture, and he looks very grim. The man [or person] in the background is chastising him for something.
>
> "The man is probably a musician and his teacher or instructor is rebuking him for the mistakes he did in the performance earlier.
>
> "In the past, this musician never lived up to his potential. He has a wonderful gift of music but he lacks the discipline. His instructor knows this and has been very frustrated from the very beginning.
>
> "The instructor wants his student to do the best he could possibly do. He is merely frustrated that this gifted and talented musician is 'throwing' his talent away.
>
> "The musician, on the other hand, does not care for music. He merely wants to live his life as he pleases, and not follow the step [sic] of his father. He, at this point, is thinking that he can't wait to leave the room so he could go out and have some fun.

"The instructor will continue to chastise him and will continue to push him into studying more. Perhaps in time, he will stop needling him.

"The musician will one day rebel from the wishes of his family, and follow his own desires."

The central theme of this story is one that is common in adolescents—namely, the struggle between older and younger; parent and child—in which the child feels pressured to follow in the parent's footsteps but prefers to take his or her own direction. However, in addition to the recounting of this recognizable conflict, there are some more personally idiosyncratic aspects of the story. The first is the fact that the opening focus is on a character who cannot be seen in the picture, that is, a character who comes entirely from the mind of the storyteller. Only after presenting this character does the storyteller shift her attention to the one figure who *is* clearly portrayed in the picture. This is an unusual reaction to the picture and seems to speak to the existence of an important figure who occupies the recesses of the storyteller's mind and whose salience, psychologically, is of equal or greater importance than the figure portrayed, with whom, we assume, the storyteller identifies.

Quickly, we learn that this instructor/authority chastises and rebukes the central character for not living up to his potential, for not making use of his musical talent. Then, suddenly, there is a significant "addition" to the conflict: The storyteller advises us that the hero does not want to follow the "step of his father." Although this unprepared-for mention of the father may refer to a third character, it seems highly likely that the reference is to the chastising teacher, and that the mention of "father" is a slip, highlighted by some disruption in the storyteller's immediately preceding thought processes, as seen in the use of the word "step" rather than "steps" or "footsteps." Either way, it is now made clear that the teacher's chastising and pushing for the student "to do the best he could possibly do" significantly involves the father.

Another idiosyncratic aspect of the story is the reference to "being very frustrated from the very beginning," with the suggestion that there has been disharmony between the instructor/father and the student since early in life, and that the importance of living up to one's potential (as determined by the adult) has been a long-standing source of conflict.

Autobiographical Material

With these thoughts in mind, we turn to the life story of the storyteller. Marie is the oldest child of parents from an ethnic minority background.

The opening paragraph of her autobiography recounts her parents' description of her as a "difficult baby," born prematurely:

> "It was reported to me that I was an extremely fussy baby—one who refused to drink her milk, one who slept very lightly, and cried easily during the night."

This was in contrast to the children born after her, who caused no problems.

We see, in this opening comment, a theme that resonates with the idiosyncratic remark in her story—"frustrated from the very beginning." It is as though this family tale—that Marie was always a difficult child for the parents, not eating, not sleeping, not performing up to potential—has been firmly ingrained and seeks expression as part of an explanation of the nature of the relationship between self and authority.

The theme of talent having been early identified also appears in her autobiography:

> "I remember my Dad telling me when I was really young that when I grew up I was going to go to college and succeed."

In her story, the instructor knew from the beginning that his student had a wonderful potential.

The remainder of her autobiography focuses entirely, and exclusively, on school.

> "I grew up with the idea that academics were extremely important, and that education was the only means to move up in the world."

Marie writes that prior to beginning school, her mother had taught her to write the alphabet in print and in script, so that the kindergarten teacher was impressed. She refers to doing well in elementary and junior high school, being encouraged by her parents. Her father, however, seems to have played an especially important role from very early on, as indicated in the previous quote.

It was during junior high school that Marie recalls feeling great pressure from her family to do well so that she could go to a special high school for talented science students. Again, the focus is on this "step" as her father's goal:

> "My father had extremely high hopes for his daughter to go to this prestigious science high school."

When she was not accepted into her first-choice school, there was a great deal of stress in the family, with her father wanting her to go to her second-choice school "merely because it was a science high school." However, Marie convinced her father to wait 1 year so that she could take the entrance exam again; this time, she was accepted into the first-choice science school.

Marie recalls being unhappy about the amount of academic pressure at this school, which resulted in her being cut off from her former friends and social activities.

> "There were many times I resented going to such an achievement-oriented high school because I felt that I was missing out on a lot. My junior high school friends, for example, often invited me out to go to the movies, and I had to decline the offer because of the tremendous amount of schoolwork. I often resented my parents for pressuring me to go to this high school."

Here again, the narrative themes coincide with those of the story. The instructor focuses continually on the talent of the student, rebuking him for not working hard to make the most of his potential, while the student wants to follow his own desires, and wants to go out and have some fun. This struggle continues throughout the story, as it continues throughout the autobiography. The story, however, suggests that at some point in the future, the student will rebel and break away from the family's wishes—a possibility that is foreshadowed in the autobiography when Marie refused to accept the placement in a second-choice school simply because it was the type of (science) school toward which her father directed her. Taking a different direction from that promoted by her father may also be reflected in Marie's construction of a story about a musician. It is more common, with this picture, which includes a glass beaker, to tell a story about a scientist.

It is noteworthy that when the correspondences in narrative themes between the story and subsequently written autobiography were pointed out to Marie, she was quite surprised, and indicated that she had never put much stock in projective tests such as the TAT. At the time she wrote her stories, she had no awareness of their personal significance.

Sue

TAT Story

Let us consider one final example of a story, followed by the relevant life history information of its teller. The story is told about the picture of two people sitting on a bench, near a river, with a large bridge spanning the river. The storyteller, Sue, is a female college student.

> "These two people are married, and have been for over 25 years. They have stopped at the bench, to rest and look quietly at the sunset and the passers-by. They are not speaking much now, but occasionally they look at each other, and do not look away, because there is no tension or unpleasantness between them. Yet they are sad, deeply, deeply hurting over the death of their eldest daughter. It has been 6 months since their daughter died in a very sudden accident, and their thoughts are often filled with her, and all that they have lost with her death. They have always had a strong marriage, filled with love and mutual respect. The wife has worked, but now stays at home, looking for things that please her. Her husband is only 47, and will not retire for several years. He has a successful career, but is the epitome of a family man. Their daughter was 22, just out of college—creative, exuberant, ready to tap into her potential. And she was beautiful—not stunning, but glowing and happy.
>
> "They have been trying to spend time alone together, aware of the frightening statistics about marriages that fall apart after the loss of a child. They are seeing a therapist, together and alone, trying to cope with the anger and the guilt that pervades their everyday existence. They fear for the two younger children, 18 and 16, both boys, who have had some trouble grieving openly. They have tried to encourage openness and honesty, even the expression of outright hostility. But the pain they feel is nothing they can describe, and their lives seem so empty and tedious. They think they'll survive it, and they look to each other for support and love. The husband is being careful not to get absorbed in his work as an escape, but he's never done this before, and continues to spend as much time as possible at home, with his family, or sitting quietly on park benches with his wife."

The story revolves around the death of a beautiful oldest daughter, the painful reactions of the family to this loss, and their efforts to help and support each other around this family upset. Other idiosyncratic additions to this theme are seen in the special concern expressed for the reaction of the younger boys in the family. Also, the mention of a specific age for the father, "only 47, and will not retire for several years," indicating his relative youth, as well as the number of years that they have been married, "over 25 years," and the specific age of the daughter, "22," is rather unusual. Finally, the recurring juxtaposition of the parents' involvement with work versus involvement with family is striking: "The wife has worked, but now stays home"; the husband "has a successful career, but is the epitome of a family man" and is "careful not to get absorbed in his work as an escape, but he's never done this before and continues to spend as much time as possible at home, with his family." These work–family contrasts are presented as occurring in the context of the emotional upset of the family surrounding the daughter's death, which, in addition to being painful, also involves anger, guilt, and hostility.

Autobiographical Material

With such a strong and pervasive narrative line, it should not surprise us to find a similar theme in the autobiographical material. Sue begins her autobiography by describing herself as the middle child of three and immediately adds that her parents married young and began having children right away. She describes her father as being very involved with his job, not helping with the children, but quickly adds that she "never viewed him as neglectful, and when he played with [us] it was special."

Her mother is described as being very involved with the children. Although both parents encouraged her to use her potential, it was her mother who was especially supportive.

While in grammar school, Sue had "a serious accident" that left her on crutches for several years, until surgery was performed. In high school, she was a good student and active in athletics, which her father supported; however, she was not popular with the boys. She describes herself as not being interested in "girly" things, and spending a lot of time playing with her younger brother. Despite having a group of friends, Sue recounts her school years as plagued with unpleasant experiences with peers; she was disliked, tormented, and even assaulted by classmates. No explanation is offered for the recurrence of these cruel episodes. Also, her relationship with her "pretty blond sister with many boyfriends [was] quite bad." There was a lot of competition between the two girls, who were close in age, and her older sister was always angry at her. Sue then recounts that during high school, her sister had "some severe emotional problems, and the family had come together very strongly to help her." Sue adds that she "often felt angry at her sister for causing the family so much pain" but also felt that the competition between them and the success she found at school had been a source of her sister's problems.

Sue concluded her autobiographical statement by noting that her "younger brother had a difficult time adjusting to being the only child in the house" once she and her sister went to college.

The correspondences between the autobiographical material and the story are considerable. First, there is the point of the parents' early marriage and early parenthood. The positional prominence of this information in the autobiography coincides with the prominence given in her story to the youth of the father and the length of (and therefore early occurence of) the couple's marriage. This is followed by the similar juxtaposition in the history and the story of the father who is involved more with his work than with his children but who, at the same time, was never viewed as being neglectful.

The central theme of the story—the tragic loss of the beautiful older sister and the reaction of the family—is also found in the autobiographical material. Interestingly, in the story the loss of the sister occurs as a result of a "very sudden accident," echoing the "serious accident" that Sue herself experienced, expressing, perhaps, some painful identification with this older sister or, at least, with her unhappy fate. The reactions of the family to the older daughter's plight in both story and autobiography are similar: They come together to try to cope with the problem. They recognize that there are angry, even hostile feelings about what happened with this daughter, and there is concern expressed for the younger children's reactions, who find it difficult to openly express their feelings. In the story, both these younger children are boys, reflecting, perhaps, Sue's somewhat masculine identification (she was not interested in "girly" things), as well as her brother's difficulty in adjusting to the loss of his sisters when they went to college. More central in both the story and autobiography is the theme of unexpressed hostility about the older sister, as well the guilt. In the autobiography, we learn about the source of this guilt: Sue feels she was partly responsible for her sister's problems.

CONCEPTUALIZING THE RELATIONSHIPS BETWEEN THE TAT AND LIFE EXPERIENCES

TAT and "Peak Experiences"

From the previous examples, it seems clear that the life experience narratives of storytellers are portrayed in their projective stories. We know this because we "sense" the similarity in themes, in events, in stress or salience of particular aspects of relationships, and in other features of the material. Yet, there is obviously room for question or disagreement here; the similarities between history and story sensed by one individual may not be apparent to a second reader. For purposes of credibility, one wishes for some method for determining the similarity between life history themes and those found in TAT stories which would allow for an assessment of interobserver reliability.

One approach to objectifying the similarities between autobiographical and fantasy story material is exemplified in the work of McAdams (1982b). Here, the methods developed from the TAT to assess social motives, such as the need for power (nPower), or the need for intimacy (nIntimacy) were applied to autobiographical material obtained from the storyteller. Specifically, McAdams had college students provide autobiographical memories of different types: peak experiences, great learning experiences, satisfying experiences, neutral experiences, and unpleasant experiences. These memories were then coded for themes of interpersonal intimacy and personal power by using coding schemes developed for the TAT, adapted somewhat to cover the range of content occurring in the memory protocols. The results of the coding of memories were then compared with scores for nIntimacy and nPower derived from the same subjects' TAT stories.

It was hypothesized that subjects with high intimacy or power motivation (TAT scores) would likely recall, among their more positive memories, events characterized by intimacy and power content, respectively. This hypothesis was supported. Subjects who had high nIntimacy scores provided personal autobiographical memories and peak experiences, great learning experiences, and satisfying experiences that involved intimacy concerns; subjects scoring low on nIntimacy did not provide such personal memories. On the other hand, nIntimacy scores did not predict themes of intimacy in memories that were less personally meaningful (e.g., neutral or unpleasant memories), providing an important discriminative test of the hypothesis. A similar pattern of results was found for the power motive. Subjects with high nPower scores described more positive, personally meaningful memories involving themes of power, a relationship not found with the less meaningful neutral or unpleasant memories.[4]

Although these findings do provide objective evidence that the motivational themes expressed in TAT stories are significantly related to the life history of the storyteller, there are two questions to be raised about the interpretation of the findings. First, because the data are correlational in nature, it is not possible to determine whether it is the life experience that is dictating the nature of the story told and the motives expressed, as is being suggested in the present chapter, or whether it is the current existence of the social motive that selectively determines the memories being recalled and reported. Second, even if there is a correspondence between TAT motive strength and autobiographical memories, a correspondence between specific themes in the stories and in the life history is not necessarily indicated. Themes of intimacy, or of power, as expressed in the stories may occur in quite a different context and involve very different interpersonal relationships than themes of intimacy or power in the autobiography. In such a case, the overall scores from the story and autobiography may correlate, but their referents may be quite different. One might argue, of course, that this difference in referents is not important; if it occurs, it represents a displacement of subject or object, or some other process of substitution. In this case, what we find is not "archaeological verisimilitude" between autobiographical history and TAT story but, rather, narrative identity.

Unity Thema

Another approach to demonstrating correspondences between the themes of a TAT story and the themes of an individual's life history was employed early on by Murray (1938) in his detailed analysis of the life history of "Earnst." Murray used the concept of "unity thema," which he defined as the recurring constellation of interrelated needs linked to environmental press, to which the individual was exposed on one or more occasions in childhood. These needs may be collaborating or conflicting, and the occasions of occurrence may be gratifying or traumatic. Regardless of the nature or genesis of the unity thema, "it repeats itself in many forms during later life" (Murray, 1938, p. 605). In the case of Earnst, several separate themas (e.g, oral succorance, predator, quest for provisions, and forced robbery) were identified from his autobiography and were subsumed under a single unity thema characterized as the deprivation → anxiety → aggressive quest for provision. These same thema were found to recur in the TAT stories of Earnst. A generation later, Keniston (1965) used this approach in his study of alienated college youth. This work fits well within the narrative tradition.

Script Theory

Yet another approach to studying the idea that there are recurring dynamic patterns within the life history and life productions of an individual is represented in "script theory" (Alexander, 1988; Tomkins, 1978). Tomkins (1978) designated, as the basic element of individual lives, an event that includes an affect and the object of that affect; such an event is termed a "scene." A scene has a perceived beginning and an end; the "set of scenes lived in sequence is called the *plot* of a life" (1978, p. 217).

Personality is structured in terms of the grouping, or assembling, of similar and different scenes. The term "script" refers to the rules that individuals develop in relation to these scenes; these rules determine the individual's reaction to or interpretations of experience. New experiences (scenes) are assimilated to old experiences (scenes) on the basis, for example, of similarity of objects, with the result that the affect of the preexisting scene may be attributed to the current scene. As summarized by Carlson (1986), "a *scene* tells us what is happening, and a *script* tells us what to do about it" (p. 247).

This idea of recurring thema or scripts as constituting a significant aspect of the individual's personality has been developed by Alexander (1988) into an approach to personality assessment. In this approach, the important units of personality structure may be identified from autobiographical or interview material, from such personal documents as diaries, or from such imaginative productions as TAT stories. The important task of the investigator is to identify in the material provided that which is important to the individual and which conveys the way in which the individual construes the world. This task is accomplished not by focusing on the particular content in the communications but rather by determining the principles used to organize experience. These principles are referred to as means–end sets.

To accomplish this goal, the investigator first determines which part of the material is to be studied further. This determination is made on the basis of the "principle identifiers of salience" (Alexander, 1988, p. 269). Nine such identifiers have been proposed: primacy, frequency, uniqueness, negation, emphasis, omission, error, isolation, and incompletion. Each of these has been discussed by Alexander (1988). Once these identifiers have been used to locate the salient units or sequence of "consecutive sentences which form an entity through shared content" (p. 278) within the communication, the next task is to transform the units into a form that will allow the detection of means–end commonality. This is done by rewriting the identified sequences into an abstract form. In this way, particularities of content, which might be misleading, are ignored; rather, the sequence of occurrences, the means–end relationship, and the outcome of the sequence are highlighted. Further, an examination of the identified sequences allows for judgments about the power or importance of the means–end unit in the individual's personality; the judgment is based on the frequency or repetition of the sequence in the communication of the individual. It also allows a determination of the generality of the sequence, that is, its pervasiveness, or the amount of psychological "space" that the sequence occupies in the individual's communication.

This approach of identifying the important sequences through the principles of salience and then transforming these sequences into more abstract units that may be grouped, or counted, may be used in an atheoretical manner, to "let the data reveal itself" (Alexander, 1988, p. 268)—that is, to reveal what are the most frequent and pervasive means–end sequences in the individual's communication without preconception as to what these might be. Alternatively, the approach may be used to answer a particular question of interest posed by the investigator (e.g., to discover the means–end sequences representing the individual's conceptions of authority, or of responsibility) even though the subject's communication was not necessarily focused on this question.

It is easy to see how this approach might be used to address the question of the relationship between the life story and the TAT story. If the narrative themes in the two sources of material correspond—if one reflects the other—then similar means–end sequences should be found in both. Such was the purpose of an investigation by Demorest and Alexander (1992). In this study, subjects created stories in response to photographs of faces that had ambiguous emotional expressions. The investigators then identified the scripts in the stories and related these to scripts derived from the subjects' autobiographical material. For the majority of the story scripts (62%), it was possible to make a correct match between the story script and the autobiographical script material (i.e., to match the story script with the autobiography of the individual who told the story). The authors concluded that the autobiographical scripts were critical determiners of the ways in which subjects experience, interpret, and organize ambiguous affective stimuli.

Singer and Salovey (1991) provide a review of the theoretical concepts of schema, scripts, and prototypes and of their utility in personality research, as well as their relevance to clinical practice.

Examples of Script Theory in Clinical Work

Script theory may also be used to understand various aspects of the life story itself as it is revealed at different periods of life or in different facets of the ongoing life. Carlson (1981) has used this approach to show how an early traumatic experience became a "nuclear scene" in the life of a young professional woman, Jane W. In this process, new situations are "scanned" for similarity to the old nuclear scene. Where similarities are found, the individual's reaction in the present is often determined by the dangers and disappointments of the earlier experience. That is, experiences in the person's present life are treated as analogous to the incident of the earlier, nuclear scene.[5] Over time, more and more of the person's current life experiences are taken over as analogues of the nuclear scene. Although the psychological meaning of the analogues is unconscious, they occupy increasingly greater segments of the individual's psychic life. "Initially, one's scenes dictate script formation, but over time scripts so organize experience as to dictate one's scenes" (Carlson, 1986, p. 247).

Through identifying a critical early nuclear memory and its associated scripts, Carlson (1981) was able to demonstrate the reoccurrence of these scripts in the current life of Jane W as they appeared in her autobiography, her dreams, and clinical interviews. Each of these types of "stories" could be characterized by the use of similar scripts, and thus a cohesiveness in Jane's experiences, not previously recognized, was illuminated. In a subsequent study, Carlson (1986) used the same script approach to demonstrate changes in Jane's dream stories from pre- to postpsychotherapy.

SUMMARY

The case studies in this chapter clearly demonstrate one of the main theses of this book, that stories told about the TAT include narrative themes that are significant in the life history of the storyteller. The case studies also indicate that TAT stories may provide more understanding of the emotional significance of life events than the individual can otherwise supply and may reveal links among emotions, events, and fantasies of which the individual is largely unaware. Unlike some other projective tests, however (e.g., the Rorschach), the psychological meaning of TAT stories is, in most cases, not difficult for the storyteller to discern once the consistencies between story narratives and life history narratives have been pointed out.

Empirical research studies reported in this chapter show that these consistencies between stories and life history are not just occasional, anecdotal occurrences. Using carefully constructed coding schemes, clear links have been reliably demonstrated between the story themes and the subjects' descriptions of their own life histories. There can be little doubt that the TAT provides a window on the narrative life history of the storyteller.

• SIX •

Gender Identity:
An Interpretive
Perspective

O f the various interpretive approaches to the TAT, the one that most closely approximates a true narrative was developed by Robert May to assess gender identity (May, 1966, 1975, 1980).

GENDER IDENTITY AND NARRATIVE

May's description of fantasy as "the rich and varied theater that plays in our heads all the time" (1980, p. x) orients us to his narrative mode of thinking and sets the stage for his use of fantasy (TAT) productions to study gender identity. Fantasy, which goes on in the darkened recesses of our minds, is rarely attended to; yet it is a distinctly human activity. It refers backwards in time to history and anticipates the future. In fantasy, "we interpret the events of our life and distill them into a collection of vivid tableaux which help to guide our next actions" (p. x).

Clearly, this is a narrative conception of fantasy. There is a concern with before and after, there are structures, there is intention, and there is mental activity going on outside individual awareness. Motivational forces, emotion, and conflict round out May's conception of fantasy—a conception that bears great similarity to that of narrative.

Given this conception of fantasy, it is then perhaps not surprising that the strategy May takes to study fantasy is a narrative approach. May (1980) begins his book *Sex and Fantasy* by citing two myths, which he describes as "fantasies shared by a whole culture" (p. 1). These narratives are constructed by a people to express "its important concerns and its sense of what matters in human life" (p. 1).

The first myth, from classical Greek mythology, is the story of Phaethon, the son of Phoebus, the sun god. Briefly, the tale relates how Phaethon, due to his unbridled pride, convinces his unwilling father to let him drive the sun chariot across the skies. Though his father warns him of the dangers, stressing the need for greater maturity and immortal strength to accomplish the feat—qualities not available to the youth—Phaethon persists. The boy's hubris prevails, and he embarks on the perilous ride. He flies high but then loses control of the horses. Pandemonium ensues. The chariot plunges earthward, scorching the fields, desiccating the oceans. To end this catastrophe, Zeus intervenes, strikes the chariot with lightning, and Phaethon falls to his death.

On the psychological level, this is a narrative that warns and instructs us about proper living and the dangers of excessive pride. Phaethon approached Phoebus with the request to drive the chariot in order to prove to himself and others that he was, indeed, the son of a god. He persisted in the challenge despite his father's warning to prove, one supposes, that he, who was half mortal, was nevertheless as powerful as a god.

It is central to May's thesis that this narrative is carefully constructed around a tangible trajectory: that Phaethon starts out by ascending to Phoebus' palace to prove his high social status, then climbs higher in the chariot, only to lose control and plunge down to his death. This same theme is also well-known from the myth of Icarus, who flew too high, allowing the heat of the sun to melt the wax holding his wings in place, with the result that Icarus falls to his death.[1] This structural trajectory—rising, ascending, reaching a pinnacle of height, followed then by a dramatic downfall—is seen by May as the archetypal male narrative, which he characterizes as enhancement followed by deprivation.

The second myth that May discusses is that of Demeter and her daughter Persephone. The story opens with Persephone being swallowed up into the earth and dragged down into the underworld by Hades. Demeter, her mother, is greatly pained by this and spends years in grief-filled, self-sacrificing wandering without food or comfort in her attempt to find her daughter. In her distress, Demeter makes the fields barren, threatening famine to the world. At this point, Zeus intervenes, and Persephone is reunited with her mother. With Persephone's return, there is joy and happiness, and the fields bloom full with fruit and flowers.

The focus in this myth is on emotions rather than events or actions. Again, there is a clear trajectory, or course, that these feelings run. Almost immediately, the intense emotions of loss and grief are present, followed by years of longing, searching, and unhappiness. Then, after this prolonged misery, there is a turning point: reuniting, closeness, embracing, and joyfulness. A similar narrative pattern of negative emotion followed by positive affect is seen also in the well-known fairy tales of Cinderella and Snow White. This pattern, of deprivation followed by enhancement, is considered by May to be the female archetypal narrative.

Having identified these two narrative patterns—the male pattern of enhancement followed by deprivation, and the female pattern of deprivation followed by enhancement—as central to cultural myths, May went on to explore the occurrence of these configurations in the fantasies of men and women today. Indeed, as will be discussed later, he found the same patterns to exist in the TAT stories told by today's college students. May interpreted these findings to mean that these narrative patterns which have existed over the centuries reflect something basic about the differences in male and female gender identity. Masculine identity is reflected in the narrative of enhancement followed by deprivation. Feminine identity is reflected in the narrative of deprivation followed by enhancement. What theoretical explanation could be offered for these findings?

THEORETICAL BASES FOR FANTASY PATTERNS

May's (1966, 1980) explanation for these gender-related differences in fantasy patterns is drawn from both psychoanalytic and social learning theory. Female psychology, from the psychoanalytic point of view, is characterized by activity that is directed inward. This inner orientation—sometimes erroneously referred to as passivity—comes about as the result of three factors; two of these are biological "givens," and one is the result of social conditioning. Constitutionally, the female is less active and less aggressive,[2] and female sex organs are generally not designed for the expression of active or aggressive impulses.[3] Social conditioning of females adds to this by stressing the inhibition of activity and aggression. These three factors combine to create a situation in which activity, denied overt expression, is directed inward.

In classical psychoanalytic theory (see Freud, 1924/1959), activity and aggression are intimately linked. Insofar as activity is directed inward in the female, so is aggression. This direction of aggression inward creates a situation of masochism; aggression is directed toward the self. Suffering is endured in the hope of obtaining some eventual positive gratification. Such self-abnegation, or martyrdom, for the promise of some future pleasure or reward is referred to as feminine masochism (see Deutsch,

1944). Although classical psychoanalytic theory relates masochism to sexual functioning in the female (e.g., menstruation, coitus, and childbirth, all involving pain or discomfort to a greater or lesser degree), other psychoanalytic thinkers have discussed masochism independently from sexual function or drives. Thus "moral masochism" refers to an abnegation, or denial, of the self and an inhibition of aggression directed outward, which occurs not as part of sexuality but rather to maintain an attachment to another person (see Fenichel, 1945; Menaker, 1979). In either case, whether masochism is distinctly a female characteristic as a result of biological structures and function or whether it is a mechanism that serves the social need for attachment—it is seen as the result of aggression directed inward, and it is understood as the first part of a sequence in which there is an expectation of eventual pleasure or reward. This, then, is the theoretical basis for the deprivation-followed-by-enhancement pattern for female fantasy.

The metaphor for the male pattern is also found in biological sexuality. The ascension–decension cycle of fantasy is also a biological experience of the male, repeated many times, in the sequence of phallic tumescence and detumescence. Aspects of narcissism, ambition, and pride are understood to derive from this exciting ascension of the penis, as is a sense of failure and dejection with its collapse. The external placement of the male genitals provides an external focus for (sexual) activity.

As was true in the case of the female, the social conditioning of males collaborates with biological functioning to create a position of activity directed outward. Males are socialized to overcome the environment, to be aggressive, to succeed, to be superior. The greater the emphasis on succeeding, the greater the fear of failure, or "falling down." Yet the trajectory cannot always be on the rise; some decline is inevitable. This repeated cycle of ascension–decension forms the basis for the enhancement-followed-by-deprivation pattern of male fantasy.

ASSESSING GENDER IDENTITY

On the basis of the preceding discussion, it is apparent that psychoanalytic theory considers the gender identity of an individual to consist not so much of consciously endorsed attitudes, opinions, and interests; rather, gender identity is part of a deep-seated, largely unconscious sense of oneself, and of oneself in relation to the environment. From this starting point, it is more likely that differences in the gender identity of males and females would be revealed on such projective tests as the TAT than on such measures of conscious self-report as questionnaires or checklists. These latter measures provide an indication of the extent to which an individual has learned and subscribed to existing social stereotypes regarding sex-role behaviors. But for those who understand gender identity to involve not only culturally based behaviors but also a deeper, more basic sense of self, closely derived from biological differences, such measures of surface attitudes provide only a narrow and incomplete picture of consciously endorsed attitudes toward sex roles, which may or may not be in agreement with a more deep-seated sense of maleness or femaleness.

In an attempt to develop a measure of gender identity that did not depend on obvious cultural stereotypes, May (1966, 1969) turned to the TAT. Guided both by psychoanalytic theory and the archetypal male (Phaethon and Icarus) and female (Demeter and Persephone) myths, May constructed a scoring scheme for the TAT based on the *pattern and sequence* of the fantasy story rather than on specific content or themes. He noted that the modal fantasy story of college men followed a predictable pattern: The stories typically began with a series of positive experiences or emotions, reached a climax or turning point, and ended with experiences or emotions of a negative tone. This pattern he characterized as enhancement followed by deprivation. The typical female pattern, on the other hand, he found to be the reverse: deprivation followed by enhancement.

From these observations, May devised explicit scoring criteria to reveal such gender-related differences in story patterns. The scoring process begins with identifying the "pivotal incident" (PI) in the story, defined as the dramatic turning point of the story, the central act or feeling that stands between what went before and the ultimate outcome. Once this incident (which is not scored) is identified, the story is then scored for the occurrence of units of both deprivation and enhancement. Examples of deprivation units include physical tension or pain, physical harm or injury, falling, losing control, and failure, among others. Examples of enhancement include physical satisfaction, physical accomplishment, rising or flying, success, and positive emotion, among others. (The complete set of deprivation and enhancement categories and the criteria for locating the pivotal incident are given in Table 6.1.)[4] Deprivation units that occur in the story before the PI are scored plus (+); those that follow the PI are scored minus (−).

Enhancement units that occur before the PI are scored minus (−); those that follow are scored plus (+). Because the typical male pattern is enhancement followed by deprivation, a typical male score would be negative. The typical female pattern, of deprivation followed by enhancement, would yield a positive score.

TABLE 6.1. Scoring Categories for Deprivation/Enhancement Fantasy Patterns

Categories of deprivation

 1. Physical tension.
 2. General physical discomfort, poverty, professional or vocational obscurity.
 3. Physical harm or injury.
 4. Physical exertion or striving.
 5. Falling.
 6. Physical decline or defect.
 7. Failure.
 8. Negative feelings.
 9. Unpleasant pressures.
10. Tension, dissatisfaction, generalized desire.
11. Ignorance of something important.
12. Self-sacrifice.

Categories of enhancement

 1. Physical satisfaction.
 2. Ability, physical excellence, or accomplishment.
 3. Height, rising, flying, stopping a fall.
 4. Growth.
 5. Positive feeling.
 6. Positive shift in tension level.
 7. Positive anticipation.
 8. Receiving help, affection, or concern.
 9. Success.
10. Publicity, attention, fame.
11. Revenge, retaliation, successful resistance.
12. Insight, realization.

Criteria for locating the pivotal incident

 1. A literal fall.
 2. A mistake.
 3. A high point of desire.
 4. Wishing for something.
 5. State of tension prior to the "happening."
 6. Point of decision.
 7. Intense feeling or critical action determining what is to come.
 8. Interlude between past and future.
 9. Phrases: "climax", "peak," "is going to."
10. Change in story tense (present → future).
11. "If" statements are not very acceptable.
12. Emotion or thought must be strong and clearly related to following action of outcome to be a PI.

Note. From May (1980). Copyright 1980 by W. W. Norton. Reprinted by permission.

Examples of the Assessment of Gender Identity

In Chapter 5, TAT stories from four college students were presented in conjunction with their autobiographical material. We use these stories now to illustrate the scoring method of May to determine gender identity from the TAT.

Don

Don, a senior in college, told the following story about the picture of a person standing near a flask, one hand lifted. We saw in Chapter 5 how this story contains important narrative themes from Don's own life. On this presentation, the story has been scored for the occurrence of deprivation and enhancement units, relative to the pivotal incident, which is enclosed in double brackets.

The first story Don told was about this picture of the person standing in a darkened room; to one side, there are objects that might be seen as a glass beaker and a piece of printed paper.

> "Mark Parker is a lab scientist at MIT doing independent research on genetics and DNA. He is currently hot on the trail of an amazing breakthrough sure to win him a Nobel Prize in chemistry and get him world renown. As he progresses through the final stage of his work, he notices some odd readouts on his computer printout of data. Shocked by the revelation that his great discovery may, in fact, never materialize, [[he rushes over to his equipment and pulls out the one beaker of material which is producing the faulty data, crucial to his experiment]]. As Dr. Parker stares into the beaker, he thinks about his enormous time commitment to his work and the ridicule that will come from his peers if the experiment he has staked his reputation on fails. It would be very easy for Dr. Parker to remedy the situation and get rid of the evidence and present his other findings as proof of his theory, but that would break the ethical code of research science. As he stares blankly into the offending beaker, Dr. Parker thinks of fame, glory, money, success, shame, guilt, and responsibility. As the beaker is crushed in the heat of the incinerator in the building's cellar, his only thought becomes 'I wonder if anyone will ever find out.' "

This story of Don's contains 7 units scored plus (+) and 9 units scored minus (−), yielding a total score of −2. The pivotal incident represents the moment in which a critical decision is made. There are about an equal number of deprivation and enhancement units in the story, but their sequence is important in determining the overall masculine score.

Here is a second story told by Don. The picture shows a man and woman sitting on a bench near a river, with a bridge overhead. Again, we noted in Chapter 5 the autobiographical narrative themes in this story, which we now examine using the gender-identity narrative.

> "This is Mr. and Mrs. James Smith. Their son Bill <u>committed suicide</u> [D+] almost 7 years ago, by <u>jumping off</u> [D+] this bridge. [[This is the first time they have been able to come here and really think about their son.]] They are <u>torn by emotions</u> [D-] and memories of the <u>happy times</u> [E+] they spent with their son. Their one overriding <u>fear</u> [D-] is for their youngest son, Donald, who has turned very <u>depressed</u> [D-] and has <u>trouble making friends</u> [D-] since his older brother's suicide. The Smiths are <u>extremely worried</u> [D-] that Donald may also take his own life in a fit of deep depression. The thought of losing a second son in this way tears at their souls. Donald refuses professional help and seems <u>angry</u> [D-] with his mother often. Even in this hour of stress, as his parents <u>attempt to finally accept their son's death</u> [E+], Donald is off playing baseball with his friends from college."

This story, with a total of 4 units scored plus (+) and 6 units scored minus (−), yields a total score of −2, again indicating the male pattern. The PI, enclosed in double brackets, occurs rather early in the story, but it is the clearest marker between what came before and what comes after, as seen in the change of verb tense from past to present. It is also noteworthy that the scorable units are almost entirely of deprivation, in keeping with the depressed tone of the story. Still, the overall score results in the male pattern, obtained in this case by events going from bad to worse.

DeeDee

The next story comes from DeeDee, another college senior discussed in Chapter 5. Her story is also told about the picture of the figure in the darkened room, with the beaker-like object to the side.

This story illustrates the occasional need, in scoring, to rearrange the sections of the story so that they follow a logical time sequence. In this story from DeeDee, the opening paragraph refers to what is going on at the moment, in the picture, but the paragraph that follows describes what preceded the events described in the first paragraph. Thus, for scoring purposes, the story is rearranged in chronological order. The paragraph beginning "Sarah is the daughter . . . " is placed at the beginning of the story. The last phrase of that paragraph—"that was her final act of love"—marks the pivotal incident, the point at which the story takes a new turn. The assignment of plus and minus scores is relative to the rearranged order of the three paragraphs.

"This is a [classical—word crossed out] composer of classical music from the 17th century. He is examining a gift presented to him [E+] mysteriously by an anonymous admirer of his music. She has been watching him for months and has fallen in love, but he does not know [D-] this or who she is. The note with the package merely said 'With [unloving—word crossed out] undying love and devotion, an ardent admirer.' The [note—word crossed out] mystery has intrigued him enough to drop the sheet music he has been working on, and now he stands contemplating the mysterious suitor.

"Sarah is the daughter of a count and is obligated [D+] to marry a count chosen for her by her father. But she is not in love with the [D+] count, she finds him quite dull. Her secret passion [E-] is music, and whenever she can she sneaks away from her ladies-in-waiting to hear Roberto's symphonies. She has fallen madly in love [E-] with him from [D+] afar, but does not know how to approach [D+] him, nor what would [D+] happen if she dared to break her engagement to the count. She feels [D+] hopeless, so she sent the note and gift but knows she can do no more. [D+] She must give up [D+]—[that was her final act of love and now, done, she must heed to her family's wishes.]

"Roberto will pursue this mysterious admirer with all his heart. [E+] He will hire several investigators to track her down. [E+] He has been lonely [D-] and looking for a wife with a love for music and for romance, [E+] and she is what he needs. [Eventually—word crossed out] But Sarah has moved off with her new husband and the two never meet." [D-]

With 11 plus units and 5 minus, the overall score is +6, indicating the feminine pattern. Six of the units are enhancement, whereas 10 are deprivation. Again, it is the sequence of these units that is responsible for the highly feminine score.

Marie

Marie is the college senior who, while talented, was always considered by her family to be "difficult" and who resented her family's academic pressures, preferring instead to have some social life. Here we examine the story for the gender-identity pattern.

"There is a person in the background, but the room is extremely dark so we, the observers, can only see his hand. There is also a man in the picture, and he looks very grim. The man (or person) in the background is chastising him [D+] for something.

"The man is probably a musician and his teacher or instructor is rebuking him for the mistakes he did [D+] in the performance earlier.

"In the past, this musician never lived up to his potential. [D+] He has a wonderful gift of music but he lacks the discipline. His instructor knows this and has been very frustrated [D+] from the very beginning.

"The instructor [D+] <u>wants his student to do the best</u> he could possibly do. He is merely frustrated that this gifted and talented musician is 'throwing' his talent away.

"The musician, on the other hand, does not care for music. He merely wants to live his life as he pleases, and [D+] <u>not follow the step [*sic*] of his father.</u> [[He, at this point, is thinking that he can't wait to leave the room so he could go out and have some fun.]]

"The instructor will continue to chastise him and <u>will continue to push him [D-] into studying more.</u> Perhaps in time, he will stop needling him.

"The musician will [E+] <u>one day rebel</u> from the wishes of his family, and [E+] <u>follow his own desires.</u>"

In this story, there are 8 plus units and 1 minus, for a total score of +7—a highly feminine score. The PI represents a moment of tension, or desire, preceding a change in the situation for the hero. There are seven units of deprivation, most of which occur before the pivotal incident. The two enhancement units both follow the pivotal incident.

Sue

Finally, let us consider the story of Sue, the last college student discussed in Chapter 5. Sue's story was told about the picture showing a couple seated on a bench at the river. It is interesting to compare this story with that of Don about the same picture. Both stories are about the death of a child and of the grief of the parents around this event. However, the sequence and trajectory of the two stories is quite different, yielding a strongly feminine score for Sue and a masculine score for Don.

"These two people are married, and have been for over 25 years. They have stopped at the bench, to rest and look quietly at the sunset and the passers-by. They are not speaking much now, but occasionally they look at each other, and do not look away, because [D+] there is no tension, or unpleasantness between them. Yet <u>they are sad, deeply, deeply hurting</u> over the [D+] <u>death</u> of their eldest daughter. It has been six months since their daughter died in a very [D+] <u>sudden accident</u>, and their thoughts are often filled with her, and all that they have lost with her death. They have always had a strong marriage, filled with [E-] <u>love and mutual respect</u>. [[The wife has worked, but now stays at home, looking for things that please her.]] Her husband is only 47, and will not retire for several years. He has a [E+] <u>successful career</u>, but is the epitome of a family man. Their daughter was 22, just out of college—[E+] <u>creative</u>, [E+] <u>exuberant</u>, <u>ready to tap into her potential</u>. And she was beautiful—not stunning, but [E+] <u>glowing and happy</u>.

"They have been trying to spend time alone together, <u>aware of the [E+] frightening statistics</u> about marriages that fall apart after the loss of a child. They are seeing a therapist, together and alone, <u>trying to</u> ^{E+} <u>cope</u> with the <u>anger and the guilt</u> ^{D–} that pervades their everyday existence. They <u>fear</u> ^{D–} for the two younger children, 18 and 16, both boys, who have had some trouble grieving openly. They have <u>tried to encourage openness and honesty, even the expression of outright</u> ^{E+} <u>hostility.</u> ^{D–} But the pain they feel is nothing they can describe, and their <u>lives seem so empty and tedious.</u> ^{D–} They <u>think they'll survive it,</u> ^{E+} and they <u>look to each other for support and love.</u> ^{E+} The husband is being careful <u>not to get absorbed in his work as an escape,</u> ^{E+} but he's <u>never</u> <u>done this before,</u> ^{D–} and continues to spend as much time as possible at home, with his family, or sitting quietly on park benches with his wife."

In this story, there are 14 plus units and 5 minus, yielding a total score of +9—a highly feminine pattern. Seven of these units are deprivation and 13 are enhancement. The distribution of deprivation and enhancement units is different from that of Marie. However, owing to the importance of sequence, both stories yield a highly positive, feminine score. As compared to Don's story about the same picture, it is interesting that, up to the point of the pivotal incident, the two stories of Sue and Don have the same score (+2). After the PI, however, Sue's story contains 11 positive enhancement units and 4 deprivation units, yielding a feminine score, whereas Don's includes 2 enhancement and 5 deprivation units, resulting in a masculine score. The PI in this story is that moment in the story that refers to what was before and what is now.

The distribution of deprivation and enhancement units is different from that of Marie in that each type occurs both before and after the pivotal incident.

RESEARCH STUDIES

The assessment of gender identity using the deprivation/enhancement (D/E) narrative, which allows for a masculine or feminine identity score independent from biological sex or endorsement of gender-role stereotypes, has also been used in a series of research investigations to study groups of men and women.[5] In an initial investigation (May, 1966), college students (60 females and 44 males) were asked to write stories about four TAT-like pictures.[6] Each story was scored according to the approach described above,[7] and a comparison of the scores of the men and women students was made. In this group of college men and women, when the scores were averaged over the four stories told, there was a highly significant difference ($p < .0005$) between the men and women in the direction predicted: Men showed the enhancement-followed-by-deprivation pattern; (mean score = −.24); women showed the deprivation-followed-by-enhancement pattern (mean = +.80). An examination of the stories on a picture-by-picture basis indicated that gender differences were statistically significant for three of the four pictures.[8] These differences in gender identity, as determined from the TAT, were validated in a second study (May, 1969).

Because there is some evidence that women are more likely to tell sad, unhappy stories (Murstein, 1961), May (1966) was concerned about demonstrating that what was being assessed with his approach was a narrative pattern[9] rather than the personality trait of optimism–pessimism. Using the stories about the three pictures that showed a significant gender difference, May counted the total number of deprivation units used by men and by women, as well as the number of enhancement units. From six comparisons, five indicated that males and females did not differ in the total number of either kind of expression; that is, there was no evidence that, overall, females had more sadness or unhappiness in their stories.[10] It was thus the difference in the *sequence* of deprivation and enhancement units that differentiated between males and females.

Another check was made to determine whether the findings might be explained by a tendency on the part of women to give happy endings to stories, while men give unhappy endings. To this end, only deprivation and enhancement units from the first part of the TAT stories were considered (the part of the story prior to the PI). If, in fact, it was a difference in endings that produced the results, there should be no differences between men and women in their scores for the first part of the stories. However, the results of this analysis indicated that women gave relatively more deprivation than enhancement units in the beginning of all three stories. Thus, the findings cannot be explained by happy or sad endings. Again, it is the *pattern* of the story that is important. Other possible confounding factors, such as length of stories or verbal aptitude, were also considered and ruled out. In the end, May had developed and demonstrated a reliable narrative method for assessing gender identity in college students.

In a further use of this approach with college students, Johnson (1974) asked 50 males and 50 females to write stories about a picture of trapeze artists and TAT Card 17BM (a man clinging to a rope). His results replicated May's findings, with females showing a strong deprivation-followed-by-enhancement pattern and males showing the reverse. Johnson also found that the gender-identity pattern of the students was influenced by the presence of siblings in the family. For males, the masculine identity pattern was strongest among men who had older brothers. Among the female students, those who had older siblings (male or female) had a less intense feminine pattern, while those who had younger brothers and sisters showed stronger feminine patterns.

Yet another study of college students (50 males, 50 females) found that gender identity, as assessed from TAT stories using May's approach, was related to the use of defense mechanisms (Cramer & Carter, 1978). Using a measure of defense mechanisms that had consistently shown gender differences (the Defense Mechanism Inventory; Gleser & Ihilevich, 1969),[11] it was found that gender identity was significantly related to defense choice. Females with the strongest feminine gender-identity patterns (D → E), as compared to females with weak feminine patterns, were more likely to use the feminine defense mechanism of reversal, and less likely to use the male defense of turning against the object. At the same time, males who had the strongest masculine gender-identity pattern (E → D), as compared to males with weak masculine patterns, were more likely to use the male defense of projection and less likely to use the female defense of turning against the self.

There is also evidence that the intensity of the gender-identity pattern may be enhanced by the presence of sexually salient stimulation, especially in men. Bramante (1970) recruited 60 male and 60 female undergraduates and showed half of them a romantic film (including sexual love) and half a comedy film of Laurel and Hardy. Immediately after the film, the students wrote stories about three TAT-like pictures.[12] It was predicted, and found, that the romantic film increased the differences between men and women in their gender-identity scores beyond that which was found also in the group with the comedy film. Equally important, the findings showed that the effect of the romantic movie influenced the story *pattern* differentially in men and women. For women, an increase in deprivation units occurred in the early part of the story; for men, a similar increase occurred in the later part of their stories. Thus the effect of arousal "works on the balance and position of suffering in the story" (May, 1980, p. 192). In other words, the experimental intervention influenced the *sequence* and *pattern* of the narrative.

In addition to these studies with college students, May has used his TAT approach in the study of hospitalized patients, to determine its relevance for the study of gender identity in a psychiatric population (May, 1975). In the first study of 32 acute schizophrenics, the same gender differences were found as with college students, with females scoring relatively more positively—that is, showing more of the D → E pattern than males, who showed the E → D pattern. In the second study, presence of the D → E pattern was investigated in a group of 14 actively homosexual young men who had sought psychotherapy. The narrative pattern of these homosexual men was decidedly more feminine than that of any other male group studied. In the third patient study, the presence of the gender-identity pattern was related to psychiatric diagnoses of "hysterical" or "obsessive–compulsive" character traits, with the expectation that individuals with a strong feminine identity pattern would be more likely to show hysterical traits, whereas a strong masculine pattern would be associated with obsessive–compulsive traits. The predictions were confirmed for the 27 female patients; those who were diagnosed as hysterical showed stronger D → E patterns (mean of +2.45) whereas those who were diagnosed as obsessive–compulsive showed stronger E → D patterns (mean of −1.07). Among the 22 males, only two were diagnosed as hysterical, making statistical comparisons inappropriate. However, the hysterical males did show a slightly more feminine pattern than the male obsessive–compulsives (−.50 vs. −.71).

The D/E narrative interpretive approach to the TAT for assessing gender identity has also been used with children and has revealed some interesting developmental differences. This work is discussed in detail in Chapter 11.

SUMMARY

This chapter has presented the first approach to interpreting TAT stories which is based on a perspective provided by the interpreter. This perspective for the study of gender identity is itself a narrative—one that has appeared in ancient myths—which rests on the belief that the narrative form of masculine and feminine fantasy constructions has a different pattern and trajectory. This gender-related form has been identified by Robert May as deprivation followed by enhancement (the feminine narrative) or enhancement followed by deprivation (the masculine narrative).

The use of this approach to assess gender identity through TAT stories is then described. Research studies supporting the validity of the approach are discussed. The application of the deprivation/enhancement approach is illustrated by the stories from the college students discussed in Chapter 5. By reexamining this material, we see how the same stories that were previously interpreted using the storyteller's life history as the narrative frame of reference can now be approached in terms of a very different narrative—in this case, the interpreter's narrative for gender identity. Thus, the use of different interpretive narratives provides us with different kinds of information from the same stories. In the next chapter, we will see yet another interpretive stance applied to these same stories.

• SEVEN •

Defense Mechanisms: Another Interpretive Perspective

As we have seen, stories may be highly revealing of broad narratives portraying significant events in the life history of the storyteller, as well as of narratives more clearly focused on one aspect of personality, as in the assessment of sexual identity. Most often, the storyteller is quite unaware of this personal significance or of the attitudes and motives that are being revealed in the stories.

Storytellers, like others, have some stake in not knowing what they are revealing. The procedure of the TAT facilitates this "not knowing"—the story is presumably about those characters who appear in a picture provided by the examiner. But some persons, faced with this task, will be hesitant to respond, fearing what they may reveal about themselves. Some will hesitate because they do not believe they possess sufficient imagination or creativity to produce an interesting story and do not wish to be revealed as inadequate. Others, faced with particular pictures that arouse personal conflict or doubts, may become anxious, vaguely sensing that there is a potential psychological threat involved in formulating and voicing a story.

What happens when the storytelling task arouses such hesitation? One possibility is that the anxious person refuses to tell a story, saying, "I can't" or "I can't think of anything," or, "The picture doesn't remind me of anything." Rarely does the person say, "I won't." In these brief examples of reasons given for not telling a story, we can see how mental mechanisms are used to defend the person from revealing what he or she fears to disclose. It is rare that an individual says, openly and directly, "I don't want to do this"; it is more common to hear, "I can't think of anything."

Taking this statement at face value— (i.e., believing that it is the case that he or she cannot think) the person is describing the functioning of a defense mechanism. Due to the anxiety aroused by the storytelling situation, all thought, ideas, and images that might contribute to creating a story have been blocked from awareness. Temporarily, repression has created a mental state devoid of content.

Another defensive strategy, when faced with anxiety about the request to tell a story, is seen in the individual who looks at the picture and then says to the examiner, "You probably want me to tell a story about _____." Here, storytellers *do* have some thoughts—they *can* think—but these thoughts are attributed to the examiner, who then becomes responsible for the thoughts. To escape the anxiety associated with being responsible for having these thoughts, the storyteller projects them onto the examiner.

Anxiety about telling a story may also be dealt with by a combination of these two defensive maneuvers. In using the statement, "The picture doesn't remind me of anything," the individual is protected from self-revelation. It is the picture that is at fault and causing the difficulty; the would-be storyteller is absolved from responsibility. This defensive strategy may be even more effective in alleviating the storyteller's anxiety, for it includes the first defensive maneuver ("I don't have any thoughts") but then goes on to dispel any anxiety that might result from that stance by a second maneuver which projects the entire problem to something outside of the self—namely, the picture.

These are but three examples of how, even before the story begins, the storyteller may enlist the use of defense mechanisms to protect against anxiety about self-disclosure. These prestory responses are important data, generally lost when stories are written rather than told.

However, this same attempt to void the task can appear within the story itself, written or spoken. Plots that are highly stereotyped or obviously borrowed from the media are another way in which individuals avoid self-revelation and are indicative of another kind of defensive maneuver. In this case, the storyteller is apparently complying with the instructions to tell a story but is in fact being passively resistant, not creating, but rather copying, a story. Other attempts to avoid anxiety are seen in the creation of a story that consciously mocks the storytelling enterprise. Through ridicule and denigration the storyteller hopes to be removed from any personal connection to the material; the process itself will then be shown to be worthless.

It is clear that the storytelling task itself may arouse such anxiety that a series of defensive maneuvers are called forth. But, in addition to this more general response to the task, the individual pictures may connect with conflicted feelings and wishes which, if fully recognized by the storyteller, would create considerable anxiety. So, in the process of telling the story, the expression of certain ideas may be defended against, that is, the ideas are presented in a way that does not create undue anxiety for the storyteller.

DEFENSE MECHANISMS

The concept of defense mechanism was introduced into psychology by Sigmund Freud in 1894/1962, in his paper on "The Neuro-Psychoses of Defence." As is evident from the title, defense mechanisms were originally considered part of psychopathology. This association between defense and pathology continues today, with the presence of specific defenses being considered an integral part of certain diagnoses, such as projection in the diagnosis of paranoia and repression in the diagnosis of certain hysterical conditions.

In more recent years, defense mechanisms have also been considered part of normal psychological development.[1] They function to "ward off" excessive anxiety and feelings of guilt (A. Freud, 1936/1946) and to maintain the individual's self-esteem and self-cohesiveness (Fenichel, 1945). Long-term longitudinal studies of both college and working men (Vaillant, 1977) have found that those who use mature defense mechanisms report greater happiness, marital success, and physical health at midlife, whereas those who use immature defenses are more likely to show poor adjustment to life as well as psychiatric illness. Another longitudinal study (Haan, 1974) found that adult women who made strong use of defenses were more anxious and fearful during adolescence, whereas defensive men were negativistic, extrapunitive, and covertly hostile toward adults. Also, the use of higher-level structured defenses was related to a higher IQ during adolescence and to an increase in IQ from adolescence to adulthood, whereas the use of primitive defenses was related to negative changes in intellectual ability over time.

Describing defense mechanisms as immature or mature, primitive or advanced, simple or complex, and infantile or adaptive suggests that there may be a developmental factor involved in the choice of defenses. Research evidence using a variety of assessment methods has shown that the use of the relatively simple defense of denial, although frequent in young children, decreases after early childhood (Castaneda, McCandless, & Palermo, 1956; Glasberg & Aboud, 1982; Hill & Sarason, 1966; Smith & Danielsson, 1982; Smith & Rossman, 1986). On the other hand, the use of more complex defenses, such as projection, increases through adolescence (Smith & Danielsson, 1982).

Some attempts have been made to link this developmental characterization of defenses with different types of psychopathology (e.g., Semrad, 1967; Vaillant, 1971, 1977). A problem arises with this approach, however, because the same defense that is "immature" in an adult and thus indicative of psychopathology may, in a young child, be quite appropriate and part of normal functioning (see Schwartz & Eagle, 1986). Thus the concept of age appropriate, rather than immature–mature, provides a better characterization of the developmental dimension of defense mechanisms.

Nevertheless, the fact that defense mechanisms may be ordered in terms of their simplicity–complexity and may be characterized as immature or mature raises the question whether there is in fact a developmental continuum of defense mechanism development. We return to this issue in a later part of the chapter.

DEFENSE MECHANISMS AND TAT STORIES

Over the years, clinical psychologists have noted that the use of defense mechanisms occurs in TAT stories, as in other narrative material. General guidelines for assessing defenses in stories have been provided by Bellak (1975), Henry (1956), Holt (1951), and Rapaport et al. (1946). These descriptive approaches "tuned the ear" of the listener to detecting the presence of defense mechanisms.

For several reasons, the TAT seems particularly well suited to provide information about the functioning of defense mechanisms. A defense mechanism is a form of thought process, and different defenses are defined in terms of the different forms the thought processes take. For example, in denial, thought is construed to change reality into something it is not, or to disconfirm the existence of something that is. On the other hand, in projection, thought processes are used to add or attribute some quality or motivation to objects or persons that they do not, in reality, possess. It is these differences in the formal characteristics of the thought processes involved that define the defense; these characteristics may be manifest with varying content. Although thought processes cannot be observed directly, they may be inferred from the verbal behavior that occurs during storytelling. Because defense mechanisms are rather complex mental processes, they are more likely to be revealed in relatively extended samples of thought, as compared to questionnaires that allow only a yes–no, or true–false response. The open-ended nature of the TAT story affords the opportunity for content to be expressed in a variety of forms, without restrictions on style or length. This unhampered verbal production gives us a window into discovering the thought processes of the individual, including the working of defense mechanisms.

Based on these considerations, it seemed possible that the functioning of particular defense mechanisms might be defined in such a way that they could be reliably identified in the text of TAT stories. To do this, three defense mechanisms, theoretically representing different points on a developmental continuum, were chosen for intensive study (for the developmental rationale, see Chapter 11; also see Cramer, 1987, 1991a). From both theoretical and clinical experience, it was possible to describe basic components of these defenses, which could be used to identify their occurrence in TAT stories. This tentative set of criteria for assessing the use of denial, projection, and identification was applied to a set of TAT and Children's Apperception Test (CAT) stories gathered from a group of 42 children, varying in age from 4 to 12 years old.

The results of this study, although based on a small number of children, did indicate that the use of defense mechanisms could be reliably assessed from TAT stories. The interrater reliability was found to vary between .76 and .96, indicating good agreement between two sets of different raters. Further, the results indicated that there were age differences in the relative strength of the three defenses, and these differences corresponded with theoretical predictions. The simplest defense, denial, was predominant among younger children. Projection was found to become increasingly important through middle adolescence, and identification showed a slow and gradual increase, until it became predominant in late adolescence.

A TAT Coding System for Defenses

On the basis of these results, a final set of scoring categories was established, reflecting the different components of each defense. In the case of denial, a primitive component is the failure to see what exists in reality. Another component, less extreme, is the physical or psychological withdrawal from a painful situation, thereby ignoring reality. A third component, related to ignoring reality, involves making mistakes in reality testing (as evidenced in misperception) or misinterpreting the meaning of events. Another component of denial is displayed when an event is perceived but only acknowledged in a negated form (e.g., "It didn't happen"). Less extreme than negation, but serving the same purpose of avoiding painful anxiety, is the component that involves minimizing the anxiety-arousing event or ridiculing its importance. Related to this component is the use of overexaggeration, in which the reality of an event must ultimately be denied. Another component, reversal (changing the experience into its opposite), accomplishes this same feat. A final component involves the construction of personal fantasies, akin to daydreams, to constitute an alternative reality which is then imposed upon the external world. Unfounded optimism and elation in the face of objective failure may be understood as a result of such a personal fantasy being substituted for consensual reality.

Each of these components represents a different aspect of the defense of denial, beginning with the most primitive and earliest to appear and ending with the relatively more mature manifestation. In developing the TAT system to assess the use of denial, each component was used to constitute a scoring category (see Table 7.1).

The same procedure was followed to develop the scoring system for projection. In its broadest sense, projection refers to the process of allocating inner mental phenomena to the external world. The most striking way in which this component of projection is seen occurs in hallucination, in which an internal memory-image is confused with

TABLE 7.1. Scoring Categories for Defense Mechanisms

Denial

1. Omission of major characters or objects.
2. Misperception.
3. Reversal.
4. Negation.
5. Denial of reality.
6. Overly maximizing the positive or minimizing the negative.
7. Unexpected goodness, optimism, positiveness, gentleness.

Projection

1. Attribution of aggressive or hostile feelings, emotions, or intentions to a character or other feelings, emotions or intentions that are normatively unusual.
2. Addition of ominous people, ghosts, animals, objects, or qualities.
3. Magical or circumstantial thinking.
4. Concern for protection from external threat.
5. Apprehensiveness of death, injury, or assault.
6. Themes of pursuit, entrapment, and escape.
7. Bizarre or very unusual story or theme.

Identification

1. Emulation of skills.
2. Emulation of characteristics.
3. Regulation of motives or behavior.
4. Self-esteem through affiliation.
5. Work; delay of gratification.
6. Role differentiation.
7. Moralism.

Note. From Cramer (1991a). Copyright 1991 by Springer-Verlag. Reprinted by permission.

external perception; the individual "sees" something that is not there. Another component involving this process occurs when other mental representations, such as wishes, feelings, and impulses are attributed to and assumed to exist in others; animistic thinking is a special example of this. In both these components, an internal tendency is attributed to an external object and is used to explain that object's behavior. A further component of projection involves the alteration or misperception of reality, in the direction of events appearing more negative or more ominous than they are in objective reality. As a result of this ominous alteration of reality, another component of projection may occur— namely, the development of an "explanation" for the disturbing happenings, appearing as a delusion in which circumstantial reasoning and ideas of reference contribute to the further alteration of reality.

> The belief that the world is a frightening, ominous place contributes to the occurrence of still more components of projection. On the one hand, the belief in threatening external forces leads to the attempt to protect oneself from the imagined threat. This may take the form of physical escape, the creation of protective barriers against attack, or attempts to disguise oneself. The felt need for protection may also result in a kind of wariness that includes a hyperalertness to being tricked or misled. On the other hand, the belief that one is endangered may result in attempts to disarm, capture, or destroy the dangerous other, the imagined assailant.
>
> Each of the components of projection discussed here is based on placing one's own inner mental representations onto objects in the external world. In yet another component of projection, the mental representation is not put outside the self; rather, the origin of the representation is made external. Here, the cause or responsibility for the thought is attributed to the external world. The individual is aware of having unacceptable thoughts, feelings, or impulses, but he or she attributes the source of these ideas to someone else." (Cramer, 1991a, pp. 64–65)

> In more pathological cases, the individual may experience his actions and thoughts as being under the control of another, with delusions involving magical or supernatural forces that influence behavior." (Cramer, 1991a, p. 65)

As with denial, these components of projection may be roughly ordered from most primitive to relatively more mature. As with denial, they were used to develop scoring categories to assess the use of projection in TAT stories (see Table 7.1).

Identification, a much more complex defense than either denial or projection, also can be described in terms of its components. At the most primitive level, incorporation—the individual's taking in of all, or a part, of another person (or thing), which in turn causes positive or negative changes in the individual's feelings or experiences—is a basic component of identification. A second component occurs in the introjection of important others, a process that continues the important emotional relationship with the object, relocating it from the outer to the inner world. In this process, the individual strives to be the *same* as another individual; that is, the individual strives to achieve identity with the object. A third, developmentally more advanced component, occurs when the motive is to be *like* the model. This involves the internalization of the regulations of the other, such as demands, control, guidance, prohibitions, and punishment, as well as gratification from the significant other; along with the rebellion against these regulations and against various characteristics of the other, such as behavioral patterns, motives and defenses, skills, and attitudes. Additional components of identification include imitation and learning, both of which contribute to the child's becoming more like the parent or other significant person. As with denial and projection, these components of identification were used to develop scoring categories for the defense (see Table 7.1).

RESEARCH STUDIES

With this newly developed coding system for the defenses of denial, projection, and identification, a large-scale study of defense mechanisms, using the TAT, was mounted. The purpose of this study was twofold. If the results replicated those of the initial derivation study, showing the theoretically predicted developmental differences, the concept validity of the TAT method of defense mechanism assessment would be supported. In addition, such results would add support to the theory itself (Anastasi, 1988).

Happily, the results were consistent with the initial findings. Now, with 320 individuals representing four age groups, from preschool to late adolescence, clear developmental patterns were found in the use of defenses. These findings are discussed in more detail in Chapter 11. Again, the measure of defense mechanisms based on the TAT was successful in producing the predicted results. Further, the interrater reliability was determined for each defense, for each age group separately. For denial, these reliabilities varied from .81 to 1.00, for projection from .71 to .90, and for identification from .71 to .88, indicating that the rating method reached levels of reliability exceeding the standard considered acceptable.

At this point, the TAT measure demonstrated reliability, showed theoretically predicted developmental differences, and was defined as a measure of defense mechanisms. This assertion—that defense mechanisms were being measured—would be on firmer ground if it could be shown that the measure was sensitive to situational changes which, theoretically, would be expected to influence the use of defense mechanisms.

According to theory, an important function of defense mechanisms is to maintain self-esteem. We reasoned that if an individual were placed into a situation that threatened their self-esteem, the individual should show an increased use of defenses as compared to his or her normal, "resting level," and as compared to persons who did not experience a threat to their self-esteem. Based on this reasoning, two experiments were carried out, one with children and one with college students.

For the children's study, a child's game provided the vehicle for an experimental manipulation of an experience of success or failure. The game consisted of a multilevel rollway, with a number of rollway tracks angled to transport a marble from the "start" to "finish" position; gravity determined the speed of the marble's sojourn.

This game was introduced to the elementary-school children as a test of sensorimotor coordination. Each child was told that there was a standard time to try to beat; if successful, his or her name would be attached to a large gold seal and placed on an "Honor Board," prominently located in the experimental room. On the other hand, if the child failed to beat the standard time, his or her name would not be put up on the board. (Before the conclusion of the testing session, all children were told they were successful, and all had their names put on the board.)

Prior to this game, all the children were asked, individually, to tell TAT stories. These preexperimental stories were scored for the use of defense mechanisms and were the basis for creating two groups of children who were matched for level of defense use, with an equal number of boys and girls in each group. After this matching procedure, the children in one group were all told, after the marble rollway game, that they had been successful in beating the standard time. The children in the other group were all told that they had not been successful. Immediately following this success or failure procedure, each child was asked to tell another set of TAT stories about pictures different from those seen earlier. It was predicted that the use of defense mechanisms should increase in the failure group, as an attempt to protect self-esteem, and that this increase should appear in the TAT defense mechanism scores.

The results confirmed the main hypothesis. Children who experienced failure were more likely to use the age-appropriate defenses of denial and projection than were those who experienced failure, even though their defense mechanism scores were equivalent prior to the experiment. An additional finding indicated that the experience of success was followed by a positive increase in the use of identification, a relatively mature defense for this age group. These results, then, provided evidence that changes in TAT defense scores, following experimentally produced stress, occurred as would be predicted from theory.

A second study, based on the same rationale, was carried out with men and women college students.[2] To add some modest stress to the situation, the storyteller was asked to lie down on a cot; a large video camera at the foot of the cot was focused directly on the student. The examiner was seated at the head of the cot, out of the student's line of vision. The examiner handed each TAT card to the student, whose storytelling was tape-recorded. Following the first three stories, the examiner made some neutral responses, such as "Uh huh," "OK," or "All right." However, for half the subjects, following the fourth story, the examiner became extremely critical, berating the stories for being dull, unimaginative, and lacking in creativity. This criticism continued following each story until the end of the session. For the other half of the subjects, the examiner continued her neutral responses between stories. At the conclusion of the session, each subject was debriefed.

All stories were then scored for the use of defense mechanisms. The two groups of students—criticized and uncriticized—were equivalent in their use of defenses in the first four stories told. However, following on the experience of criticism, the students whose self-esteem had been threatened increased their use of the age-appropriate defenses of projection and identification, whereas no change occurred in the uncriticized group. Again, changes in the TAT measure were consistent with predictions from theory.

The results of these two studies are consistent with the theory of defense mechanisms, which states that under conditions threatening self-esteem, people will increase their use of defenses. Implied in this theory is a further belief—that the increase in defense use will result in less psychological upset. Serendipitously, an opportunity to test this last hypothesis—and thereby again test the validity of the TAT measure—arose from a study carried out by Dr. Steven Dollinger (1985). As a clinical child psychologist, Dollinger was asked to participate in a psychological study of a group of early adolescent boys who had recently witnessed a lightning strike while playing soccer. The strike was so severe that one boy was killed and others were knocked to the ground. Among the procedures used to assess the boys' subsequent psychological status was a modified TAT in which the boys were asked to tell stories about two pictures depicting scenes with lightning. In addition, based on clinical interviews, the degree of psychological upset in each boy had been determined.

According to theory, the traumatic event of the lightning strike should increase the boys' use of defense mechanisms and, to the degree that this occurred, psychological upset should be diminished. All stories were scored for use of defenses, and these scores were correlated with the clinical ratings of psychological upset. The results indicated that the boys who had the highest scores for total defense mechanism use, as well as the highest scores for the age-appropriate defense of projection, showed the least degree of psychological upset. Again, the defense mechanisms measure produced results consistent with theory.

FURTHER DEMONSTRATION OF TAT DEFENSE ASSESSMENT

The TAT measure used in these investigations to assess defense mechanisms has been described and illustrated at length in Cramer (1991a)[3] (see also Table 7.1). In the remainder of this chapter, the use of the measure will be demonstrated by the stories from the college students discussed in Chapter 5. In addition, research use of the measure with hospitalized psychiatric populations will be discussed. In Chapter 11, we will see how developmental changes in defenses may be detected in TAT stories.

College Students

Here is one of the stories from Don, the college senior who was discussed earlier in Chapter 5.

"Mark Parker is a lab scientist at MIT doing independent research on genetics and DNA. He is currently hot on the trail of an amazing breakthrough sure to win him a Nobel Prize in chemistry and get him world renown. As he progresses through the final stage of his work, he notices some odd readouts on his computer printout of data. Shocked by the revelation that his great discovery may, in fact, never materialize, he rushes over to his equipment and pulls out the one beaker of material which is producing the faulty data, crucial to his experiment. As Dr. Parker stares into the beaker, he thinks about his enormous time commitment to his work and the ridicule that will come from his peers if the experiment he has staked his reputation on fails. It would be very easy for Dr. Parker to remedy the situation and get rid of the evidence and present his other findings as proof of his theory, but that would break the ethical code of research science. As he stares blankly into the offending beaker, Dr. Parker thinks of fame, glory, money, success, shame, guilt and responsibility. As the beaker is crushed in the heat of the incinerator in the building's cellar, his only thought becomes 'I wonder if anyone will ever find out.' "

In this story, there is no element that receives a score for denial. However, there are examples of three different components of projection: First, the statement that "ridicule will come from his peers" if his experiment fails is an example of category 1: attribution of emotions that are normatively unusual. A more neutral expression would be that the peers are sad, surprised, or disappointed; ridicule implies a hostility that is neither prompted by the picture nor explained by the preceding story. The second score for projection is based on category 3: magical, animistic thinking, as seen in the statement "the offending beaker." Here, human motivation is attributed to an inanimate object. The third score for projection comes from category 4: concern for protection from external threat, as seen in the idea that the hero must "get rid of the evidence" so as not to be found out.

There are also two scores given for identification. The first is for category 3: regulation of motives or behavior, as seen in the self-reflective comment, "I wonder if anyone will ever find out." The second score is for category 6: role differentiation, as seen in the identification of the hero as a "scientist."

The overall scores—denial = 0, projection = 3, identification = 2—show a fairly common pattern for a late adolescent male in his last year of college.

Here is a second story from Don.

"This is Mr. and Mrs. James Smith. Their son Bill committed suicide almost 7 years ago, by jumping off this bridge. This is the first time they have been able to come here and really think about their son. They are torn by emotions and memories of the happy times they spent with their son. Their one overriding fear is for their youngest son, Donald, who has turned very depressed and has trouble making friends since his older brother's suicide. The Smiths are extremely worried that Donald may also take his own life in a fit of deep depression. The thought of losing a second son in this way tears at their souls. Donald refuses professional help and seems angry with his mother often. Even in this hour of stress, as his parents attempt to finally accept their son's death, Donald is off playing baseball with his friends from college."

This story receives one score for denial, three for projection, and two for identification. The denial score comes from category 3: reversal. Although Donald is described as "very depressed and has trouble making friends," the story ends with Donald "off playing baseball with his friends from college"; the change from depression and friendlessness to playing and having friends involves a reversal of emotions and situation and occurs without explanation.

The three projection scores come from categories 1, 2, and 5. Category 1, attributions of hostile feelings, occurs in the statement that Donald is "angry" with his mother often, without any explanation of why this is so. Category 2, additions of ominous people, is seen in the statement that a son (who, incidentally, does not appear in the picture) is "depressed." Category 5, apprehensiveness of death, is seen in the older brother's suicide.

The two scores for identification come from categories 2 and 3. Category 2, emulation of characteristics, is seen in the concern that Donald may also take his own life, just as his older brother had. Category 3, regulation of motives or behavior, is seen in the negative form in that Donald refuses to allow his parents to influence his behavior.

Thus, although Don's two stories have different themes and content, the relative use of defense mechanisms is quite similar. The scores for the second story are nearly identical with those from the first story.

Let us now look at the story from DeeDee, a female college senior, also discussed earlier in Chapter 5.

This is the story DeeDee told:

"This is a [classical—word crossed out] composer of classical music from the 17th century. He is examining a gift presented to him mysteriously by an anonymous admirer of his music. She has been watching him for months and has fallen in love, but he does not know this or who she is. The note with the package merely said 'With [unloving—word crossed out] undying love and devotion, an ardent admirer.' The [note—word crossed out] mystery has intrigued him enough to drop the sheet music he has been working on, and now he stands contemplating the mysterious suitor.

"Sarah is the daughter of a count and is obligated to marry a count chosen for her by her father. But she is not in love with the count, she finds him quite dull. Her secret passion is music, and whenever she can she sneaks away from her ladies-in-waiting to hear Roberto's symphonies. She has fallen madly in love with him from afar, but does not know how to approach him, nor what would happen if she dared to break her engagement to the count. She feels hopeless, so she sent the note and gift but knows she can do no more. She must give up—that was her final act of love and now, done, she must heed to her family's wishes.

"Roberto will pursue this mysterious admirer with all his heart. He will hire several investigators to track her down. He has been lonely and looking for a wife with a love for music and for romance, and she is what he needs. [Eventually—word crossed out] But Sarah has moved off with her new husband and the two never meet."

This story receives three scores for denial, one for projection, and four for identification. The three scores for denial all occur in category 4, statements of negation. The first example occurs when DeeDee writes, "With unloving . . . "; however, she crosses this out and negates the negative emotion ("unloving") by changing it into "undying love." The second example occurs when it is stated that Sarah, the heroine, "does not know . . . what would happen if she dared to break her engagement. . . . " This "not knowing" denies the rather obvious result—that her father would be furious. Finally, there are three other places where DeeDee begins to say one thing but crosses it out and substitutes a new phrase: "classical" becomes "composer of classical music," "note" becomes "mystery," and "eventually" becomes "but . . . the two never meet." Although no one of these is a strong example of denying a fact or feeling, it is noteworthy that this occurs three times and that, in the last case, one has the rather clear feeling that "eventually" was going to lead in a different direction than that taken after the word is crossed out—all this contributes to a third score for category 4, of denial.

DeeDee's story receives one score for projection, in category 6, themes of pursuit; "Roberto will pursue . . . [and] . . . track her down." For identification, two of the scores are in category 3, regulation of motives or behavior, as seen in the father choosing her husband (she "is obligated to marry a count") and in the partial rebelling against this "she sneaks away. . . . " The other two scores for identification occur in category 6, role differentiation, in the designation of a "composer" and a "count."

As compared to the first two stories from Don, DeeDee's story shows a greater use of denial and a lesser use of projection. When this pattern is found in college students, it is more likely to occur with women; men are more likely to show a greater use of projection.

Here is Marie's story, also discussed in Chapter 5.

"There is a person in the background, but the room is extremely dark so we, the observers, can only see his hand. There is also a man in the picture, and he looks very grim. The man (or person) in the background is chastising him for something.

"The man is probably a musician and his teacher or instructor is rebuking him for the mistakes he did in the performance earlier.

"In the past, this musician never lived up to his potential. He has a wonderful gift of music but he lacks the discipline. His instructor knows this and has been very frustrated from the very beginning.

"The instructor wants his student to do the best he could possibly do. He is merely frustrated that this gifted and talented musician is 'throwing' his talent away.

"The musician, on the other hand, does not care for music. He merely wants to live his life as he pleases, and not follow the step [sic] of his father. He, at this point, is thinking that he can't wait to leave the room so he could go out and have some fun.

"The instructor will continue to chastise him and will continue to push him into studying more. Perhaps in time, he will stop needling him.

"The musician will one day rebel from the wishes of his family, and follow his own desires."

The defenses shown here are less typical for a woman, with no scores for denial, three for projection, and four for identification. Two of the projection scores occur in category 1, attribution of emotions that are normatively unusual, as seen in the description of the foreground man as "very grim" and the background figure, whom the storyteller says cannot be seen, as "chastising." The third projection score occurs in category 4, concern for protection from external threat. This results from the storyteller's need for self-justification: "The room is extremely dark so we, the observers, can only see his hand."

The four scores for identification occur in two categories. Category 3, regulation of motives or behavior, is scored once for the instructor who will "push him into studying more" and once for the musician who will "one day rebel from the wishes of his family." Category 6, role differentiation, is scored once for the mention of "musician" and once for "teacher."

The last story from a college student comes from Sue, previously presented in Chapter 5.

"These two people are married, and have been for over 25 years. They have stopped at the bench, to rest and look quietly at the sunset and the passers-by. They are not speaking much now, but occasionally they look at each other, and do not look away, because there is no tension, or unpleasantness between them. Yet they are sad, deeply, deeply hurting over the death of their eldest daughter. It has been 6 months since their daughter died in a very sudden accident, and their thoughts are often filled with her, and all that they have lost with her death. They have always had a strong marriage, filled with love and mutual respect. The wife has worked, but now stays at home, looking for things that please her. Her husband is only 47, and will not retire for several years. He has a successful career, but is the epitome of a family man. Their daughter was 22, just out of college—creative, exuberant, ready to tap into her potential. And she was beautiful—not stunning, but glowing and happy.

"They have been trying to spend time alone together, aware of the frightening statistics about marriages that fall apart after the loss of a child. They are seeing a therapist, together and alone, trying to cope with the anger and the guilt that pervades their everyday existence. They fear for the two younger children, 18 and 16, both boys, who have had some trouble grieving openly. They have tried to encourage openness and honesty, even the expression of outright hostility. But the pain they feel is nothing they can describe, and their lives seem so empty and tedious. They think they'll survive it, and they look to each other for support and love. The husband is being careful not to get absorbed in his work as an escape, but he's never done this before, and continues to spend as much time as possible at home, with his family, or sitting quietly on park benches with his wife."

This story is scored twice for denial, twice for projection, and three times for identification. The denial scores come from category 1, omission, for failure to mention the bridge, which is prominent in the picture, and from category 4, statements of negation, for the statement "there is no tension or unpleasantness between them."

The projection scores come from category 2, additions of ominous qualities, "a very sudden accident," and category 5, apprehensiveness of death, as seen in "the death of their eldest daughter."

Two of the identification scores come from category 3, regulation of motives and behavior; both of these are indications of self-reflection. There is "guilt that pervades their everyday existence," and the husband is "careful not to get absorbed in his work as an escape." The third score for identification comes from category 6, role differentiation, in the mention of a "therapist."

Psychiatric Patients

This approach to assessing the use of defense mechanisms with TAT has also been used with hospitalized psychotic and severe neurotic and character disorder patients. In one study (Cramer, Blatt, & Ford, 1988) the TAT stories of 90 hospitalized patients, obtained shortly after admission, were scored for the use of denial, projection, and identification according to the coding system discussed in this chapter. It was found that the level of defense use was meaningfully related to the level of patient pathology; the more primitive the level of defense use, the lower the level of psychological functioning. For example, the use of the lower-level defenses of denial and projection was related to independent ratings of greater psychopathology and poor interpersonal relationships, whereas the opposite was found for patients using the higher-level defense of identification.[4] In a follow-up study after 15 months of treatment, there was a decrease in the use of defense mechanisms, and this was associated with a reduction in psychiatric symptoms (Cramer & Blatt, 1990).

A further study of defense use by psychiatric patients, as assessed from TAT stories, found further confirming evidence for this coding system (Hibbard et al., 1994). The diagnoses of the patients, who were from an acute psychiatric unit of a Veterans Administration hospital, were about evenly divided among depression, bipolar disorder, schizophrenia, and posttraumatic stress disorder. As compared to a contrast sample of college students, the patients showed a greater relative use of denial and projection and a lesser use of identification. Further, the TAT analysis showed that within each defense, the patients demonstrated a greater use of the lower-level components of each defense, as compared to the college students.

SUMMARY

This chapter addressed the issue of how storytellers protect themselves from revealing or acknowledging feelings, wishes, or thoughts that might arouse excessive anxiety. The protective maneuvers, referred to as defense mechanisms, can be seen in TAT stories and can be systematically assessed using a reliable coding scheme. The development and the rationale for this coding scheme are discussed and research studies demonstrating its validity are described.

This interpretive perspective is then applied to the TAT stories from the college students discussed in Chapter 5. Research studies with psychiatric patients, in which defenses are assessed from the TAT and related to other clinical variables, are described at the end of the chapter.

STUDIES OF CLINICAL PATIENTS

EIGHT

The Storyteller's Narrative

This chapter looks at the narrative themes of two patients who were hospitalized for psychiatric illness in a small psychoanalytically oriented long-term treatment center. In both cases, we will see how the patients' own narrative themes are expressed through their stories. Further, because each patient told stories on more than one occasion, we have the opportunity to see how these themes are modified over the course of treatment. Following this demonstration, I will approach these stories using two of the interpretive perspectives discussed in previous chapters—namely, the perspective of defense mechanisms and that of gender identity.

CASE 1: MS. F

The patient is a 41-year-old woman, noticeably short and plump, who had been experiencing psychological problems for many years and had been hospitalized on a number of occasions. These hospitalizations were characterized by extremely regressive behavior, involving histrionic self-abuse that was not life threatening. Although she had held a responsible job for most of her adult life, she became increasingly unable to function and was admitted to the open, psychodynamically oriented psychiatric hospital for intensive treatment.

Her course in the hospital may be divided into three periods, as described later. During each of these occasions, she was given a full battery of psychological tests, including the TAT. During each period, she was also the subject of an intensive clinical case conference at which the various professional staff members who were responsible for her treatment provided a detailed description of her development while in the hospital. These various sources of information were used to formulate a psychiatric diagnosis.

The patient's *first period* in the hospital extends from her initial admission until her discharge 18 months later. During that period, she was tested with the TAT after 4 months in the hospital and was discussed at a case conference the following month. The *second period* extends from her second admission to the hospital, 10 months after the first discharge, until 12 months later, when she moved from the hospital to supervised apartment living, continuing as an outpatient. During this second period, she was tested with the TAT shortly after admission and reviewed at a case conference the next month. The *third period* continues from the time she began supervised apartment living until 12 months later, when she was discharged from hospital care. At the beginning of this third period, she was again tested with the TAT and discussed at a clinical case conference.

According to the report of her female therapist during the first period, the patient presented herself as having numerous physical and psychological complaints, often appearing quite immature, proclaiming helplessness and inability to care for herself. Initial therapeutic work was directed to the ways in which she used these various symptoms in a defensive manner to cover the person underneath. A second focus of the therapy revolved around the issue of who, in the end, was responsible for her—who was supposed to take care of her. It was the patient's perspective that the therapist and the hospital were completely responsible for her and her care; the therapist provided an alternative viewpoint—namely, that it was the patient who would need to assume control of her life. The patient's response to this disruption of her view was to regress, indicating her unwillingness to be responsible for herself.

However, after being in the hospital for about 3 months, a gradual shift in her outlook was noticeable. She began to realize the burden that her helpless stance put on others, and she had some recognition that she relied on physical problems to validate her helpless behavior.

Shortly after this period, the first psychological testing was done. At the clinical case conference held the following month, the patient was diagnosed as Axis I, schizoaffective disorder, bipolar type, and Axis II, mixed personality disorder. Treatment continued until the first discharge from the hospital.

The patient fared reasonably well back in her home community for about 6 months. Then, she experienced several personal losses. Following these stressful experiences, the patient became increasingly agitated and regressed and was readmitted to the inpatient psychiatric hospital. She was tested, including the TAT, at this time and was evaluated at a clinical case conference the next month. The diagnosis was Axis I, schizoaffective disorder and Axis II, borderline personality disorder. The possibility of a sleep disorder was also considered. For most of this second period of treatment, the patient had a new, male therapist. Much of the therapy time was taken up with her complaints about this development, yet she seemed, at the same time, unwilling or unable to transfer from this therapist to another; the more relevant issue appeared to be the patient's fear of abandonment. Therapy sessions revolved around repetitive negotiations about working with a male versus a female therapist, with the patient eventually agreeing that she would work with the male until a female became available. At the same time, there was a lessening of her psychosomatic symptoms. In a sense, there was a shift during this time from a focus on the physical to a focus on the interpersonal realm, where the conflict now seemed to reside. Eventually, the issue of staying or going receded, and the patient was able to work through issues relating to her losses, expressing appropriate mourning. She also became less symptomatic. Toward the end of this second period, the therapist took a 1-week vacation. Subsequent to this absence, and knowing that the therapist would be leaving the institution shortly, the patient decided that she would change therapists. Toward the end of this period, the patient shifted back to her original therapist in the hospital and moved to a supervised apartment near the hospital, continuing treatment as an outpatient.

At the beginning of the third period, the patient was again tested, including the TAT, and she was discussed at a clinical case conference. The diagnoses were consistent with those made previously, with an added emphasis on depressive features. The shift back to her original therapist appeared to indicate a wish, on the part of the patient, to let go of her symptoms and take charge of her life. She experienced the therapist as someone who supported her getting better and not having a life career as a mental patient. The patient did well, and 1 year after the beginning of the third period, she was discharged from the treatment program, continuing privately with the female therapist.

The patient was tested on three occasions, corresponding to the three periods in the hospital treatment program. The stories were told to the examiner and recorded verbatim. The first occasion (Time 1) occurred after 4 months in the hospital. The second occasion (Time 2) occurred on the patient's readmission to the hospital. The third testing (Time 3) occurred as the patient resumed work with the original therapist and moved to an apartment outside the hospital.

I begin with the stories told at the first testing (Time 1), looking for the story lines that characterize the patient's narrative at that time. Then,

I compare these stories with those told at the second and third testing occasions (Times 2 and 3) to note the changes that occurred.

The Initial TAT Stories

TAT Card 1,[1] Time 1

"Okay, the boy has been playing the violin and he's supposed to practice more, but he doesn't want to, and he's just staring at it, wishing it would go away so he wouldn't have to play it anymore and he can go outside and play. Like he wants to be good at it but he doesn't want to spend all his time practicing it, he's like ambivalent. Is that enough? (?) Well he'll halfheartedly play for another half hour. And, it'll be time to eat and he will have missed going outside to play."

TAT Card 5, Time 1

"Oh, it could tie in with the one with the boy with the violin. She's looking in to see if he's practicing and to tell him he has to practice for one more half hour or he can't have supper. Or, it could be someone who heard a noise in the room and came down to see what it was, but she couldn't find anything. And she doesn't look too pleased though. I like the CAT better. It has animals and stuff."

TAT Card 14, Time 1

"Wow. I never saw this card. He couldn't sleep and he's standing by the window waiting for it to be morning and the day's getting lighter and he's glad the night's over. On one hand . . . on the other hand it's dusk and he didn't bother turning on the light. He doesn't want to go through another night so he's contemplating jumping. Or, he's a grown up violinist and he still hates it. He's going to Juilliard and they want him to practice more and he's had it. (*feeling?*) One part is feeling hopeful 'cause day has come and it was a rough night, and the other one is feeling despair and frustration and anger and wants to jump. But somehow the window gives me more like . . . the light outside the window . . . gives me more a feeling of hope than concentrating on all the black. He could be somewhere like in a beach town watching sunset. That's about it. Is that enough?"

TAT Card 13MF, Time 1

"Well this is a lot of . . . what it is he can't take her anymore 'cause she just won't get out of bed. He doesn't understand why she just can't get just . . . like can't get up and get dressed and just go on with her life and he's had enough and he doesn't know how to deal with her anymore. Or, going more extreme, he just killed her. He didn't mean to and he's like really ashamed of what he's done. Or, another story could be she'd . . . it's his first prostitute he's seen and he's . . .

you know, went to . . . and he's really ashamed and he got on his clothes and he'll probably leave the money on the books or something and he's going. But, I think the first one the most."

TAT Card 12M, Time 1

"The old man and the younger man have been on the outs for a really long time and there was never words to get back together, and now he sees his son or his grandson resting and he wants to just touch him and be close again. Or, he got there too late and the boy's already dead and he couldn't make amends. It's hard to tell because you can't see the older man's face. Or, he could even be in some kind of therapy and he was just hypnotized."

TAT Card 2, Time 1

"Well, she wants to better herself from living and working on a farm and she's going to school and she's really serious about learning a trade and leaving this back-breaking world of work. It's her brother and her mother in the picture. Her mother's still having children . . . Probably have a large family and not a lot of food to go around and she wants to escape into another life or another way of life. That's it."

TAT Card 18GF, Time 1

"She's making her tell her something but she doesn't understand what she wants to know and she says, '*Tell* me.' And she says, 'I don't know.' And she keeps saying, 'Tell me' over and over. She doesn't know and now she's gotten so mad that she's choking her."

TAT Card 12F, Time 1

"The old lady can't accept the fact she's old and she still thinks she looks like she did when she was younger. And the woman up front is like her imagined self and the one in the back is her real self. (*feeling?*) Reminiscent and a little schitzed out because she doesn't know which is . . . which one she is, the old person or the younger person. But, with time she grew like more express . . . expressive 'cause the young woman has a very flat affect. The woman in back seems to have more the look of youth and animation in her face."

First we will examine the story lines from this patient's narrative, as they are revealed in her initial TAT stories. Several prominent interrelated themes recur in these stories, illustrated in more detail later. First, there is a repeated attribution of responsibility for action to someone else. In conjunction with this helpless stance, there is an overarching portrayal of passivity coupled with a regressive wish for gratification without effort.

A subtheme occasionally occurs in connection with this passivity, when it serves to provoke aggression in someone else. Finally, and consistent with the other themes, the stories provide evidence for a strong regressive component in the patient, seen both in the wish to be as a child and in the references to oral gratification.

The patient begins her storytelling on Card 1 with a clear statement of attribution of responsibility for activity. The only way in which the boy will be able to stop playing the violin is if "*it* would go away," or if someone would indicate it is "time to eat"; there is no suggestion that the boy, himself, could assume the responsibility for making a decision about playing or not. This theme occurs again on Card 14, in which nature is made responsible for the boy's feelings; he is hopeful "'cause *day* has come"; "the *light* outside the window gives me more a feeling of hope." Again, the origin of the boy's feelings is placed outside himself, as is the reason for his practicing: "they" want him to "practice more." Yet another example of this occurs in the story about Card 12M, in which the patient, unable to decide whether the character in the story is resting or dead, attributes her difficulty to the way in which the picture is drawn: "you can't see the older man's face." It is also noteworthy that in two of the cases (Card 1 and Card 12M), this attribution of responsibility entails a type of thinking that borders on being pathological. In the first case, attributing responsibility to an inanimate object (the violin) involves animistic thinking, whereas the latter example, "It's hard to tell because you can't see the older man's face," involves circumstantial reasoning. Both these types of thinking are often associated with a paranoid disorder.

The second prominent story line is the repeated sense of passivity and avoidance of effort. In Card 1, the boy wishes but does not act. He wishes the violin would go away, he wants to be good but does not want to practice, he even misses going outside to play. This passive stance of the storyteller is seen in the perseveration of the opening story in the responses given to the next two cards (Cards 5 and 13). Rather than making an effort to create new stories, the patient told the same story two more times, thereby passively complying with the examiner's instructions to make up a story for each card. Although most storytellers understand that a different story is required for each card, this patient adopts a passive solution that requires the least amount of effort—simply keep telling the same story. The story told about Card 14 also carries this passive image: "He *didn't bother* turning on the lights," although it is dark; he is "*waiting* for it to be morning." The wish to avoid work is also seen in the story about Card 2. She is going to school to learn a trade *so as* to avoid "this back-breaking world of work." The motivation here seems primarily to avoid work (mentioned twice) rather than to grow up and develop; there is the rather naive assumption that going to school and learning a trade will not involve work.

Passivity continues as a main theme in the story told about Card 13MF. The woman "won't get out of bed"; she "can't get up and get dressed"; she can't "go on with her life." This shutdown of movement is also seen in the story about Card 18GF, in which one woman persistently foils the attempts of the other by assuming a position of "not knowing." In both these stories, the passivity of one character provokes an aggressive reaction in the other.

The regressive theme occurs both in direct references to wanting to be as a child and in the unusual mention of food and eating in the stories. Some conflict around this regressive pull forms the central plot of the story told about Card 12F, in which the woman wants to continue to be as she was when she was younger; in fact, she cannot decide whether she is a child or an adult. The preference for being like a child is also seen in the comment made at the end of Card 5: "I like the CAT better. It has animals and stuff." References to food, eating, and possible oral deprivation occur in the stories about Card 1, "it'll be time to eat"; on Card 5, "he can't have his supper"; and Card 2, "not a lot of food"—comments that are unusual in adult stories.

Changes in the TAT Stories over the Course of Treatment

Let us consider now how these stories changed over time. The stories from the three testing occasions are presented consecutively for each of the eight TAT cards, followed by a discussion of the prominent themes and changes that occurred.

TAT Card 1

Time 1. "Okay, the boy has been playing the violin and he's supposed to practice more, but he doesn't want to, and he's just staring at it, wishing it would go away so he wouldn't have to play it anymore and he can go outside and play. Like he wants to be good at it but he doesn't want to spend all his time practicing it, he's like ambivalent. Is that enough? (?) Well he'll halfheartedly play for another half hour. And, it'll be time to eat and he will have missed going outside to play."

Time 2. "Oh . . . He has to play the violin in order to go outside and he hates the violin, and he's sitting there waiting and waiting hoping his mother will say it's okay, he doesn't have to play now and he can go out and play and that's it. He never really wanted to have violin lessons. She picked it. Is that enough? (?) He's gonna go out . . . no, he's not gonna go out. He's gonna sit in front of the violin until he plays it and he can't come to dinner until he's done his practicing."

Time 3. "I don't know. I think he's grown up and he's looking back to when he was little, and he has this wonderful guitar, uh, violin

... violin lessons and he just didn't want to play and he like gave it up but now a grownup, he like wishes he practiced so he would have been ... uhm ... a violinist. He feels as a grownup ... he feels regret and as a kid ... like I don't want to do this anymore."

Looking at these three stories about the same TAT card provides some interesting insights into changes that occurred over the treatment period. As noted earlier, at Time 1 there is an attribution of responsibility and motivation to an *object* outside the self, which is close to animistic thinking: The boy is "wishing it would go away," as though the responsibility for movement and intention resides in the violin, not in the boy. The story is also characterized by the wish for gratification without effort, leading to a situation of ambivalence and passivity. Finally, the ending is unusual, with the focus on eating. In all, the story is striking for its regressive qualities—attribution of intention to an object, wish for effortless gratification, and focus on oral gratification.

At Time 2, the ambivalence about the violin is gone. Now, there is a clear expression of *not wanting* to play, and a clarity that it is the mother who is responsible. Also, there is a clearer connection between the boy's own behavior and the consequences that follow: He "has to play the violin *in order to* go outside"; "he can't come to dinner *until he's done* his practicing." There is still the passivity noticed at Time 1—"he's gonna sit ... until he plays it" and "he's sitting there waiting and waiting"—with the responsibility for action given to the other (mother). On the other hand, there is a glimmering of a self-motivated act—"He's gonna go out"—which almost occurs but is aborted, and there is some attempt to assume control over oral regressive tendencies—"He can't come to dinner until he's done his practicing."

At Time 3, there is a distinctly different flavor to the story. There is a new capacity for self-reflection and self-observation; the hero can look at himself from the outside and from the perspective of an adult. There is also a recognition of one's *own* responsibility, without blaming the mother. Further, there is a recognition that *activity* could have led, or could lead, to adult competence: "he like wishes he practiced so he would have been ... uhm ... a violinist." There is also an indication of some wish for change from the passive stance: "like I don't want to do this anymore." Finally, the hated violin has become a wonderful guitar. However, this misperception may be an indication of denial, in turning the hated object into something it is not. If so, this misperception is indicative of regression. The two hesitations around the nature or identity of the instrument—"guitar, uh, violin" and "he would have been ... uhm ... a violinist" are interesting. The uncertainty around continuing to perceive the instrument as a violin *might* be thought of as a rejection of the false, forced attempt at an identity, whereas the change to a "wonderful guitar" may represent a move toward a new self, which, however, is not yet firmly established.

TAT Card 5

Time 1. "Oh, it could tie in with the one with the boy with the violin. She's looking in to see if he's practicing and to tell him he has to practice for one more half hour or he can't have supper. Or, it could be someone who heard a noise in the room and came down to see what it was, but she couldn't find anything. And she doesn't look too pleased though. I like the CAT better. It has animals and stuff."

Time 2. "Well, she's looking into the study and doesn't like what she sees. And whoever was in the study really made it into a mess and didn't clean up after themselves and she's really pissed and she's not gonna clean anymore—each one takes care of their own shit. Will the tape be censored cause I said shit? (*no*) There is an FCC code. ( ) Okay. And eventually she winds up doing all the work anyway and is a whole martyr about the whole thing."

Time 3. "She's very nervous and she's expecting company and she's going from room to room to make sure everything looks just right, like the flowers on the table and she's looking in to make sure everything's all right. (?) Nobody's going to come."

Consideration of these three stories again provides information regarding the changes that are occurring with this patient, which is consistent with some of the observations made from the stories about Card 1.

At Time 1, the patient begins with some perseveration from the previous story about Card 1 as well as with the theme of eating—unusual in an adult and indicative of regressive tendencies. This quality of the patient is further demonstrated in the highly unusual, personal statement of preferring a child's test: "I like the CAT better. It has animals and stuff."

At Time 2, the issue of responsibility for one's behavior comes clearly into focus. First, there is a recognition that failure to take responsibility enrages the other person, as was seen at Time 1 in the stories about Cards 13MF and 18GF. Second, there is some slight recognition that this stance—shitting on the other—is hostile. Significantly, the patient experiences great anxiety about this hostility, resulting in paranoid-like ideation: "Will the tape be censored cause I said shit? There is an FCC code." However, these gains in psychological maturity are fleeting, for the story ends with an abrogation of responsibility and a derogatory attitude toward the one who was used and who *does* the work.

At Time 3, there is again a very different quality to the story. The focus now is on providing for others, with anxiety attendant upon the possibility of responsibility and interpersonal intimacy. This anxiety is handled through obsessive–compulsive defenses, illustrated in the "checking" and making sure that "everything's all right." The basis for the anxiety—the fear of rejection—is clearly indicated in the last sentence of the story.

TAT Card 14

Time 1. "Wow. I never saw this card. He couldn't sleep and he's standing by the window waiting for it to be morning and the day's getting lighter and he's glad the night's over. On one hand . . . on the other hand it's dusk and he didn't bother turning on the light. He doesn't want to go through another night so he's contemplating jumping. Or, he's a grown up violinist and he still hates it. He's going to Juilliard and they want him to practice more and he's had it. (*feeling?*) One part is feeling hopeful 'cause day has come and it was a rough night, and the other one is feeling despair and frustration and anger and wants to jump. But somehow the window gives me more like . . . the light outside the window . . . gives me more a feeling of hope than concentrating on all the black. He could be somewhere like in a beach town watching sunset. That's about it. Is that enough?"

Time 2. "Ah, he's gonna jump. . . . What came before, just the black nothingness. He wants to jump into the light. And afterwards he's flying through super white light rather than being in the dark, dark pit."

Time 3. "He was walking the street and walking the streets, and he found this vacant, almost demolished building and he like climbed the steps way up to the top, and he's just standing there staring out into space and he just doesn't know . . . he just doesn't know what he's going to do next, like he feels alone and desperate, and he doesn't know what to do and he's trying to find different things that are comfortable. One of the things he's thinking is the possibility of jumping. I don't know if he's going to because he doesn't know if he's going to."

At Time 1, the story is characterized by passivity, consistent with that noted in the other Time 1 stories. This passivity is seen both in the perseveration (now for a third story) of the violin theme and in the story, as discussed above. The man does nothing to change the darkness in the room, and responsibility for activity and feelings is attributed outside the self.

At Time 2, the story indicates greater psychological disturbance than previously. Perhaps the male figure and the blackness of the card arouse emotions connected with the recent losses she experienced while living in her home community. In any case, the story has a quality of autistic fantasy, with an eerie lack of contact with reality, which provides a pathological flavor. The fusion of abstract symbolism with concrete referents occurs in the expressions "jump into the light" and in the unearthly image of "flying through super white light." It is also significant that, as noticed earlier, there are no consequences to his behavior; jumping is not followed by a fall.

As noted for the two previous cards, at Time 3 there is a noticeable difference in the story. There is much more activity this time; he was "walking . . . and . . . walking"; he "climbed the steps way up to the top." Also, we see here the first indication of the storyteller spontaneously recognizing and describing inner feelings: "he feels alone and desperate." However, the regressive pull toward inactivity and physical gratification has not completely disappeared, as seen in the rather peculiar statement that he is "trying to find different things that are *comfortable*." The ending is also regressive in the sense that the storyteller attributes responsibility to the other, in this case, the character in the story: "I don't know if he's going to because he doesn't know if he's going to."

TAT Card 13MF

Time 1. "Well this is a lot of . . . what it is he can't take her anymore 'cause she just won't get out of bed. He doesn't understand why she just can't get just . . . like can't get up and get dressed and just go on with her life and he's had enough and he doesn't know how to deal with her anymore. Or, going more extreme, he just killed her. He didn't mean to and he's like really ashamed of what he's done. Or, another story could be she'd . . . it's his first prostitute he's seen and he's . . . you know, went to . . . and he's really ashamed and he got on his clothes and he'll probably leave the money on the books or something and he's going. But, I think the first one the most."

Time 2. "She's dead. He's upset. He came into the room . . . bedroom and she was lying there nude in bed and he thought that was really neat. And he went over to get ready to join her in the bed and he leaned down and she was dead, and he's . . . he's a little freaked out about the whole thing. And I'd say they weren't a married couple, they were in an affair, 'cause it's a single bed, it's not a double bed."

Time 3. "Oh, he killed her. She picked him up, and he came and he just got really intense and he killed her, and now he's upset because he usually doesn't . . . he's not like a serial killer or anything. He feels remorse and said, 'Oh, my God, what did I do?' He had done it earlier in the night. He's just finally getting the courage to be dressed and to leave, but he can't believe what he did, but he killed her."

At Time 1, the main theme again is passivity; the woman will not get out of bed and will not go on with her life. This passivity enrages the other person: "he's had enough." There is also a connection made here; the woman's passive aggression provokes aggression in the other: "he just killed her."

At Time 2, the female has now become completely passive (dead). It also becomes clear that this passivity serves as a defensive maneuver in that it precludes interpersonal, or sexual, intimacy. Noteworthy also is the circumstantial reasoning at the end of the story: "I'd say . . . they were in an affair, 'cause it's a single bed, it's not a double bed."

By Time 3, there is a clearer delineation of responsibility for the situation: "*he* killed her"; "*she* picked him up." Also, the basis of the anxiety surrounding an intimate relationship becomes clearer; there is a fear that the emotions involved will be overwhelming, leading ultimately to death.

TAT Card 12M

Time 1. "The old man and the younger man have been on the outs for a really long time and there was never words to get back together, and now he sees his son or his grandson resting and he wants to just touch him and be close again. Or, he got there too late and the boy's already dead and he couldn't make amends. It's hard to tell because you can't see the older man's face. Or, he could even be in some kind of therapy and he was just hypnotized."

Time 2. "He's dead too. It's an old priest over him, giving him his last rites."

Time 3. "He hypnotized him. This old guy is some kind of hypnotist or something and . . . uhm . . . he hypnotized the person to find out the secret."

At Time 1, there is another example of attribution of responsibility to another, this time presented in the context of rather peculiar logic. The storyteller states that she cannot tell whether the boy is resting or is dead "*because*" she cannot see the older man's face. There is also the continuation of death precluding interpersonal intimacy.

At Time 2, the story is a perseveration from that told about the preceding card, indicating both passivity on the part of the storyteller and the role that passivity plays in avoiding intimacy.

At Time 3, although the main character is still passive, he is no longer dead. Rather, the issue has become one of being under the control of another person, who wants "to find out the secret"—a theme expressed to Card 18GF at Time 1. As discussed below, this theme may refer to the patient's experience with her therapist.

TAT Card 2

Time 1. "Well, she wants to better herself from living and working on a farm and she's going to school and she's really serious about learning a trade and leaving this back-breaking world of work. It's her brother and her mother in the picture. Her mother's still having children . . . probably have a large family and not a lot of food to go around and she wants to escape into another life or another way of life. That's it."

Time 2. "Well, two women are interested in the same man. He's like, what movie was it? I forget, but, um, anyway, they're two different types, very two different types . . . one's an older woman, who's like, really been around, really knows that's going on and the woman's like very innocent schoolgirl who it . . . They're both seduc . . . seductive in their own ways. She, by her innocence and the other one by her worldliness."

Time 3. "She grew up on this farm, you see, and she doesn't want to be like another generation farmer. She wants to go on to school but she realizes once she makes that step away, she's like really leaving it for good."

At Time 1, the ambivalence about becoming independent versus remaining passive is portrayed in the situation of going to school to learn a trade *so as* to avoid "this back-breaking world of work," as discussed above. There is also a contrast between the farm girl and the educated girl. As in the stories about Cards 1 and 5, there is another reference to food and fear of deprivation: "not enough food to go around."

At Time 2, the contrast between two types of females is brought into clearer focus and is reminiscent of a similar comparison expressed in the story about Card 12F at Time 1. The story focuses on the contrast between the innocent schoolgirl and the worldly wise woman.

At Time 3, there is more capacity for self-reflection, as seen also in the story about Card 1 at this time. Here, on Card 2, this capacity is seen in the recognition that activity (making "the step away") means separation (from childhood, from immaturity).

TAT Card 18GF

Time 1. "She's making her tell her something but she doesn't understand what she wants to know and she says, '*Tell* me.' And she says, 'I don't know.' And she keeps saying, 'Tell me' over and over. She doesn't know and now she's gotten so mad that she's choking her."

Time 2. "Oh no! She's trying to make her come back to life, and, she loves her in some sort of capacity. I don't know what kind of way and they've been really close for a long time and, she's, she doesn't know whether she wants to come back to life or not."

Time 3. "These pictures are so disturbing. She's choking her. She can't take her anymore. She's just choking her. She loves her but she can't take her anymore so she's choking her."

At Time 1, the story again portrays the passive position of the patient and the experience of coercion. The passivity is carried out through a stance of mental incapacity. Again, as in the story about Card 13MF, this passivity enrages the other, who chokes her.

At Time 2, the quality of the affective relationship between the two women in the story has changed, but the passive position is still present. The life (activity) of one character is made the responsibility of the other: "She's trying to make her come back to life. . . . " Significantly, activity (living) is connected to emotional closeness, about which the heroine is uncertain. The anxiety around intimacy is expressed in the peculiar verbalization, "She loves her in some sort of capacity."

It seems likely that the themes expressed in the stories from Time 1 and Time 2 reflect a change in the patient's perception of her original female therapist. Initially, the therapist's efforts were experienced as controlling, demanding, and coercive, and the patient felt her refusal to take an active part in the therapy was angering the therapist. However, after a period of productive treatment, the patient perceives the therapist differently. There is some understanding that the therapist cares for the patient, but that the form of this caring is different from what the patient had imagined. Rather than "taking care of" the patient in some infantalizing fashion, the therapist urges the patient to assume an active role in finding and developing her life.

At Time 3, the story reverts back to the theme expressed at Time 1, in which the heroine, through passivity, provokes aggression in the other. Given that this story was told after a period of conflict in which the patient wished to return to her previous female therapist but instead was assigned to a new male therapist, the story may be seen as a commentary on the patient's experience of that "rejection." The woman who "loves her but can't take her anymore" is likely the patient's explanation of why she was shifted from the female to the male therapist, and it fits with her more general theme of sensing that her passivity enrages others.

TAT Card 12F

Time 1. "The old lady can't accept the fact she's old and she still thinks she looks like she did when she was younger. And the woman up front is like her imagined self and the one in the back is her real self. (*feeling?*) Reminiscent and a little schitzed out because she doesn't know which is . . . which one she is, the old person or the younger person. But, with time she grew like more express . . . expressive 'cause the young woman has a very flat affect. The woman in back seems to have more the look of youth and animation in her face."

Time 2. "The woman in the back is obviously very old and she's looking and reminiscing about what she was like when she was younger. And that's the woman in the front and, I don't know . . . by looking through her eyes she could be young again."

Time 3. "This woman in the front, the younger woman, has just like a scary, secret part of her and that's what the old lady is, and she tells her all horrible things and tells her to do all horrible things and makes her feel awful, and even now, you can tell by the younger woman's eyes she's being controlled by the older woman. Is that it?"

At Time 1, the story revolves around the confusion between the wish to be a child and the difficulties of being an adult. Again, the passive–active issue is expressed, in that the child-self is "flat" (i.e., passive and inactive) whereas the adult has the possibility of activity, "animation."

At Time 2, there is a clearer differentiation than at Time 1 between the child-self and the adult-self. It also becomes clearer here that by maintaining a childish way of looking at the world—meaning, probably, passive and dependent—it is possible to remain a child.

The story told at Time 3 indicates a real shift. Now it is no longer the old woman longing to be (like) the younger woman. Rather, the old woman has been introjected into the younger woman, and this is the bad introject who controls—that is, is responsible for—the young woman's negative behavior and feelings. It is this negative introject that is "the secret," perhaps illuminating the previous references to secrets (Card 18GF, Time 1; Card 12M, Time 3). Most generally, this story portrays the continuing confusion in the patient's identification, for she identifies with the child, who is being controlled by the bad female adult, rather than identifying with the adult who must integrate the child and the childish longings into the self. There is also an indication of why she does not identify with the female adult, who is connected to scary, horrible events and feelings. As in the previous story, it is possible that the portrayal of the older woman refers to her experience of the female therapist she has just reacquired. The end of the story provides yet another example of paranoid ideation: "even now, *you can tell by the younger woman's eyes* she's being controlled by the older woman."

Considering these stories as a whole, we can see how the storyteller's narrative themes are revealed. The repeated story lines—of attribution of responsibility for activity, incapacitating passivity and avoidance of effort, the regressive pull to childlike immaturity, and strong oral needs—indicate to us the important underlying psychological problems in this patient.

The continuation of these themes over a period of years suggests the stability of such narrative themes in the individual personality. At the same time, the modifications in the way the themes are expressed—especially the qualitative change that is noted in a number of the stories told at the end of this period—are generally consistent in demonstrating more mature or adaptive solutions to the earlier problems. A comparison of the three storytelling occasions also reveals the development of some capacity for self-reflection, self-observation, and the description of inner feelings, as well as continuing identity confusion. From the narrative themes in these TAT stories, it is possible to construct a useful clinical description of the patient.

Defense Mechanisms

It is also interesting to look at these TAT stories from the interpretive perspective of the use of defense mechanisms. Particularly in a patient who shows so many immature, regressive features at the time of the initial testing, we might expect that there would be a tendency to use the developmentally earlier defenses of denial and projection. In fact, this was the result when the Time 1 stories were scored for defense mechanisms. At that initial testing, the defense scores were as follows: denial = 8, projection = 11, and identification = 6. By Time 2, however, the use of all three defenses had decreased: denial = 4, projection = 7, identification = 3. At Time 3, the use of denial had decreased even further, denial = 3, whereas the use of projection was at its highest, projection = 14. The use of identification had also increased: identification = 5. What is noteworthy about the identification score at Time 3 is that although numerically it is similar to Time 1, the later score is obtained through instances of self-reflection rather than indicating instances of behavior being regulated by another.

As an example of the use of denial at Time 1, let us consider the story told by the patient about Card 12F. This story, which shows the greatest use of Denial of all the stories told at that time, is, significantly, about the confusion in identity between being young and old, youth and adulthood. The first occurrence of denial appears in the statement, "The old lady *can't accept the fact* she's old"; this is scored for denial 5, denial of reality. The next occurrence is, "*she still thinks she looks like she did when she was younger*"; this is also scored for denial 5. The next occurrence is, "*she doesn't know which is–which one she is*," again an example of denial 5. The last occurrence is the statement, "*The woman in back seems to have more the look of youth . . .* "; this is scored for denial 3, reversal. This story thus receives a total denial score of 4.

As an example of the use of projection at Time 1, let us consider the story told about Card 12M. The first occurrence is in the statement, "The old man and the younger man *have been on the outs for a really long time*"; this is scored projection 1, attribution of feelings that are normatively unusual. The next occurrence is, "the boy's already *dead*," which is scored projection 5, apprehensiveness of death. This is followed by, "It's hard to tell *because you can't see the older man's face*"; this is scored projection 3, circumstantial thinking. Finally, the statement, "he was just *hypnotized*," is scored projection 3, use of hypnosis. The story receives a total projection score of 4.

For an example of the use of identification, let us consider the story told about Card 1 at Time 3, a story that revolves around the question of forming an identity. The first occurrence of identification is in the statement, "*He's looking back to when he was little,*" which is scored identification 3, self-reflection. The second occurrence is, "*He feels as a grownup,*" which is scored identification 2, emulation of characteristics. Finally, "*he feels regret*" is scored identification 3, self-criticism. The story receives a total identification score of 3.

The change in these defense scores over the three testing occasions is consistent with the description of the patient's course in hospital. At Time 1, she was described as presenting herself as given to regressive behavior and a helpless, childlike attitude, demanding that others care for her. The use of less mature defenses, and especially the defense of denial, is consistent with this picture. At Time 2, significant characterological changes had occurred as a result of the first treatment period. This is consistent with the overall lower use of defenses, but the relative use of immature and mature defense at the point of readmission to the hospital is similar to that at Time 1. At Time 3, the patient is embarking on a significant change in her life, leaving the hospital and moving to an outpatient apartment. She has recently concluded an ongoing conflict with her male therapist by returning to the original therapist. As discussed earlier, the therapist may have been perceived as having left the patient because she was angered by the patient's passivity. The defense scores at Time 3 are compatible with this formulation. There is both an absolute and relative decrease in the immature defense of denial, consistent with the patient's moving out of the dependent position of being a hospital patient. There is a marked increase in the use of projection, which is consistent with a developmental advance as well as with the hypothesized "explanation" for the therapist's behavior. The slight increase in the use of identification is also consistent with psychological development, especially in the self-reflection shown.

Gender Identity

It is also possible to look at these TAT stories from the perspective of May's deprivation/enhancement (D/E) approach to assessing gender identity. When Ms. F's stories are approached in this way, the following scores are obtained: Time 1: +.50; Time 2: +.17; Time 3: +.43. On each occasion, her scores are just slightly in the feminine direction, with little change over the course of treatment.

CASE 2: MR. M

We turn now to the TAT stories of a second, male patient. Mr. M was 26 years old at the time of his admission to the hospital. Clinically, he was more disturbed than Ms. F. There was evidence that serious psychological difficulty had existed since at least high school, and probably before, although Mr. M's parents had steadily ignored and failed to recognize the patient's illness, seeing him instead as lazy and spoiled. The patient had been hospitalized for short periods on a number of previous occasions, following psychotic breaks in which grandiose delusions were prominent. Recently, he had been experiencing severe panic attacks occasioned by intense fears of separation.

On admission, he was noted to engage in unusual bodily movements, akin to posturing or psychotic stereotypy. His thought processes were characterized by loose associations and cognitive slippage. Staff observations noted that he was quite vulnerable to affective disruption and to what he perceived as interpersonal impingement. Staff members noted, for example, that he was unable to continue sitting at a table if another person also sat at that table. This vulnerability to being overstimulated by the presence of another person sometimes resulted in psychological disintegration and disorganization. At other times, feelings of sadness or anger could produce similar disintegration. Attempts to control this through obsessive intellectualization were not always effective. The clinical diagnosis at admission was schizophrenic disorder, chronic undifferentiated; the diagnosis was changed at the clinical case conference 1 month later to a principal diagnosis of separation anxiety disorder, as well as schizoaffective disorder.

The Initial TAT Stories

Here are Mr. M's TAT stories at the time of his admission to the hospital.

TAT Card 1, Time 1

"Well, here's a boy looking at a violin. The boy has gotten to his seat recently and is trying to decide whether to play the violin. The boy decides he has enough inspiration so that he stands up and starts to try to play the violin. (*feeling?*) He is feeling the insecurity of not knowing whether he can play the violin very well. And he is also feeling the hope that he can, which is what is leading him in his attempt to try."

Although the general plot expressed here is not especially unusual, the story strikes one as different in several noticeable ways: First is the unusual verbalization, "gotten to his seat recently." This is the first in a series of references to the physical position or location of the hero of the story. This concern for physical position is seen also in the statement, "he stands up."[2] The story is also noteworthy for the isolation of the hero. There are no other characters involved or even mentioned. Also, there is a stilted use of language: "He is also feeling the hope that he can, which is what is leading him in his attempt to try." Together, one gets a feeling of someone who is physically uncomfortable in his own skin, resulting in awkwardness and rigidity in moving through life.

TAT Card 5, Time 1

"This is a woman who is standing in the doorway of her clothes closet. She just got in there and she is surprised because she is wondering if someone else is in the room, so she is checking to see if anyone else is in the room. (?) She is feeling startled because she thought she had her own time of privacy."

As in Card 1, the story opens with a statement about the physical location of the main character: "standing in the doorway of her clothes closet." This is an unusual perception of the TAT picture; the woman is seen as having moved into a small space, rather than the more usual scene of her looking or moving into a large space. Anxiety about the possible presence of another person continues the issue of isolation noted in the first story. Again, we see an example of peculiar verbalization in the statement: "her own time of privacy."

TAT Card 14, Time 1

"This is a person who is looking out the window of a building that's in a ghetto. An urban place. The person comes from a financially very disadvantaged family and is both getting some fresh air as well as yearning to be someplace else."

Again, there is an emphasis on location: "looking out the window of a building that's in a ghetto. An urban place." Here, the patient begins with the most restricted indication of place, the window, then locates this in its place, the building, which is then located in the ghetto, which is then placed in the larger urban environment. There is further evidence in this story of the use of stilted language: "financially very disadvantaged."

TAT Card 13MF, Time 1

"This is a picture in which a woman on a bed has just died and her husband, who is standing up in the picture, has realized that his wife has just died and is in terrible tears of the first time beginning the mourning process."

Again, the story begins with a focus on the physical position of the characters: "a woman on a bed," and a husband "who is standing up." Perhaps as a result of the intimacy implied in the picture, the patient closes the story with a peculiar verbalization that borders on being a word salad: "terrible tears of the first time beginning the mourning process."

TAT Card 12M, Time 1

"This is a picture of two people who are in the outdoors. One of . . . the woman is sitting . . . lying down and the man is hovered over her and he is going to check her in some way with his right hand, but he hasn't done it yet, he is in process of being about to. And a woman seems asleep or very calm and ready to be checked in whatever way the man intends to check her."

This is now the fifth story of five that begins by noting the physical location of the characters. Placing the characters in this picture out of doors is unusual, as is the sitting position of the character (mis)perceived as female. Overall, there is an extremely frozen quality to this story, giving an almost catatonic feeling to the production.

TAT Card 2, Time 1

"This is a picture of things going on in the 19th century, on a farm. There is a man with a horse who is taking care of farming the ground and there are two women who are standing by. One has very little interest in what he is doing. She is standing by a tree, daydreaming. And the closer woman, who has a book in her hand, has just finished thinking for a while about her studies and she can't decide whether she likes the man for his knowing of the toiling of the . . . of the farm. She would much rather immerse herself in the ideas and subject matter of her book . . . her books."

Again, this story contains the theme of interpersonal isolation. Although there are three characters mentioned, they have no interaction and little or no interest in each other. There is also another peculiar verbalization in the statement: "for his knowing of the toiling of the farm."

TAT Card 18GF, Time 1

"This is a picture of two people: a mother and a son, and the . . . er . . . what's the mother doing . . . uhm. The mother, in fact, seems to be hurting the son. She has tension on her face and there is anger on her face and she is squeezing the . . . face of her son. That's it."

Here is the second time in which there is a misperception of the sex of the character depicted; both the people in this picture are usually seen as female. There is also another example of an unusual verbalization: "squeezing the face of her son."

One may now hypothesize that the aggressive potential of Cards 12M and 18GF led to a breakdown in the patient's reality testing, as seen in the misperception of the sex of the figures. Whereas the aggressive impulses are frozen in a catatonic-like stance in the story about Card 12M, they break through in Card 18GF.

TAT Card 7BM, Time 1

"Here are two people: two men, who are . . . have just been confronted with a legal question. And they are both trying to develop some ideas and some insight into the question that they have been posed, and they are in the process of thinking about it and communicating with one another verbally about it and that's what they are doing."

This story is noteworthy for its wordiness, in contrast to a lack of action. It also contains another unusual verbalization: "communicating with one another verbally about it. . . . "

Taking an overview of the stories from Time 1, they are remarkable for what they do not tell us about the patient and for what they do. The patient's responses are more like picture descriptions than stories. There is little in the way of a personal story line that might reveal to us something about the underlying narrative of this man. At the most, we note a concern with delineating and separating locations and people, consistent with a concern around boundaries. Information about this patient from his clinical record relates this concern to his fragile sense of self and his fear of separation, as well as his fear of narcissistic obliteration. Rather than expressing aspects of a well-formed narrative, the stories are noteworthy for the lack of a personal narrative.

At the same time, along with the persistent concern about location and position, the stories have a superficial and static quality, as if the characters were frozen. It is this quality of the stories that is most revealing and might be considered the main "story line" of this patient—an attempt to locate his psychological self in terms of physical positions and locations. This aspect of the stories reminds us of the bodily posturing noted on admission to hospital. In addition, the sexual misperceptions on two cards and the unusual perceptions on others, along with the peculiar verbalizations, all speak to the presence of serious psychopathology.

Defense Mechanisms

Scoring these stories for the use of defense mechanisms produced the following results: denial = 3, projection = 7, identification = 0. Significantly, the three denial scores all result from misperceptions, which is indicative of a very primitive level of denial. The projection scores all occur in connection with female figures involved with potential or actual aggression. To have such a low identification score in an adult is quite unusual but well reflects the psychological status of this severely disturbed man, who lacks a sense of identity or cohesion and is continually vulnerable to psychological disintegration.

Gender Identity

Scoring these same stories using May's D/E system yields a slightly positive score of +.43, which is somewhat in the feminine direction.

The TAT Stories 18 Months Later

At the time of the second storytelling, the patient was described by his therapist as showing a greater readiness to be active and instrumental in his functioning. He was also described as beginning to experience himself as a participant in interpersonal relationships. Confusion around gender identity was being revealed in therapy; ambivalent longings for closeness to a man led to a feminine identification. The diagnosis made at a clinical conference at this time was schizoaffective disorder, in remission.

Here are Mr. M's stories 18 months after admission.

TAT Card 1, Time 2

"A boy was given a Christmas present of a violin which he wanted very much because he wanted to learn to play the violin. In this picture, the boy is looking at the violin and is con . . . um . . . can't think of the word . . . contemplating getting . . . asking his parents for lessons for the violin. The parents complied because they're happy to see that their child has an interest . . . their son has an interest and he sets about to begin lessons learning how to play the violin."

There is a noticeable change in this story, as compared to that told at Time 1. Now, there are other people present who provide the possibility of interpersonal gratification, whereas before the boy was completely isolated, with no other characters mentioned. In the present story, the hero's wishes are gratified by others, who give him both the violin he wants and the lessons he asks for.

TAT Card 5, Time 2

"There's a woman who is inviting some guests over for dinner and there are members of her family and she wants to see if the living room . . . this is a picture of the living room . . . if she wants . . . this is a picture of her looking at the living room and she's making sure that everything is in place for her guests, that everything's in order and put in the proper place and the woman is satisfied with that and her guests come over . . . members of her family come over and they have a nice dinner together."

As with Card 1, this story differs markedly from that told at Time 1; now the story is filled with other people. The theme revolves around the imminent interaction with others. It presents the story line of what families do, which will reappear in subsequent stories. At the same time, anxiety around this situation is handled through obsessive–compulsive behavior: "making sure that everything is in place for her guests, that everything's in order and put in the proper place. . . . "

TAT Card 14, Time 2

"There exists a housing project or a building in the middle of the storm in a bad part of New York City and, uh, it's a very dilapidated and run down and poor project . . . housing project and, uh, the person who lives there doesn't like living there and the people . . . the person there doesn't like . . . and, uh, the person is sitting at the . . . at his window. In the picture, the person is sitting at his window, wishfully thinking how nice it would be to get out of the slum and, uh, in the course of time, he does but it takes a great deal of effort to keep his mind on his studies so that he can be trained, in some way, to get a job and leave the slum so he doesn't leave the slum immediately."

The story begins with the stilted phrase: "There exists . . . ," apparently an attempt to locate or place the story in some category (e.g., the category of things that exist). The story continues with this need to place the story, by locating the "building *in the middle of a storm in a bad part* of *New York City*." In contrast to the earlier story, there is now some indication of the feelings of the hero, who "doesn't like living there" and who is "wishfully thinking." The story ends with a good example of the use of the defense of identification: "in the course of time, he does but it takes a great deal of effort to keep his mind on his studies so that he can be trained . . . to get a job."

TAT Card 13MF, Time 2

"It can happen that when people in families get sick in a mental way, sometimes the parents don't know how to help the person who's sick

so in this picture, there is a woman lying on her bed in a great deal
of severe mental illness and the father is quite scared and wiping his
brow of the sweat because he doesn't know what to do to help his
daughter. The woman is his daughter, and, uh, in the end the father
is able to get to the right doctors to get some advice on how he can
be helpful and beneficial to the . . . his daughter's recovery."

Here again, the story begins by placing it in a category—the category
of things that can happen. The plot again refers to "families." In contrast
to the story of Time 1, and similar to Card 1 (Time 2), the family is now
involved in providing nurturance and interpersonal gratification. The
autobiographical reference to parents who do not know how to help a
family member with mental problems, but finally get to the right doctors
is noteworthy, as is the stilted verbalization: "sick in a mental way."

TAT Card 12M, Time 2

"When people are sick in a physical way, sometimes they can . . .
sometimes families can be aware of that, that a member of the family
is sick in a physical way. In this case, there's a woman on a bed who
doesn't feel well and conjectures she has some temperature and the
man standing up is his . . . her father also and he's about to feel her
brow to see if he can detect whether there is any temperature and,
in fact, there is some temperature and, in the end, they get the
antibiotics, the penicillin to, uh, heal her in her sickness, a bacterial
infection."

This story begins with a perseveration of the stilted expression of the
previous story, now expressed as "sick in a physical way." The contrast
between the idea expressed in this story—families *can* be aware of *physical*
illness—and that in the previous story—families do not know how to
respond to *mental* illness—again has an autobiographical referent. As at
Time 1, the misperception of the male as being female continues and is
seen additionally in the confusion: "the man standing up is *his* . . . *her*
father. . . . " Although the language continues to be rather stilted, there
is also the possibility for gratifying interpersonal interaction to occur.

TAT Card 2, Time 2

"It used to be that when farmers had farms and had families, they
did a great deal of manual labor because they didn't . . . they did a
great deal of manual labor in making their farms function because
they didn't have the modern, electrical equipment. In this picture,
there's a farmer who is using his horse to till the soil of his farm and
his daughter is going away from the farm with some schoolbooks in
her hand and, uh, she expects to read the books because she's not a

... a person very much interested in farming. She wants to do more intellectual, education things rather than be a ... rather than do manual labor to help the farm."

The story begins with yet another example of placing or positioning the story into a category—here, things that "used to be." The theme of families continues. There is also a rather interesting avoidance of stating directly the adult role, or identity, of being a farmer. The patient begins to say "rather than be a farmer" but cuts this short and substitutes an impersonal expression of the same idea: "rather than to do manual labor to help the farm." This reminds one of the clear expression of the difficulty in becoming a working adult that was expressed in the story about Card 14 (Time 2). The avoidance of personal statements is also seen in the preceding sentence. The patient aborts the direct statement of what the character is or is not: "she's not a ... " is shifted into a more impersonal mode "a person very much interested in farming."

TAT Card 18GF, Time 2

"It would be helpful if I could know what it is the picture of, on my part. Uh, family members ... families get ... the different members of the immediate families get angry at one another from time to time and, in this picture, there's a teenaged fellow who is being berated or blamed by his mother for not being properly genial or properly, uh ... oh, genial is a good word ... caring, but, uh, not disrespectful but being inadequately a nice interpersonal person and in the end, the mother is able to convey to her son what she feels ... how she feels about things and, uh, the son is able to absorb what she's saying and they bring the relationship to a peaceful level, even if he doesn't entirely agree with what she ... his mother is saying."

Mr. M now responded to this card, which produced a highly disturbed story at Time 1, with an attempt at an intellectualizing defense, which is unsuccessful: "It would be helpful if I could know what it is the picture of, on my part." The theme of families occurs again, and there is greater control over the aggressive feelings aroused by the picture. The story contains further examples of peculiar verbalizations: "being inadequately a nice interpersonal person." The theme of this story centers on the expectations of the family for "proper" behavior. In this context, we may reconsider the increased references at Time 2 to families and how families are, and whether these references in the stories indicate a superficial attempt to have the kind of ideas that one is "supposed" to have. The story ends with an example of incorporation or introjection, which is an early stage of the defense of identification: "The son is able to *absorb* what she is saying." It is also noteworthy that the hero is able to differentiate between himself and the mother: "even if he doesn't entirely agree with what she . . . his mother is saying," and that this separation does not threaten disintegration.

TAT Card 7BM, Time 2

"When sons and daughters grow up, parents often look at them in somewhat different ways sometimes from the way they were as children and when they become adults, they have a sense of the world around them and sometimes in a political way, and it's something that they begin to develop when they're younger but they don't have the adult capacity and sense for thinking and, in this picture, there's a father who's of a mature age who is talking to his son about politics and the father is trying to learn whether his son has some valuable thoughts about politics and the son is trying to convey to his father some of the thoughts he has and, in the end, they both agree that they each have some interesting things to share with one another, interesting thoughts to share with one another's concepts."

The story again begins with the ways that families are but continues the story line of psychological differentiation. There is also the story line of interpersonal gratification, although in this context peculiar verbalizations continue: "they . . . agree they . . . have . . . interesting thoughts to share with one another's concepts." The theme of the story revolves around the question of how identification develops. However, there is a noticeable reversal in that it is the father who is trying to identify with the son.

Overall, these stories are quite different from those told at Time 1. The therapist's description of Mr. M at the time of the second storytelling portrayed important positive changes. Much of the therapeutic work involved helping the patient to establish an inner, psychological world and to understand that this world determines how he feels and what he does. In therapy, Mr. M showed an increased ability to talk about his experience and was somewhat more open in revealing his fears about dependency, autonomy, and separation.

These changes in the patient, as well as those discussed earlier, are reflected in the stories told at Time 2. The capacity for greater openness is seen in a looser, more relaxed style of storytelling, with less of the static, frozen quality of his earlier stories. One consequence of this relaxed control is that the stories appear more troubled. In an attempt to control the anxiety associated with experiencing feelings, Mr. M relies on attempts at intellectualizing or obsessive–compulsive defenses, which frequently result in peculiar verbalization. Positive changes are seen in the increased presence of (other) people in the stories and, thus, we assume, in the patient's inner world. There is evidence of interpersonal gratification, as well as anxiety around such interaction. In addition to the greater articulation of inner feelings, there is a recognition that personal development is possible.

Defense Mechanisms

There is a noticeable change in the defense scores for these stories at Time 2. Whereas the use of denial and projection continues at about the same level (denial: Time 1 = 3, Time 2 = 5; projection: Time 1 = 7, Time 2 = 5), there is a dramatic change in the use of identification (Time 1 = 0, Time 2 = 9). This change is consistent with positive development, noted in the therapy, in the creation and stabilizing of an internal world in the patient.

Gender Identity

Given the therapist's description of Mr. M's confusion around gender identity and his attempt at this time to solve this conflict through a feminine identification, as well as the evidence of confusion about the sex of figures on the TAT cards, we might expect a deviant pattern in the patient's gender-identity scores this time. When the TAT stories from Time 2 are evaluated using May's D/E system, the average score of +2.25 is strongly in the feminine direction, consistent with this expectation, and quite different from his score (+.43) at Time 1.

SUMMARY

This chapter has provided an in-depth study of two patients with problems serious enough to require hospitalization. An extended discussion of clinical pathology and course in the hospital is presented for each patient, along with a complete TAT protocol of eight stories for each. These stories were told shortly after admission to the hospital and again after a period of treatment.

A detailed analysis of each story is provided. The focus in this chapter is on the narrative themes that are revealed and found to be consistent across stories. Changes in these themes over time, associated with treatment, are discussed. In addition, the stories are assessed from the perspectives of gender identity and the use of defense mechanisms, and changes on these dimensions are related to changes in the narrative themes.

NINE

The Anaclitic/Introjective Perspective: Two Personality Organizations

Over time, a striking consensus among personality theorists has developed, suggesting that people may be characterized by two distinctly different orientations toward the environment and the self. One of these is organized around a concern for others and an attachment to them; the other is focused on a concern for self-definition and on autonomy from others. These two orientations have been variously termed "communion" and "agency" (Bakan, 1966), "surrender" and "autonomy" (Angyal, 1951), Freud's *"leben und arbeiten"* (Freud, 1930/1961)[1] or "libidinal and aggressive instincts" (Freud, 1926/1959), and, among the motivational researchers, "intimacy" (McAdams, 1980, 1985) and "power" (Winter, 1973).

THE ANACLITIC/INTROJECTIVE PERSONALITY ORGANIZATION: THEORY

Within contemporary psychoanalytic writings, a similar distinction has been made between the anaclitic and introjective personality organization. Blatt (1990) and Blatt and Shichman (1983) have drawn a carefully described process of personality development in which the two basic dimensions of personality organization—the capacity for interpersonal relatedness and the development of self-definition—are seen as central. Healthy development requires an integration of these two dimensions.

> These two developmental lines normally evolve throughout the life cycle in a complex dialectic transaction. An increasingly differentiated, integrated, and mature sense of self is contingent on establishing satisfying interpersonal experiences, and, conversely, the continued development of increasingly mature and satisfying interpersonal relationships is contingent on the development of more mature self-definition and identity. Meaningful and satisfying relationships contribute to the evolving concept of the self, and a new sense of self leads, in turn, to more mature levels of interpersonal relatedness. In normal personality development, these two developmental processes evolve in an interactive, reciprocally balanced, mutually facilitating fashion from birth through senescence. (Blatt, 1990, pp. 299–300)

Each of these personality organizations utilizes different types of defense mechanisms. Individuals primarily concerned with interpersonal relatedness, to the neglect of self-definition, use mainly avoidant defenses (e.g., denial). Individuals primarily invested in self-definition, with a neglect of relatedness, use counteractive defenses (e.g., projection). Avoidant defenses function to avoid recognizing the existence of conflict or anxiety. Problems and associated affect are kept out of consciousness and not acknowledged. Counteractive defenses convert or transform unacceptable feelings or thoughts in ways that permit partial but disguised expression.

In normal development, the two modes—relatedness and self-definition, anaclitic and introjective—evolve in an integrated fashion "so that the individual develops an active commitment to interpersonal relatedness and a viable sense of self." This process, however, can be disturbed by biological and environmental causes, with the result that one mode is exaggerated at the expense of the other. Mild exaggerations result in different character styles; extreme exaggerations are associated with psychopathology.

Patients who become preoccupied with relatedness at the expense of the development of self (who, statistically, are most often female) frequently appear needy, and demanding of care and attention. If the developmental disruption has occurred early in life, such patients appear infantile and focused on becoming part of a dyad in which they are accepted and cared for. Denial is their primary defense. If the disruption occurred somewhat later in development, the patients appear hysterical, placing themselves as part of a triad in which they are concerned about being attended to and loved by one parent while they are in competition with the other. Repression is their primary defense.

In contrast, patients who become preoccupied with establishing a sense of self at the expense of interpersonal relatedness (who, statistically, are most often male) direct their interest toward things rather than people. They emphasize thoughts and accomplishments rather than feelings and relationships; self-reproach and guilt are common. If the disruption leading to the excessive focus on the self began early in life, a paranoid pathology may be evident in which the concern is to ensure a separate self rather than being merged or fused in a symbiotic relationship. At a somewhat higher level of development, the concern about self-definition may underlie obsessive–compulsive pathology—concerns about mastery, control, and possessions. At yet a higher developmental level, the concern will be more about self-worth than mastery, as occurs in introjective, guilt-ridden depression. The reverse of this—endless exhibition and seeking of praise in order to defend against feelings of guilt, shame, and worthlessness—occurs in phallic narcissistic pathology (Blatt, 1990).

Pathologies of the first type—warped and overstated attempts to establish and preserve gratifying interpersonal relationships—are termed "anaclitic" and include the infantile and hysterical syndromes. Pathologies of the second type—warped and overstated attempts to establish and preserve a convincing sense of self—are termed "introjective." These include the paranoid, obsessive–compulsive, introjective depressive, and phallic narcissistic disorders (Blatt, 1990, p. 312).

Research studies with both clinical and nonclinical samples have found that depressed individuals may be identified as being either anaclitic or introjective. Some depressives show an exaggerated concern with relatedness and are characterized as being highly dependent, whereas others show a preoccupation with self-definition and are characterized as being self-critical. The former, the anaclitic depressives, and the latter, the introjective depressives, have each been found to report different life histories and to be vulnerable to different types of environmental stressors.

The anaclitic/introjective distinction has also been found to predict response to psychotherapy. Although both anaclitic and introjective patients show change following a course of treatment, they change in different ways and appear to benefit from different forms of treatment (Blatt, 1990). Anaclitic patients, who are concerned about interpersonal relatedness, were found to benefit more from face-to-face psychotherapy than from on-the-couch psychoanalysis; change in these patients occurs in the quality of their interpersonal relationships and conceptions of people. Introjective patients, who are concerned about self-definition and autonomy, benefited more from psychoanalysis than from psychotherapy; change in this group occurs in the quality of their cognitive processes, with diminished thought disorder and fewer pathological behaviors. In other words, patients were found to change along the dimensions that were most salient to their personality organization.

Given the difference between these two personality configurations, with different needs, concerns, foci, and defenses, we might expect that the TAT stories of anaclitic and introjective individuals would reflect some of these differences. If we approach TAT stories with the two configurations in mind—if we adopt an anaclitic/introjective interpretive stance—we will be sensitive to the occurrence of certain types of thematic material and certain types of defenses.

For the anaclitic configuration, we will look for themes indicating concern for, or a focus on others—on interpersonal relatedness and attachment. We would expect to find themes concerned with gratification or the lack of gratification. We would also expect story lines characterized by demandingness, neediness, and indications of wanting care and attention, within an infantile dyad; themes involving narcissistic triads would be indicative of a higher level of anaclitic development. Attempts to avoid recognition of conflict and anxiety should be present, and defenses would be expected to be of the avoidant kind (e.g., denial and repression).

For the introjective configuration, we would expect to find themes about self-definition, autonomy, and identity. Concerns about mastery, control, possessions, and self-worth should be expressed. An emphasis on mental processes and accomplishments, with an absence of references to emotions and relationships, would be expected. Defenses would be anticipated to be of the counteractive kind—projection, intellectualization, rationalization, and reaction formation; paranoid-like thinking may be present. Story lines expressing shame or guilt may be present, or these emotions may be defended against through narcissistic exhibitionism and praise seeking.

CLINICAL EXAMPLES

Let us look now at some sample TAT stories from individuals who have, on the basis of close clinical analysis, been independently determined to have primarily an anaclitic personality configuration (one female, one male) or an introjective personality configuration (one male, one female).[2] These individuals were, at the time of telling the stories, experiencing psychological problems severe enough to require hospitalization. Each was a patient at a small, open, psycho-analytically oriented hospital. Each was clinically evaluated shortly after admission and again after approximately 15 months of intensive treatment. Each of these patients were independently determined to have improved significantly over the course of treatment.[3] Because these patients provided TAT stories on admission to the hospital and again some 15 months later, it is possible (1) to identify anaclitic or introjective themes in their stories and then (2) to look for changes in these themes related to psychological improvement.

For each patient, stories are provided for TAT Card 5 (a middle-aged woman is standing on the threshold of a half-opened door looking into a room), to be able to compare responses to the same stimulus picture. In addition, a second TAT story is given for each patient which demonstrates particularly clearly the anaclitic and introjective story lines.

Ms. I: Anaclitic

The first set of stories comes from a young woman in her late teens with a primarily anaclitic personality configuration. On admission to hospital, her diagnosis was uncertain; she showed hysterical, obsessional, and paranoid symptoms. A preliminary diagnosis of chronic depression with serious borderline features was made.

Following in the footsteps of her older sister's promiscuity, which led to her mother throwing the sister out of the home, the patient at age 16 had given birth to a child. The baby was placed for adoption; the patient probably suffered a postpartum psychotic reaction at that time.

At admission, Ms. I reported feeling empty, passive, and helpless. She presented as a little girl, placing responsibility outside herself and search-ing for responses from others. With her therapist, she was clinging and excessively sought of his attention and time. She was described as showing a grasping helplessness, continually dissatisfied that her needs were not being met. Despite her demands for attention from her therapist, she was rather isolated in the patient community.

Here is her initial story about TAT Card 15, a woodcut drawing of a gaunt man with clenched hands standing among gravestones.

TAT Card 15, Time 1

"I am cold and alone, please God help me. I see all these dead people here and I'm dead too. I want to be alive. I am all alone . . . I've come out to the graveyard to tell you my sorrows. . . . He goes back to his lonely room, lonely empty room. Waits. . . . He becomes someone. He can go out and talk to people. He finds what he likes and does it. He can say hello and get to know people and he isn't alone anymore."

This production contains a number of anaclitic story lines. The story begins with a needy, defenseless individual pleading for help from another. The repeated main theme of a wished-for attachment predominates, along with the story lines of neediness and wish for gratification. The focus is on finding another person to provide care and attention, with the main character assuming a passive position in the dyad. When that need is not met, there is a retreat, or avoidance of the conflict. The more positive ending to the story illustrates anaclitic wish fulfillment: The hero is successful in establishing an attachment to others.

When Ms. I told a story about this same card after approximately 15 months of treatment, there are some notable changes.

TAT Card 15, Time 2

"This is a graveyard. That is very icy. Gravestones look like ice cubes. I wouldn't say he was praying, he might be but maybe he's thinking about himself. He's got skeleton like fingers. He isn't angry but he is feeling maybe resentment or remorse—he's really into himself—all hunched up."

Although there is still an aura of deprivation in the focus on the coldness of the scene,[4] the hero has shifted away from asking for gratification from another. Although there is still some conflict around this issue, it is handled through denial ("I wouldn't say he was praying"). The hero now focuses on himself. There is evidence of awareness of inner feelings, although here, too, we see the use of denial ("he is not angry"). Most striking is the overall shift from looking to others for gratification to a focus on the self and personal emotions; that is, a shift from an excessively anaclitic orientation to an awakening of the introjective developmental line.

Although the story told at Time 1 to Card 15 was reasonably well formulated, the stories that were told earlier in that same testing session were quite scattered. The patient complained that she was unable to tell stories, that she could not "play this" (i.e., tell a story), that she could not make up a story "unless maybe I look like that or something." In response to the examiner's question about her difficulty, she had the thought, "Maybe I can't because I'm afraid"; that is, she had some sense that her inability to think of a story might serve a defensive purpose. What we seem to see in action here is the malfunctioning of the defense of repression, which is so pervasive in the patient that most of her thoughts are blocked from consciousness, leaving her, indeed, without any ideas from which a story could be created.

This phenomenon is seen in Ms. I's initial story about TAT Card 5.

TAT Card 5, Time 1[5]

"Can't really make up a story. I don't know, I don't know what she is thinking. I'm supposed to relate to it or something. I can't, too many things, I can't. I don't want to. ( ) She looks angry and not too pleased . . . she is barging her way in . . . I just can't speak, nothing comes out. Nothing flows. I can't tell you what first comes to my head, it is not the pictures, it is me. I can't talk to people. Come on down to supper, give me another one. It will be the same with all of them . . . I can't. I just want to go back to my room, not that I like it there. ( ) That's all I see. (?) I don't know. Bunch of kids, her children or child. I don't know. (?) I don't know, I don't know what they're doing. Maybe she's opening the door and saying what are you doing, but I don't know. But I don't know what. I don't know. (?) I don't think I can. I never could write or tell stories. (?) I do not know, the kids say leave us alone. I don't know what she does after that. I don't know what they are playing at. ( ) Two little kids, a brother and sister are naked. Their mother is horrified. She says 'what are you doing?' They say they're playing . . . which never happened to me. Mother says angrily, 'put your clothes on and never do that again,' and they do it. (?) I just did not think of it."

The overwhelming communication in this production is one of helplessness. The patient repeatedly complains of her inability, her neediness, and inappropriately tries to enlist an attachment to the examiner by asking him to accompany her to dinner. She expresses the wish to deal with this stress through avoidance, by retreating to her room. Only through the repeated questioning and prompting of the examiner does a story finally emerge. The focus is on an angry woman, a mother, who barges her way into a room in which she finds a naked boy and girl. Given the mother's "horrified" reaction, the suggestion is that the children are involved in some kind of unseemly activity—possibly sex play—which the mother admonishes them never to do again.

This story demonstrates not so much the story lines of an anaclitic personality but, rather the typical avoidant defenses used in situations of stress and anxiety. We see in this story both the use of repression and, when that is not effective in warding off the anxiety-arousing thoughts, the use of denial. Immediately, and then repeatedly, Ms. I complains that she cannot think, she cannot talk, she has no ideas. Rather than viewing the complaint as being oppositional, this avoidant response to the storytelling task may be better understood as an example of the massive use of repression, which blocks not only conflict-laden ideas but thinking in general.

As the story unfolds, we discover the source of the anxiety: The picture, which shows only a single adult woman, has aroused conflicted feelings about some illicit behavior. As these ideas emerge, indicating weakness in the repression defense, the lower-level avoidant defense of denial comes into play. Ms. I introduces "kids" into the scene but immediately denies knowing what they are doing. She further denies knowing what the mother does after the kids say "leave us alone." She denies knowing what the kids are playing at, but the idea that they are naked emerges anyway. The use of denial then becomes personal, when Ms. I spontaneously denies the possibility that she, herself, had ever experienced anything like that.

The patient's response to Card 5 some 15 months later, as was the case with Card 15, indicates a marked change.

TAT Card 5, Time 2

"This mother is kind of stern. She is coming up to check, maybe she knocked on the door, wants to know what her daughter is doing. Maybe she's telling her not to use the telephone."

This time, there is no blocking, no difficulty in formulating a story. There is evidence of greater impulse control: The mother no longer barges in but knocks on the door. There is still an implication of suspicion on the part of the mother, but the "misdeed" is more socialized, and at a higher developmental level. Rather than infantile sex play, the daughter is on the phone. In both stories, however, the mother interferes with the child's gratification.

Mr. F: Anaclitic

We turn now to the stories of a man in his early 20s who was evaluated as having an anaclitic personality configuration. This configuration is less common in males, statistically, and is incongruent with gender stereotypes. For this reason, we might expect an anaclitic male to have special difficulties in the area of identity formation.

Mr. F, at the admission conference, was diagnosed as a schizophrenic character disorder with depressive and paranoid features. He described himself as always having felt marginal, different from others, lonely, and the object of ridicule. As a child, he was involved both in beating up younger children and in being beaten up. His mother, described as being cold and probably a chronic paranoid schizophrenic, was very protective of the patient. His father was described as largely withdrawn, afraid of precipitating psychotic episodes in the mother. The clinical staff noted that Mr. F appeared angry, violent, and hateful but also soft and vulnerable. His overlearned verbal skills provided him a facade of rational, clear thinking, but in emotionally arousing situations he became vague and disorganized.

He came to his therapy appointments regularly, and by not wanting to leave the sessions, showed a tendency to cling to his female therapist.

Early in the therapy, he complained about being oppressed, but later he criticized the therapist for not urging him to be sufficiently active.

Here is Mr. F's story about TAT Card 1, told shortly after admission.

TAT Card 1, Time 1[6]

"It is a kid. He is looking at a violin and he is contemplating whether to pick it up and experiment with it. He is wondering where he can find out where to tune it. He is afraid of asking someone. He goes to the library and looks in the file under violin. He takes out numerous books on techniques for playing this instrument. Then he goes off on his own and isolates himself and studies the books thoroughly. For days and days out he practices until he feels he can play it. One day he decides he is an accomplished violinist because he developed techniques that were not accepted, which did not fit in with any other orchestra or whatever because his music was so exotic. He put the violin down on the table and splits. No, he puts the violin down on the table and contemplates ways of relating to these people who rejected him musically."

One of the main story lines of this production revolves around the unmet interpersonal needs of the hero. He needs help, but he is afraid to ask and no one offers. He tries to solve his problem through withdrawal—isolation and self-soothing. But as a result of this isolation and absence of interpersonal relatedness, he becomes unacceptably different, and again his needs for attachment are unfulfilled. Once again he attempts to deal with the pain of rejection through withdrawal, but, with a wish-fulfilling ending, there is a shift now to thinking about ways in which his interpersonal needs might be met.

Although the story both opens and closes with concerns around interpersonal relatedness, it also contains themes about self-definition, that is, introjective themes that are more characteristic of males. Thus, there is a focus on individual accomplishment, mastery, mental processes, and narcissism. The presence of these introjective concerns in the central section of the story, bound on either side by anaclitic themes, may well be expressing the identity conflict of a man whose personality configuration is gender incongruent.

Some 15 months later, a very different story was told by Mr. F, in which the main theme revolves around interpersonal relatedness and gratification.

TAT Card 1, Time 2

"A child sitting there in a rather dimly lit room in the lower East Side contemplating playing the violin. His grandfather just died and left him a Stradivarius as an heirloom to remember him by. The kid always admired his father's, no, grandfather's impressive talent, and having an admiration for that and inclination to music and interest in participation and interest in music theory, he studied violin and became a musician. When he passed away, he left it to his grandson."

Now, there are familial connections: grandfather and grandson, grandson and his grandson. Significantly, the vehicle for establishing relatedness is a prized possession; actual people do not relate. Nevertheless, this relatedness does provide gratification and does contribute to the hero's success.

At the same time, there is a notable skipping of generations in the arena of relatedness and the use of denial to remove any attachment to the father. The death of two grandfathers and the absence of the father suggests a possible conflict between the wish for relatedness and attendant hostility.

Again, in addition to the anaclitic themes, which now indicate positive gratification as compared to the unfulfilled wishes of the previous occasion, there are, in the central part of the story, introjective themes. There is a focus on accomplishment and individual effort that leads to mastery. Although there is a small amount of emotion expressed ("admiration"), the storyteller retreats from that expression into a description of emotion-free intellectual processes ("inclination to music," "interest in music theory"). The absence of living relationships is noteworthy.

This intermingling of anaclitic and introjective themes is most striking in the story Mr. F told about TAT Card 5 on the first testing occasion.

TAT Card 5, Time 1[7]

"Can't think of anything for this one. It's a woman living in a home. She has a family and she's very close to nature. One day she opened the door to a room she rarely went to and discovered a potted flower plant . . . still growing. She resented this . . . finding this. She was completely outraged at this . . . the plant's being cultivated indoors in a pot lacking the gift of sunlight and minerals of the earth. Not being able to reproduce offspring because the flowers are captivated in the vase which presents the seeds from falling into the soil. She took the vase out into a field of lilies in the valley and finds a barren spot of fertile soil in which to plant the flowers. She gently removes the flowers from the soil in the pot. Very carefully doing so not to injure the roots. She transplants the flowers into the soil and she walks . . . she leaves the valley enlightened. (?) She was enlightened by seeing these flowers go outdoors in the sunlight, soil and gasses. That's what it needs for a healthy life. (?) She goes back home."

This story strikingly conveys the two lines of development—anaclitic and introjective. The need for nurturance, sustenance, nourishment, and careful attention—all anaclitic themes—is intertwined with the problems of growing, producing, becoming self-sufficient and autonomous. Only through interpersonal gratification can the organism grow, flourish, and attain self-definition. Yet, even in isolation, the drive for survival, growth, and reproduction exists separately from the control of others. The story portrays the anger around unmet needs, a hyperconcern for the lack of gratification, and an excellent illustration of the dyad in which one member is entirely responsible for the satisfaction and well-being of the other. The extreme neediness of the plant is repeatedly stressed—its lack of sunlight, nutrients, suitable environment, and fragility. Significantly, the dyad cannot be represented as being between two people but, rather, is presented symbolically, between a person and a plant, reminiscent of the relationship between the boy and the violin in Mr. F's story to Card 1, Time 2.

The story also contains a number of examples of loose associations and idiosyncratic use of words, indicative of an underlying thought disorder. This aspect of the story is discussed in Chapter 10.

On the second occasion of storytelling, a very different picture emerges.

TAT Card 5, Time 2

"This reminds me of my parents' home in Connecticut. The furniture is Early American. There's usually flowers on the table. It's not unusual to see a middle aged woman popping her head through the door; if one wants to take the chance of being harassed and staying there (?) (*confused*). They may find themselves entwined in a mass of hurricane . . . no, holocaust of, (*sighs*) insanity that exists under that roof. Having lived there for 8 years, this woman reminds me of my mother. She is very suspicious and was always popping my head in and asking questions. I am sorry."

This story is less symbolic, focusing on the behavior of real people. The perpetrator of the negative deeds, unknown in the story told at Time 1, is now clearly identified as the mother. A paranoid-like concern for being ill treated and having one's autonomy or self-worth challenged is expressed, followed by a confused attempt to use ideational processes to handle the anxiety associated with feelings about the intrusive mother. The concern about the lack of autonomy continues throughout the story, culminating in a confusion between the mother and son ("*she* . . . was always popping *my* head in . . . "). On this second occasion, at which marked clinical improvement was noted, the introjective themes predominate in the stories of Mr. F.

Mr. B: Introjective

Our first introjective patient is a man in his early 20s. On admission, he described fears of "falling apart" or going "over the edge." The initial diagnosis was a narcissistic character disorder with borderline and obsessive features. He was noted to be extremely anxious, with an unformed, fragmented identity. In clinical interviews, he expressed concerns about revealing material that would produce strong shame or guilt. Attempts to defend against this brought ineffective, obsessional-like defenses into play. Much of his energy was spent in censoring and doubting his feelings. His discourse often lacked coherence and was characterized by the intrusion of tangential material.

Here is Mr. B's initial story about TAT Card 14 (the silhouette of a figure in a dark room against a bright window).

TAT Card 14, Time 1

"I have two stories. First, someone committing suicide. Second, someone going from darkness to light . . . getting it together. I think that's what it is more than the first. Like passing out of depression into sunlight."

Although the topic of the story is ostensibly about a highly emotional topic—depression and suicide—the description is devoid of affect. Instead, emotion is controlled through the use of obsessional defenses, as seen in the dividing up into categories ("two stories"), and the concern for sequence ("first . . . second"). The main theme of the story focuses on the evolution of the self, from death to life, and on attaining some kind of cohesive self-definition ("getting it together"). Mental processes—symbolism—are used to express emotional issues: darkness equals depression, light equals living. However, indicative of some confusion in his thought processes, there is also a meld of the concrete, the abstract, and the symbolic and a confusion of the metaphor ("passing out of depression into sunlight"). There is an overly intellectualized quality to the story, which becomes more like an allegory than a tale about a real person.

Here is Mr. B's story about the same TAT card after 15 months of treatment.

TAT Card 14, Time 2

"This is, let's see, this is someone wandering around an old mill in the dark and, uh, the guy sees a window and opens it and looks out. It's really grungy inside the mill. Dark and depressing. Outside there's a beautiful view and when he sees how beautiful it is outside he decides to go outside the mill."

There is a very different quality to this second story. The rigid categorizing and ordering of the earlier story has given way to a relatively free-flowing tale about a real person. The use of muddled symbolism is gone, as is the concern about suicide. Overall, there is a decreased self-focus. The depressive affect is now externalized and projected onto the environment. The contrast between the "grungy," "dark and depressing" inside and the "beautiful view" outside has qualities of reaction formation as well as, perhaps, self-reference. These typically introjective defenses are functioning more effectively, allowing for a more alive, related, and realistic production. As in the first story, there is an absence of relationship with others.

Here is Mr. B's first story about Card 5.

TAT Card 5, Time 1

"That must be someone's mother. She's looking in the room and she sees her son playing doctor with a little girl. She is amazed and she goes in . . . she looks like a severe kind of mother. She gives him a lecture. The sort of mother that would fuck up the kid . . . telling him it is dirty."

The theme of this story is reminiscent of that of the anaclitic female patient, Ms. I. A stern, harsh mother intrudes on the physical (sex) play of two children. Although the mothers in both stories admonish the children not to engage in this behavior, it is only in the introjective story of Mr. B that the issue of shame and guilt is raised: the mother's words "fuck up the kid"; she makes him feel "it is dirty." Significantly, the responsibility for this shame is projected onto the mother: The boy is guilty, not because of his behavior but because of the mother's actions. The story line of "playing doctor" reflects a narcissistic, exhibitionistic component, and the intrusion of the mother raises issues around control and autonomy.

On the second testing occasion, Mr. B told the following story.

TAT Card 5, Time 2

"I am analyzing myself while I am making up stories, it's terrible. That's someone else's mother, I guess it looks like a mother and the phone's ringing and she's looking for her husband to tell him who it is on the phone, that he's wanted on the phone. (?) She answers the phone, I don't know if I really understand. You said to make a start and a finish, and I didn't really make any finish to the story. (?) He gets up, he's tired after work, he grimaces, and drags himself to the phone."

The story begins with an immediate reference to self-definition ("I am analyzing myself . . . ") followed by a self-reproach ("it's terrible"). The main theme of the story, however, shows a significant shift. As in the case of Ms. I, the theme shifts from the mother's criticism of sex play to the mother's concern about the telephone. For Mr. B, this also involves a shift from mother as a controlling adversary to mother as helper. Also, for Mr. B, the imported other figure is now an adult male rather than a little boy, suggesting some change in self-image. Resentment around the mother's muted interference with the male's autonomy is still present, expressed through the man's negative reaction to her intrusion into his solitude. Feelings of self-doubt and inadequacy are expressed directly ("I don't know if I really understand . . . I didn't really make any finish to the story"), and in the form of an obsessive concern about structure and order ("You said to make a start and a finish").

Ms. K: Introjective

Finally, let us consider the stories of Ms. K, who was considered by the clinical evaluators to have an introjective personality configuration—a situation, as in the case of Mr. F, that is gender incongruent.

Ms. K was in her mid-20s when she was admitted to the hospital. She described herself as experiencing an increased sense of futility, depression, and detachment; she became extremely confused and was unable to function at work or to manage the daily tasks of living. At admission, her condition was diagnosed as decompensation in a long-standing, severe obsessive character disorder, with depressive and masochistic features.

Although depressed, in her withdrawal she appeared as if in a rage; she feared she could become violent. She evidenced considerable confusion over her sexual identity, hiding her femininity and fearing intimacy. She expressed the hope that she might find herself and become a woman.

Here is her story about the same TAT Card 14 as used in the illustration of the introjective male, Mr. B.

TAT Card 14, Time 1

"This is a boy, sitting, standing by his window at night. He is wondering why he must be alive . . . why he cannot find a way of being and a way of acting that satisfies him and how people who have found such a way ever did find it. He has no answers . . . that's all."

As with Mr. B, Ms. K's story displays strong self-focus coupled with a kind of obsessive concern about why things are the way they are. There is an emphasis on mental processes ("wondering why he must . . . ," "why he cannot," and how others "ever did find it") as well as on looking for answers; there is no expression of emotion in the story. The entire theme revolves around the attempt to establish a self-concept, with the concern of how to act and how to be. Although the character wonders about other people, it is primarily in the service of self-definition; relationships with others are missing from the story. Nevertheless, there is the indication that the "answers" may be found through interpersonal relatedness, an anaclitic theme. We thus see the intermingling of introjective and anaclitic themes, with the emphasis on the introjective line of self-definition on this first testing occasion.

Here is Ms. K's story about the same card 15 months later.

TAT Card 14, Time 2

"Looks like he is climbing out the window. This isn't going to be a very interesting one either. Are you writing that down too? That's not part of it. All ready? This is a house in a city and there are others very close to it. This man is looking out his window to the yard of the next house where there's a party. Everyone there is dressed nicely . . . talking and gay . . . looks colorful and lively. He's thinking it would be fun to be at that party. He's wondering if he had a party, what sort it would be and who would come. He might spend a long time at the window. I suppose that is the end of that one."

There is a dramatic shift in this story, from the previously self-absorbed, inner-directed preoccupation to an outwardly focused interest in others. In addition, the story is filled with positive emotion, stemming from interpersonal relatedness; there is also an expression of longing for relationships with others. There are still indications of the use of obsessive mental processes to handle anxiety ("he's wondering if . . . what sort . . . who . . . ") as well as self-reproach ("this isn't going to be a very interesting one either") and a hyperalert concern about control ("Are you writing that down too? That's not part of it. All ready?"). Nevertheless, the focus has clearly moved from self-definition to a wish for relationships with others, that is, from the gender-incongruent introjective configuration to the gender-congruent anaclitic personality organization.

A significant shift in the problem of self-definition and identity is also seen in the stories about Card 5.

TAT Card 5, Time 1

"This is a child's room and the child's mother is looking in . . . to see what he's doing. This is something that she does often and it annoys him increasingly. He, he feels that she expects him to be busy with something all the time. Sometimes he would like to just sit and look out the window or look at the floor. Sometimes he is tired and would like to sleep. He never allows himself to do these things. Without thinking about it he believes that he mustn't let her find him idle."

TAT Card 5, Time 2

"There's a little girl in this room who's playing . . . making up a story in her mind. She's engrossed in her game and doesn't see her mother who's just opened the door and is looking at her. While she's playing she feels suddenly that there's somebody else in the room. Becomes self-conscious and ends her game. She pretends to be doing something else because she wants all her games and her stories to be her own. So if her mother asks her what game she's playing she'll tell her something else."

The most striking change in this story is that Ms. K has changed the sex of the child she imports into the picture; the little boy of Time 1 has become a little girl. Further, this heroine is now involved in her *own* mental processes ("engrossed in her game") rather than being focused on the mother's dictates. Although an uneasy awareness of the possibility of mother's control is present ("she feels suddenly that there's somebody else in the room"), the child is now successful in warding off the interference and in maintaining her autonomy ("she pretends to be doing something else because she wants all her games and all her stories to be her own"). This is accomplished through the use of counteractive defenses ("she'll tell her something else").

If we assume that the child of each story represents the patient and her self-concept, the two stories then indicate a change in her sexual identification from male to female and an increased sense of self-definition and freedom from outside control. The phrase in the second story—"becomes self-conscious"—is highly meaningful, referring not only to a kind of uneasiness but also to the awareness of a self that has the capacity to act autonomously—to "end her game." That this is accomplished through maneuvers designed to hide, disguise, and mislead the mother is an example of the use of introjective defenses. Overall, the shift from an almost robot-like boy, driven from without, to a playful girl who protects her thoughts and her activities to keep them as her own provides a remarkable description of the "unsticking" of development along the introjective line.

GENDER IDENTITY

In our discussion of these two personality configurations, we have made use of the concept of gender incongruence. It is of interest, then, to determine whether the concept of a personality organization that is gender congruent or incongruent might be related to the TAT measure of gender identity. We would expect patients who are identified as gender incongruent to show D/E patterns in their stories that are characteristic of their opposite sex (i.e., a male anaclitic patient to show the feminine D → E pattern, and the female introjective to show the E → D pattern). On the other hand, the gender-congruent patients would be expected to show the patterns typical for their sex.

To explore this possibility, the TAT stories of Ms. I, Mr. F, Mr. B, and Ms. K were evaluated according to May's D/E approach to assessing gender identity from the TAT (see Chapter 6). Although the patients did not tell stories to the pictures typically used to assess gender identity—the trapeze and the rope climber—we can examine the story that each patient told about TAT Card 5 at time 1 and again at time 2. Although this TAT card is not typically used in studies of gender identity, as we will see, the method is strong enough to pick up meaningful patterns and differences among the four individuals.

Let us consider first the story of the anaclitic female, Ms. I, now scored for deprivation and enhancement.

Ms. I: TAT Card 5, Time 1

"Can't really make up a story. I don't know, I don't know what she is thinking. I'm supposed to relate to it or something. I can't, too many things, I can't. I don't want to. (?) She looks angry and not too pleased
. . . she is barging her way in . . . I just can't speak, nothing comes out. Nothing flows. I can't tell you what first comes to my head, it is not the pictures, it is me. I can't talk to people. Come on down to supper, give me another one. It will be the same with all of them . . . I can't. I just want to go back to my room, not that I like it there (?) That's all I see. (?) I don't know. Bunch of kids, her children or child. I don't know. (?) I don't know, I don't know what they're doing. [[Maybe she's opening the door and saying what are you doing]], but I don't know. But I don't know what. I don't know. (?) I don't think I can. I never could write or tell stories. (?) I do not know, the kids say leave us alone. I don't know what she does after that. I don't know what they are playing at. (?) Two little kids, a brother and sister are naked. Their mother is horrified. She says 'what are you doing?' They say they're playing . . . which never happened to me. Mother says angrily, 'put your clothes on and never do that again,' and they do it. (?) I just did not think of it."

Score: +2

This story, discussed earlier in the chapter from the interpretive stance of the anaclitic/introjective personality organization, is considered here in terms of the gender-identity narrative. The PI occurs about midway through the story, when the mother opens the door to the children's room. Prior to this, there are three units scored plus for deprivation; following, there are two more deprivation units scored minus, and one enhancement unit scored plus, for a total score of +2, indicating the feminine pattern, consistent with the subject's biological sex and personality organization.

Next, let us look at the story of the anaclitic male, evaluated for gender identity.

Mr. F: TAT Card 5, Time 1[8]

"Can't think of anything for this one. It's a woman living in a home. She has a family and she's very close to nature. One day she opened the door to a room she rarely went to and discovered a potted flower plant . . . still growing. She <u>resented</u> this . . . finding this. She was completely <u>outraged</u> at this . . . the plant's being cultivated indoors in a pot lacking the gift of sunlight and minerals of the earth. Not being able to reproduce offspring because the <u>flowers are captivated in the vase which prevents the seeds from falling into the soil</u>. [[She took the vase out into a field of lilies in the valley]] and <u>finds a barren spot of fertile soil in which to plant the flowers. She gently removes the flowers from the soil in the pot.</u> Very carefully doing so not to injure the roots. She transplants the flowers into the soil and she walks . . . <u>she leaves the valley enlightened</u>. (?) She was enlightened by seeing these flowers go out doors in the sunlight, soil and gasses. That's what it needs for a healthy life. (?) She goes back home."

Score: +5

Looking at this story now from the gender-identity perspective, we note the PI occurs when the woman takes the potted plant outside into the field. Before that, there are three deprivation units; afterwards, there are two enhancement units, yielding a total score of +5, which is a highly feminine pattern for this man. This finding indicates that the patient's gender identity is consistent with his anaclitic personality organization, although both are incongruent with his biological sex.

Now, let us look at the story about the same picture from the introjective male.

Mr. B: TAT Card 5, Time 1

"That must be someone's mother. She's looking in the room and <u>she sees her son playing doctor</u> with a little girl. She is amazed and [[she goes in]] . . . she looks like a <u>severe</u> kind of mother. She <u>gives him a lecture</u>. The <u>sort of mother that would fuck up the kid</u> . . . <u>telling him it is dirty</u>."

Score: −5

In this story, the PI again occurs when the mother goes into the room. Prior to that, there is 1 enhancement unit.[9] After the PI, there are 4 deprivation units, yielding a total score of −5. This masculine pattern is consistent both with the patient's personality organization and biological sex.

Finally, let us consider the introjective female.

Ms. K: TAT Card 5, Time 1

"This is a child's room and the child's mother is looking in . . . to see what he's doing. This is something that she does often and [[it annoys him increasingly.]] He, he feels that she expects him to be busy with something all the time. Sometimes he would like to just sit and look out the window or look at the floor. Sometimes he is tired and would like to sleep. He never allows himself to do these things. Without thinking about it he believes that he mustn't let her find him idle."

Score: −4

In this story, the PI occurs relatively early in the story, representing an intense feeling that prepares us for what is to come. Prior to that, there is 1 deprivation unit; afterwards, there are 5, yielding a total score of −4, a highly masculine pattern. As in the case of the other gender-incongruent patient, Ms. K's gender identity is found to agree with her introjective personality organization, not with her biological sex.

In order to determine that these findings were not accidentally due to stories told about a single TAT card, six more stories told by each patient to an identical set of TAT cards[10] were evaluated. The resulting scores, averaged over seven different stories, are reported in Table 9.1.

The results based on this larger sample of stories were consistent with the findings reported above. The anaclitic female patient had a positive feminine pattern (mean = +3.33) and the introjective male patient had a negative masculine pattern (mean = −.60); the gender-identity scores of these two patients were gender congruent. However, the anaclitic male had a positive feminine pattern (mean = +3.17), whereas the introjective female had a negative masculine pattern (mean = −2.00).

These very interesting results show that patients who are gender incongruent in their anaclitic/introjective personality organization are also gender incongruent in their TAT fantasy patterns. Of course, one might argue at this point that the D/E approach is actually a measure of the anaclitic/introjective personality organization rather than gender identity, because both of the anaclitic patients had positive (feminine) scores, whereas both of the introjective patients had negative (masculine) scores.

One way of investigating this possibility is to look at the D/E scores of these four patients after 15 months of treatment. Because all these patients were considered to be improved, we might expect that, as part of their psychological improvement, those whose gender identity was initially incongruent would show some change toward becoming gender congruent. At the same time, we would expect that the gender identity of initially congruent patients would remain congruent.

As may be seen in Table 9.1, this is exactly what happened. Based on the stories told about the same seven TAT cards after 15 months of treatment, the gender-identity score of the anaclitic female remained positive and that of the introjective male remained negative. On the other hand, the anaclitic male changed from a feminine score of +3.17 to a masculine score of −.83, whereas the score of the introjective female changed from a masculine −2.00 to a feminine +2.80.

To summarize thus far, we have seen how two different interpretive approaches to the TAT—anaclitic/introjective and gender identity—provide different kinds of information about the patients. Although the interpretive frameworks differ, we also see how they can be combined to support each other and to enrich our understanding of the individual patient.

DEFENSES

We may now apply a third interpretive approach to the same stories. In the process of interpreting from the anaclitic/introjective perspective, mention has been made of the use of defense mechanisms. If we systematically apply the perspective of defense mechanism interpretation (discussed in Chapter 7) to these stories, some interesting findings emerge.

In addition to the two stories discussed in detail above, each patient also told stories about five other TAT cards. This provided a set of stories based on identical stimulus cards (TAT Cards 1, 5, 15, 14, 10, 13MF, and

TABLE 9.1. Gender-Identity Scores of Anaclitic/Introjective Male and Female Patients: Time 1, Time 2

	Time 1	Time 2
Anaclitic female	+3.33	+1.20
Anaclitic male	+3.17	−0.83
Introjective male	−0.60	−0.86
Introjective female	−2.00	+2.80

12M) for each patient, from each testing occasion. These stories were evaluated for the use of the defenses of denial, projection, and identification (see Chapter 7) and then were related to the anaclitic or introjective personality configuration. Because stories were available from two points in time, it was also possible to determine the change in defense use after treatment. Based on the full set of stories, the use of defense mechanisms as related to the anaclitic/introjective personality organization, to biological sex, and to treatment was assessed. The findings appear in Table 9.2.

As may be seen from Table 9.2, the two anaclitic patients show the greatest use of the defense of denial, as would be predicted from theory (Blatt, 1990; Blatt & Shichman, 1983). This is especially true at the time of the first evaluation. The anaclitic patients also show the largest decrease in the use of defenses, due in part to the decreased use of denial but also to the noticeable decrease in the use of Identification. Interestingly, projection (a typically male defense) decreases in the female anaclitic at Time 2 but increases in the male anaclitic.

A marked decrease in identification is also seen in the two gender-incongruent patients. Ms. K, the introjective female, shows a decrease from 9 to 5; Mr. F, the anaclitic male, shows an even greater change, from 16 to 5. As discussed in the preceding section, these two patients also showed dramatic changes in their gender-identity scores between the two testing occasions. Further, Ms. K was noted to change the sex of the character she imported into TAT Card 5, from being male at Time 1 to being female at Time 2. It is tempting, then, given the conceptualization of these two patients as having gender-incongruent personality organizations, to put these different sources of information together and to

TABLE 9.2. Defense Mechanism Scores of Anaclitic/Introjective Male and Female Patients: Time 1, Time 2

	Denial	Projection	Identification
Anaclitic female			
Time 1	8	10	9
Time 2	4	5	1
Anaclitic male			
Time 1	7	11	16
Time 2	3	16	5
Introjective male			
Time 1	1	9	9
Time 2	1	5	10
Introjective female			
Time 1	1	5	9
Time 2	4	9	5

interpret the decrease in identification as reflecting a change in a false identity.

The decrease in identification in Ms. I, the anaclitic female, might also indicate a change in a false identity, although this need not be gender identity. Indeed, the highly dependent, clinging, attachment-seeking behavior shown by Ms. I when first in the hospital suggests the presence of a very primitive, almost merged "identity" at that time—an identity that needed to be discarded for growth to occur.

Of course, the results from four individual patients may be highly idiosyncratic. Fortunately, we are not limited to these individual cases in our investigation of defenses and defense change as related to gender and the anaclitic/introjective personality organization. In a large-scale study of 90 hospitalized patients who were independently evaluated as having primarily an anaclitic or an introjective personality configuration, changes in the use of defense mechanisms were evaluated from TAT stories told shortly after admission and again approximately 15 months later (Cramer et al., 1988; Cramer & Blatt, 1990; Cramer & Blatt, 1993; see Chapter 7 for a more complete description of this study). The results of this investigation were quite similar to those found with the four patients just discussed. The entire group of patients showed a decrease in total defense use from Time 1 to Time 2. Further, the gender-incongruent patients—the anaclitic males and introjective females—showed a significant decrease in the use of identification after 15 months of treatment, while the gender congruent patients, did not show this decrease in identification. Interestingly, both anaclitic and introjective male patients showed a decrease in the use of denial, a feminine defense, whereas the females in both groups showed a slight increase. Again, the use of combined interpretive perspectives enriches our clinical understanding.

SUMMARY

In this chapter, another interpretive perspective for TAT stories has been described and illustrated. Two types of personality organization—the anaclitic and the introjective—have been described and differentiated, and the themes, concerns, and defenses characteristic of each have been indicated. Using this interpretive perspective, the TAT stories of four patients, previously identified as having either an anaclitic or an introjective personality organization, were used to illustrate how the characteristic themes of each may be expressed in the stories, and how these themes may change after intensive treatment. For each patient, stories about the same TAT card were provided, both making it possible to see differences in the narrative responses of the two personality types to the same picture.

Alternative interpretive perspectives—the assessment of gender identity and of defense mechanisms—were also used to examine these same stories. It was demonstrated that predictions made from one interpretive perspective could be supported by findings based on a second perspective, providing an enhanced view of the psychological functioning of the patient and supporting the validity of the individual approaches. The reliability of these findings based on four individual patients was supported in a larger research study of the anaclitic/introjective personality organization.

• TEN •

The Interpreter's Perspective: TAT and Psychopathology

This chapter considers several different approaches that may be taken by the interpreter of TAT stories to assess the presence of psychopathology in the stories. The approaches are derived from clinical theory and observation, as well as from empirical studies of patients with psychological disorders. Several of the perspectives are entirely qualitative, whereas others rely on a systematic coding scheme to assess pathology. Examples are provided showing how two different perspectives may be applied to the same TAT stories.

QUALITATIVE AND FORMAL ASPECTS OF THINKING

One of the earliest, most complete discussions of the use of the TAT to describe, discern, and diagnose psychopathology is that of Rapaport et al. (1946; see also the revision of this work [1968]). In an extremely thorough examination of the TAT, the authors provided a rationale and approach to interpreting protocols that has informed the clinical practice of numerous psychologists who have been trained in this tradition. In extensive discussion, the issues of ideational content, memory organization, defenses, and strivings are all considered, along with the expected reaction to individual TAT cards. Considerable attention is given to the formal characteristics of the story structure and content. There is also a detailed section on diagnostic indicators, with particular attention given to depression, obsessive–compulsive symptoms, affective lability, paranoid indications, and schizophrenic process. This type of analysis provided a framework for clinicians to highlight such aberrant aspects of the stories as peculiar verbalizations, disturbances in the frame of reference, peculiar turns in the content, and the use of overelaborate symbolism, features found in many of the TATs of clinical patients studied at the Menninger Foundation. In all, it is an approach that heightens the sensitivity of the clinician to nuances and aspects of thought processes underlying the story production which are often significant indicators of psychopathology. An excellent and detailed example of the use of this general approach is provided by Rosenwald (1968) in his analysis and interpretation of 10 TAT stories told by a 30-year-old man who was experiencing significant psychological problems. The importance of formal characteristics of TAT responses for diagnosis has also been discussed by Hartman (1949), Holt (1958), Murstein (1961), and Schafer (1958).

Examples

As examples of these qualitative characteristics, consider the following two stories, which were told by patients in a long-term intensive treatment psychiatric hospital. Each story was given in response to TAT Card 14, which shows the silhouette of a man (or woman) against a bright window; the rest of the picture is totally black.[1]

From a female patient who was independently diagnosed as having severe character pathology:[2]

> "This is a man who has felt very dark and confused, but now finds himself to be at the threshold of what he thinks is enlightenment. No, I do not know whether it is enlightenment or not. Well, the metaphor, the light of day."

The thought processes of this individual demonstrate a fusion of the concrete properties of the picture with symbolic processes. The physical stimuli—darkness, and a man standing at a lighted window—are transformed into a symbol of being at the threshold of enlightenment. But the storyteller becomes confused about this symbolism and reverts to the concrete "light of day" with an unsuccessful attempt to use intellectualization ("Well, the metaphor") to contain anxiety. This confusion of the storyteller is, in fact, first revealed in the opening statement, in which the physical properties of the picture (darkness) have been merged with the (projected) psychological state of the storyteller ("felt very dark"). For a similar fusion of concrete with symbolic, see the story told by Mr. B about this TAT card in Chapter 9.

The reaction of another female patient to the same TAT card contains some of the same formal elements, along with circumstantial reasoning and occasional loss of the frame of reference for the task. This patient was diagnosed as psychotic.

> "About three things come into my mind. A man lives in New York and on the Lower East Side in a tenement type building. It is a hot summer night and, his body is not right, he is sitting on his window ledge. The air is hot in the room, listening to the sounds of the city. The position of his body is not right for that. Or, I could make it very symbolic. Wait a minute, something about the position of the body, it's not clear but suggests that, someone who is about, who has felt he has lived in loneliness or darkness in his own head seeing enlightenment inside, draws back, looks at it in hesitation, sort of undefined. I am sure it is supposed to be like that. Another one, I thought he was going to jump out the window. That suggests to me a skyscraper, but a skyscraper would not have a window like that open. It would have to be really high to kill himself. He was going to jump out the window but decided not to. I wonder how somebody would feel, just all shaky about his close call."

After the somewhat unusual opening statement ("About three things . . . "), indicating an attempt at obsessional control, the story begins in a typical enough manner, but as the storyteller's attention begins to be focused on the figure sitting on the ledge of an open window, with possible suicidal overtones, there is an unexpected, peculiar intrusion into the story—"his body is not right." This becomes an obsessive preoccupation, which contributes to circumstantial reasoning: "The position of his body is not right for that." There is, of course, nothing about the figure's body position that would or would not indicate whether he was listening to sounds of the city. The patient's thought processes then slide into an attempt at symbolism, but once more the preoccupation with the body intrudes. Again circumstantial reasoning appears, now linked with symbolism, in which the dark and light of the picture are transformed into psychological darkness and enlightenment within the mind of the character, who now looks inward rather than out through the window. This unusual thought process is then followed by a disturbance in the frame of reference: "I am sure it is supposed to be like that."

The storyteller then extricates herself from this pathological story and begins a new one. This time we see more clearly the nature of the concern behind the preoccupation with the body position—namely, that the figure is about to commit suicide. From that pathological concern, the storyteller again demonstrates circumstantial reasoning—if he is going to jump, it must be a skyscraper—which is then denied through further circumstantial reasoning—if the window is open, it cannot be a skyscraper. The story concludes by displaying another loss of the frame of reference, with the intrusion of the storyteller's own concerns into the narrative.

From the interpreter's perspective of analyzing thought processes, the decision that these two stories are indicative of psychopathology is based not so much, if at all, on the basis of peculiar or bizarre content. Rather, it is the quality and form of thinking revealed in the stories that marks them the product of a disturbed or confused mind. It is the mixing, merging, and shifting from the concrete to the abstract, from outer reality to inner psyche, the confused attempts at symbolism and the obsessive preoccupation with an idiosyncratic concern that mark these stories as products of pathological thought processes.

THE BORDERLINE PERSONALITY DISORDER

Since the time of Rapaport et al.'s (1946) work, psychoanalytic theory has changed to include a greater emphasis on psychodynamic developmental issues, a focus on self psychology, and an integration of the theory of object relations. At the same time, and in conjunction with these theoretical developments, a focus has developed on new or different pathologies. I refer here to the borderline personality disorder (BPD) and the narcissistic personality disorder (NPD). The concept of borderline disorder initially referred to those pathological conditions that fell somewhere between neurosis and psychosis (i.e., not normal or neurotic but not "insane"). Earlier designations of these patients have included "ambulatory schizophrenic," "latent schizophrenic," "schizophrenic character disorder," and "pseudoneurotic schizophrenic."

Currently, on the basis of numerous clinical and research studies, the central, defining characteristics of the BPD, as seen within psychoanalytic theory, have been characterized as "(1) intense affects (anger and depression), (2) consistent lapses in impulse control, (3) social adaptiveness, (4) transient, circumscribed psychotic episodes, (5) primitive drive-laden thinking on projective tests, and (6) erratic interpersonal relationships due to their inconsistent self-identity" (Kwawer, Lerner, Lerner, & Sugarman, 1980, p. 13).

According to the description provided in the fourth edition of the *Diagnostic and Statistical Manual of Mental Disorders* (DSM-IV; American Psychiatric Association, 1994) the essential feature of the BPD is instability in mood, interpersonal relationships, and self-image. Mood may shift from normal to dysphoric or to inappropriate intense anger, with a lack of control and characteristic impulsivity. Relations with others, although frequently intense, are equally likely to be changing and shifting, with the idealized other becoming the hated villain. A deep identity disturbance may be seen in confusion around gender identity and long-term goals or values, as well as in feelings of emptiness and boredom and difficulties in being alone.

From a psychoanalytic perspective (see Kernberg, 1967, 1975, 1976; Kwawer et al., 1980), the etiology of the BPD is to be found in the early years of life. Rather than emphasizing the oedipal period and libidinal drives for understanding pathology, as was characteristic in earlier theory, the focus has shifted to the pre-oedipal period and to the importance of very early experiences for the development of sense of self and sense of other. From this developmental perspective, the individual with a BPD suffers from a defect in psychological development, especially in ego development, with a resulting difficulty in tolerating anxiety.

To understand the BPD, psychoanalytic clinicians focus on the issue of disturbance in object relations, including problems in maintaining the boundaries between self and others, resulting in distorted interpersonal relationships. Again, the BPD individual appears to be arrested at an early level in the development of object representations, such that the distinction between self and other is not clearly formed. This, in turn, results in a fluctuation between extreme dependency on the one hand and a fear of merging on the other. Instead of differentiation and integration, representations are split based on affective valence such that the part identified as the good self and the part identified as the good other become one constellation, while the bad self and bad other become a second entity. This mechanism of splitting is the primary defense of the BPD. Nevertheless, despite this defect in ego functioning, there is a "specific, stable, pathological personality organization; their personality organization is not a transitory state fluctuating between neurosis and psychosis" (Kernberg, 1967, p. 24). Rather, the underlying pathology is overlain with a "pseudoadaptive facade" (Kwawer et al., 1980, p. 24).

In this perspective (Kernberg, 1967; Sugarman, 1980), the BPD refers to a stable character organization. Thus, one does not see the extensive ego disturbances that are present in the psychotic patient. On the surface, the thinking of the BPD appears appropriate, but this may be accomplished through superficial responses to external cues, using mundane, ordinary themes. In contrast, when the BPD individual begins to draw on internal, personal material to develop themes, the adequacy of reality testing may seriously deteriorate. Nevertheless, we do not expect to find a true thought disorder in this group of patients. Ego weakness, which is manifest at times of stress, is seen in the difficulty these individuals have in tolerating anxiety. On psychological tests, there may be a shift toward primary process thinking, which is not seen in more structured situations or in overt behavior. This often occurs around such conflictual material as aggressive imagery, which may induce a temporary loss of reality contact.

The BPD individual also experiences problems with boundaries—boundaries between self and others, and between internal and external worlds. At these times, there is "a loss of distinction between inner experience and external reality with a subsequent tendency to overinfuse external reality with one's own affective colorations of it" (Sugarman, 1980, pp. 42–43).

Boundary disturbances also produce jumbled descriptions of experiences that seem to run together and lack clarity. BPD individuals appear not to impose order on the world but, rather, wait for the world to provide whatever order they experience.

Two Interpretive Perspectives for the BPD

Because the BPD is a relatively newer diagnostic category for whom the use of the TAT as a diagnostic instrument has been less discussed in the published literature, two interpretive perspectives for the TAT stories of this group are presented here in some detail, along with a variety of example protocols.

The first of these psychoanalytically informed approaches to studying the BPD with the TAT has been suggested by Sugarman (1980). Working with the theoretical descriptions of the borderline personality organization as developed by Kernberg (1967), Sugarman illustrated how the various aspects of the borderline organization may be manifest on psychological tests. His focus is on evidence for ego weaknesses, disturbance in affective organization, use of primitive defense mechanisms, and psychopathology of object relations. A second approach to studying the BPD is that of Westen (1991a), who has focused on the assessment of four dimensions of object relations as revealed in TAT stories. Each of these approaches is presented below, and is illustrated with stories from hospitalized patients.

Sugarman's Assessment of the BPD

In a detailed discussion, Sugarman (1980) has indicated a series of ways in which aspects of the borderline personality disorder are manifest in TAT stories. In the following discussion, these are underlined, discussed, and illustrated with TAT stories from BPD patients.

The BPD individual often experiences difficulties with integrating affect and thought. In turn, this may produce problems in controlling and modulating emotional expression, resulting in unexpected emotional eruptions. On the other hand, many individuals with BPD are *inhibited in the expression of emotions*, and their TAT stories will thus have a paucity of emotional expression.

In the following two stories, told by a female patient with a borderline personality disorder,[3] denial is used repeatedly to prevent the expression of any emotions. The storyteller attempts to focus on the absence of "facts" as an explanation for this paucity of expression, but it is clear from the content of the stories that it is the emotionally charged ideas (suicide, marriage, disgust, sex) that are being denied.

The first story was told about TAT Card 14:

> "A man sitting on a window. I could not by any means tell you what is going to happen or what happened, maybe he is going to jump out the window or maybe he is going to close the window and go back to the room. I cannot because I do not know all the facts."

The same patient told the following story about TAT Card 13MF:[4]

> "I do not know if they are married or not and I do not know if they feel disgust or if he is covering his eyes and I do not know if they just had intercourse or not. I cannot. I have no idea. . . . This is like judging people and I find it very hard to judge people without knowing them. It is unfair in all instances."

Depression of the anaclitic type, which is frequently present in the BPD, is seen in TAT themes of loss, as well as in themes of weakness, helplessness, emptiness and abandonment, or, alternatively, in a blatant, almost callous denial of depression. Also, there is a *lack of an independent sense of self-directedness*; characters react to other characters only in a passive fashion, with a strong dependence on and concern with the other, on whom one's fate depends. In general, there is an ineptness in experiencing, modulating, and expressing dysphoric affect.

The following story, told by a female psychiatric patient[5] gives a sense of this helplessness in relation to the environment, as well as some of the other formal aspects of pathological thinking. The story is told to Card 15, which depicts a drawing of a gaunt man with clenched hands standing among gravestones. The patient's ineptness in expressing dysphoric affect is seen in the repeated use of the peculiar expression "too shy to die."

> "May I comment on the picture? The mood of the picture is almost too imposing or extreme to stimulate very much. Very ghoulish picture, and melodramatic. This man is a Charles Addams character in a German graveyard. Graveyard in East Berlin, also in West Berlin. It was in both at one time. Now the wall is here but the ghouls underneath are all the same. Charles Addams placed this man here,

and the man is too shy to die, so he is simply standing there. The way Charles Addams drew him made it impossible for him to associate with life except through the death he is too shy to experience. So he stands there thinking in German, repeating the German word for cold over and over to himself."

Almost the very first comments from this woman focus on her feelings of helplessness in regard to the environment; it is because of the nature of the picture, which overwhelms her, that she is unable to say very much. (This situation, however, is described with somewhat contradictory logic: Because of the extreme overstimulation, she is understimulated.) Even the existence of the character in the picture and his location are the responsibility of another: the cartoonist who created him and "placed him" in the graveyard. The absolute weakness of this character is made clear; not only can he not live and move, he is also too weak and too unable to express emotion ("shy") to die. And even the responsibility for this absence of ability to live or to die is made the responsibility of someone else (the cartoonist). The only activity this character is capable of is a stereotyped repetition of a word signifying his emotional state of cold-ness, emptiness, and loneliness. The closed-loop circuit of hopeless-ness/helplessness that characterizes some BPD individuals is well exem-plified in the statement, "The way Charles Addams drew him made it impossible for him to associate with life except through the death he is too shy to experience."

The TAT stories of BPD individuals may also reveal the *pathology of internalized object relationships,* as seen in frequent themes of *object loss and subsequent despair.* The despair appears to be more for the loss of the object, per se, than for the loss of the object's love. Relationships are described as superficial; there is little sense of genuine interpersonal encounter. For a TAT card in which only one character is depicted, it is rare that other, nondepicted characters are introduced, suggesting a lack of object constancy; the object is experienced as existing only when it is concretely present.

For example, the following story was told about TAT Card 1 by a male patient with a BPD diagnosis:[6] The story has also been discussed in Chapter 9, as an example of an anaclitic personality configuration.

"It is a kid. He is looking at a violin and he is contemplating whether to pick it up and experiment with it. He is wondering where he can find out where to tune it. He is afraid of asking someone. He goes to the library and looks in the file under violin. He takes out numerous books on techniques for playing this instrument. Then he goes off on his own and isolates himself and studies the books thoroughly. For days and days out he practices until he feels he can play it. One day he decides he is an accomplished violinist because he developed techniques that were not accepted, which did not fit in with any other orchestra or whatever because his music was so exotic. He put the violin down on the table and splits. No, he puts the violin down on the table and contemplates ways of relating to these people who rejected him musically."

This story revolves around the complete absence of emotional relationships with others and the inability of the hero to establish any kind of contact with others to help him. It portrays his subsequent aberrant development and his anger about this, feeling that it is others who have rejected him. The story ends with the hero still enmeshed in this conflict.

In conjunction with abandonment, TAT stories of the BPD individual portray characters as *deliberately hurting and taking advantage* of the protagonist. *Pre-oedipal aggression* is seen in story content in which there is an emphasis on oral phenomena, envy, and deprivation. There is a tendency to *experience others as exploitative, noncaring and often abusive*, as in the following story about Card 15 from a BPD man:

"This is an elderly man come to his wife's grave. Sort of a sneer on his lips now, looking down and remembering the fact that he did her in. No remorse, sort of a cold narrow person, presume possibly that he killed her because she was the opposite. Sort of like *My Last Duchess*. Do you know the poem *My Last Duchess*? She was greater in spirit than he and he envied this. She could be free in love and spirit and he could not, drew him to poison her or something. Now he has grown older. He does look unhappy. Sneer but maybe regret. Maybe he needs her now. His own miserliness made him poor indeed. But not a great wealth of feeling there. A thin brooding, sneering still and not much future for him. . . . Face seems, see the cheeks, face drawn narrow, narrow chin, flat, selfishness of flesh, as if he had none to spare. Thin in feelings, nothing underneath, derisive feeling but little else."

The story begins with a clearly noncaring, abusive character ("he did her in"; "a cold narrow person"). Accompanying the theme of object loss is a callous denial of despair ("no remorse") with the peculiar logic that he killed her *"because* she was the opposite." This action, however, is explained as being due to envy ("he envied this") which has eventuated in oral aggression (the "poison"). Significantly, the envy is about her ability to express emotions, in contrast to his inhibition ("she could be free in love and spirit and he could not"). The story then shifts in tone, with some recognition of the object loss ("maybe he needs her now") and some depression ("he does look unhappy"). There is a sense of emptiness in the physical description of the man; the paucity of genuine emotions continues ("not a great wealth of feeling there"). The story also contains several peculiar verbalization in which physical dimensions are used to express emotional states: "a cold *narrow* person," "a *thin* brooding," "*thin* in feelings."

In the TAT stories of BPD individuals, the descriptions of *characters tend to be unidimensional*; characters are seen as all bad or all good, all powerful or all weak, all nurturant or all frustrating, related to the use of the primitive defense mechanism of *splitting*, which is the major defense of the borderline personality disorder.

Here are stories told about TAT Card 12F by two BPD patients. The picture shows the portrait of a young woman in front and old woman, grimacing, in the background.

> "There's a preponderance of witches and devils and spooks. The woman behind looks like she's senile. She's holding back laughter. She's very weird. And the woman in the foreground holds herself very erect looking at something. They don't look in any way connected. The older woman in the back looks like she comes from a small village a few hundred years ago. One of the town's busybodies. The woman in the front looks much more modern. I do not see any outcome or plot line developing."

> "The picture in the background, the character in the background represents one facet of the young man's personality. I guess that facet would be insanity. Oh, the character in the background looks foolish and simpering. He or she, uhm, I can't tell, it has no look of understanding or recognition of an external reality, the young man who is looking in the opposite direction from the picture in the background and he does not even realize that this side of him exists. He has lots of ambitions and hopes for the future and but, ah, he will be dragged down and have to struggle with the insanity that's within him."

In the first story, the split is between an old woman with a multitude of negative affective attributes who is placed at a considerable distance in time, as compared to an up-to-date modern woman who shows considerable affective control. The function of splitting is well portrayed in the storyteller's remark, "They don't look in any way connected." The effect of the defense on the thought processes of the storyteller is further demonstrated in the closing sentence, which illustrates how splitting prevents the two images from being integrated to form a single story.

In the second story, the two characters are perceived as being male—an unusual perception. The description of splitting, between insanity on the one hand and healthy ambition on the other, is placed more clearly within one individual in this story. At the same time, the unconscious nature of the function of the defense mechanism is illustrated in the statement, "he does not even realize that this side of him exists." Nevertheless, there is a clear sense of conflict between the two split-off self-representations.

A more extreme example of this *splitting* is seen in the following story from a female BPD patient about a card taken from the first Harvard Psychological Clinic edition of the TAT (see Chapter 2). The picture is a woodcut, showing line drawings of two old men in front view, one above the other.

> "A man has just decided to willfully kill or eliminate that within him that represents goodness. The demands of his emotions are in conflict with his desires. He does this and finds himself half a man. (?) I see a willful murder of this thing, if you like, pushed down, submerged."

The split between good and evil, emotions and desires, is concretely portrayed here. The good-self, good-emotions constellation, which stands alone, unintegrated with the rest of the personality, is physically split off, leaving the other half behind.

The use of *projective identification,* a second primitive defense characteristic of the BPD, occurs when the good or bad self-representation is projected onto the other, followed by some fusion between the self and that (projected) aspect of the other. In turn, this may result in a situation of *simultaneous hate and fear of being attacked,* as seen in TAT stories in which there is a focus on others attacking and hurting the protagonist.

The following story was told about the schematic drawing of one old man above the other. It was told by a patient who was diagnosed as psychotic but is included here for its clear illustration of projective identification.

> "Two giants I do not know. Do not get anything from it. They are not enemies they are friends. But there is this little spirit that keeps telling them that the other guy is going to kill them. They are trying to get the spirit. But the spirit keeps telling them this thought. They kill each other. The spirit gets away."

Here, there is complete confusion around the location of the murderous impulse. Each character believes it to reside in the other. The hostile emotion shifts from one character to the other and is finally located in both, when they both kill each other.

Another story from a BPD patient, told about TAT Card 18GF, again illustrates the situation in which each character perceives the other to be as the self. The hatred of each is projected onto the other, one of whom must then become the feared attacker. The situation cannot be resolved until one becomes the victim of the other.

> "Never can quite decide what these two are doing. Looks like one woman is strangling the other one. These are two women who live together in house for some time who, despite being together in the house, they've always been apart . . . like two metal rods which don't bend in any way. They have forced this sort of relationship on each other and can't get out of it except when one dies. Finally this solution of death became necessary . . . so forceful that it seemed the only solution. And so this one woman strangled the other. And afterwards was still not free. That's the end of that."

Projective identification, with both *hate and fear of being attacked*, is expressed in a different way in the following two stories. The first is told by a male BPD patient about TAT Card 15:

> "There is a storm brewing. It's dark, wind blowing, cold, bleak. There is thunder in the background. The scene is ominous, foreboding, and there is a sense of the place as doomed. This man has come to this spot to remember how someone dies. It's not important who dies, or how, but the importance to this man and to me is not, throughout his life he recognizes that he will be able to continue to struggle against his hostile environment, knowing that he may not live to see the end of the struggle. That kind of expresses it. If I can remember what I have said, I have completed what I started out to say. I think I am finished. He is taking responsibility knowing he may not be able to resolve it. This is a moral idea, a fight to preserve civilization, freedom, a sense of individuality, a sense of independence."

The second story, previously discussed in Chapter 9, is told by a male BPD patient[7] about TAT Card 5, which depicts a middle-aged woman looking into a room in which there is a pot of flowers.

> "It is a woman living in a home. She has a family and she is very close to nature. One day she opened the door to a room she rarely went to and discovered a potted flower plant still growing. She resented this, finding this. She was completely outraged at this, the plant's being cultivated indoors in a pot lacking the gift of sunlight and minerals of the earth. Not being able to reproduce offspring because the flowers are captivated in the vase which prevents the seeds from falling into the soil. She took the vase out into a field of lilies in the

valley and finds a barren spot of fertile soil in which to plant the flowers. She gently removes the flowers from the soil in the pot. Very carefully doing so not to injure the roots, she transplants the flowers into the soil and she walks, she leaves the valley enlightened. She was enlightened by seeing these flowers go outdoors in the sunlight, soil and gasses. That is what it needs for a healthy life. She goes back home."

In both these stories, there is an initial indication of hostility on the part of the protagonist: In the first story, the man is thinking about how someone dies; in the second, the woman is outraged. Interestingly, both these stories then shift to using nature to carry out the theme of a hostile environment, which hurts the protagonist. In the first story, the theme is played out, via nature, on a somewhat grandiose scale; in the second it is expressed in the focus on a single small plant. There is a merging, or projective identification, between the protagonist and the environment in both stories, with the environment held responsible for potential doom and destruction. The stories also contain some peculiar verbalizations— going to a spot "to remember how someone dies," "a pot lacking the gift of sunlight," not being able "to reproduce offspring" because the flowers are "captivated in the vase," and becoming "enlightened by seeing these flowers go outdoors in the sunlight"—the latter expression again demonstrating the fusion of physical and psychological characteristics, in the use of the words "enlightened . . . in the sunlight."

Both of these stories also illustrate another characteristic of the TAT stories of BPD individuals, which is related to the use of splitting as a defense. The difficulty of the BPD individual in integrating affectively polarized self-representations and object representations (i.e., splitting) results in a poorly integrated superego, with the consequence that *moral issues then are highly personalized and affect laden*. This is seen in both of the above stories: the intensely moralistic concluding statement of the first story and the moral outrage of the second story.

Finally, let us consider a story from a female BPD patient that illustrates the use of *projective identification*.

"Oh my god, I know this one too. I was originally torn between deciding whether the woman was hurting the person or whether she's a very rigid person lifting up someone who's been hurt. She has a tension in her face I don't think she knows about. Is at the limit of her strength and is forcing someone to understand her. Great deal of pain in her face, she doesn't recognize vindictiveness in her. May be determinedly angry, but I don't think so. Other person will ask to be let go of, at which point she'll back away quickly and in a dazed fashion. Other person who goes quietly upstairs to his or her room for the night. The woman will not really understand her impulse of the moment and will be frightened and withdraw afterwards. Younger will become very frightened of this new attitude and become more scared of him or herself. (?) Could be a young boy as servant. Don't think she could be so unconscious of her motivation if it were another woman. If it were another woman she would be very angry and determined. No ambiguity."

Here, there is confusion about where the "hurting" resides—in the first women, or in the second. There is a recognition of this split-off part of the personality, which is then denied. This is followed by considerable confusion around the location of aggressive impulses and the fear of these being expressed. First these feelings are placed in one character, then in the other; both characters are implicated with similar descriptions.

To summarize, from this psychoanalytic perspective, one would expect the TAT stories of persons with a BPD to contain a number of the following characteristics: The expression of emotion may be inhibited, with the result of a paucity of emotional display. Dysphoric affect may be poorly modulated or ineptly expressed. Anaclitic depression will be seen in themes of weakness, helplessness, emptiness, and abandonment, or in a blatant denial of depression. Characters may lack independence and self-directedness, being instead passive, dependent, and reactive to others. There may be evidence for pathological object relationships, characterized by loss, superficiality, unidimensionality, and the absence of others, or by exploitation, lack of caring, and abusiveness. Themes involving pre-oedipal aggression—an emphasis on oral phenomena, envy and deprivation—will be common. The defenses of splitting and projective identification may produce themes in which there is simultaneous hate and fear of being attacked, as well as highly personalized and affect-laden moralistic statements.

Westen's Approach to Object Relations

The distortion of object relations in the borderline personality disorder has been the focus of work by Westen (1991a, 1993, 1995), who has developed an interpretive perspective to use with the TAT. Again, this represents a shift in psychoanalytic theory, away from an emphasis on the drives and their vicissitudes toward a concern with the internal representations of significant others, the quality of affect in relationships with others, the capacity for and quality of emotional investment in relationships and in moral standards and values, and the understanding of interpersonal motivation. These dimensions of interpersonal experience have been found to be especially relevant in understanding the nature of the BPD. In Westen's approach, the storyteller's developmental level is assessed along each of the dimensions.

Based on theoretical descriptions, clinical observations, and research, Westen (1991a, 1991b) first devised an interpretive scheme to assess various developmental levels of object relations. The Social Cognition and Object Relations Scale (SCORS) consists of four scales designed to assess different dimensions of object relations; within each dimension, five levels are defined, from relatively primitive to relatively mature (see Table 10.1).

The first scale, Complexity of Representations of People, was designed to assess three phenomena that normally occur in the process of development: the increasing capacity for differentiation between self and others; the increasing perception of self and others as having stable, multidimensional dispositions; and the increasing representation of self and others to include complex motives and subjective experience. At the most primitive level (level 1), people and perspectives are not clearly differentiated. At the most mature level, there is evidence of understanding the complexity of the interaction of temporary and enduring psychological experience, in which dimensions of personality are perceived as interacting with each other and with the environment.

The second scale, Affect-Tone of Relationship Schemas, refers to the emotional quality of the representations of people and relationships, ranging from malevolent (level 1), in which the person expects relationships to be destructive, to benevolent (level 5), in which the person expects relationships to be safe or enriching. In contrast to the other three scales, this scale does not assume a developmental progression across the levels described.

The third scale, Capacity for Emotional Investment in Relationships and Moral Standards, was designed to assess the development from a narcissistic stance (investment in others based on need gratification; level 1) to relationships with others based on mutual love, concern, valuation of specific attributes, and the concern for moral standards (level 5). The scale integrates ideas from cognitive-developmental theory/research with those from object relations theory and clinical observation.

The fourth scale, Understanding of Social Causality, also was designed to integrate what is known from developmental research on ideas about social causality with clinical observations of borderline patients' confused attributions of people's intentions. At the lowest level, social causality is poorly understood; it is illogical, with inappropriate, unlikely, or absent explanations of interpersonal behavior. At the highest level, there is an understanding of the way in which complex psychological processes, including unconscious motivation, contribute to the thoughts, feelings, and behaviors involved in interpersonal interactions.

Westen (1991b) provides examples of TAT stories from a female BPD

TABLE 10.1. Social Cognition and Object Relations Scale (SCORS)

Complexity of Representations of People

Level 1. People are not clearly differentiated; confusion of points of view.
Level 2. Simple, unidimensional representations, focus on actions; traits are global and univalent.
Level 3. Minor elaboration of mental life or personality.
Level 4. Expanded appreciation of complexity of subjective experience and personality dispositions; absence of representations integrating life history, complex subjectivity, and personality processes.
Level 5. Complex representations, indicating understanding of interaction of enduring and momentary psychological experience; understanding of personality as system of processes interacting with each other and the environment.

Affect-Tone of Relationship Schemas

Level 1. Malevolent representations; gratuitous violence or gross negligence by significant others.
Level 2. Representation of relationships as hostile, empty, or capricious but not profoundly malevolent; profound loneliness or disappointment in relationships.
Level 3. Mixed representations with mildly negative tone.
Level 4. Mixed representations with neutral or balanced tone.
Level 5. Predominantly positive representations; benign and enriching interactions.

Capacity for Emotional Investment in Relationships and Moral Standards

Level 1. Need-gratifying orientation; profound self-preoccupation.
Level 2. Limited investment in people, relationships, and moral standards; conflicting interests recognized, but gratification remains primary aim; moral standards developmentally primitive and unintegrated or followed to avoid punishment.
Level 3. Conventional investment in people and moral standards; stereotypic compassion, mutuality, or helping orientation; guilt at moral transgressions.
Level 4. Mature, committed investment in relationships and values; mutual empathy and concern; commitment to abstract values.
Level 5. Autonomous selfhood in the context of committed relationships; recognition or conventional nature of moral rules in the context of carefully considered standards and concern for concrete people or relationships.

Understanding of Social Causality

Level 1. Noncausal or grossly illogical depictions of psychological and interpersonal events.
Level 2. Rudimentary understanding of social causality; minor logic errors or unexplained transitions; simple stimulus–response causality.
Level 3. Rudimentary understanding of the role of thoughts and feelings in mediating action; logical, relatively sophisticated situational causality.
Level 4. Expanded appreciation of the role of mental processes in generating thoughts, feelings, behaviors, and interpersonal interactions.
Level 5. Complex appreciation of the role of mental processes in generating thoughts, feelings, behaviors, and interpersonal interactions; understanding of unconscious motivation processes.

Note. From Westen et al. (1991a). Copyright 1991 by the American Psychological Association. Reprinted by permission.

patient and a nonpatient female of similar background. Each of the four
TAT stories from each woman is evaluated along the four scoring
dimensions, with explanations for the choice of scoring level.

The scales have been shown to correlate with social adjustment, as
rated by clinicians and by the subjects themselves, and with scores on the
same scales assessed from interview data. The affect-tone scale has been
shown to correlate significantly with similar measures from interview
data, free-response personal descriptions, and questionnaires (conver-
gent validity). The scale did not correlate with conceptually unrelated
measures, demonstrating discriminant validity (Barends, Westen, Leigh,
Silbert, & Byers, 1990). The scales have also been successful in predicting
membership in criterion groups and scores on related personality measures. In addition, they have been successful in differentiating adolescents
and adults with a borderline personality disorder from other psychiatric
patients and from normal comparison subjects. Summaries of research
using these four scales, with both clinical and normal populations, appear
in Westen (1991a, 1991b, 1993) and in Westen, Lohr, Silk, Gold, and
Kerber (1990). A discussion of the theoretical background as derived
from psychoanalysis and social cognition theory appears in Leigh,
Westen, Barends, and Mendel (1992). The use of the scales in developmental studies is discussed in Chapter 11.

Recently, Westen has revised the SCORS, replacing the 5-point scales
with a Q-sort procedure (the SCORES-Q), in order to provide greater
differentiation among the complex and interrelated dimensions being
assessed.[8] The Q-sort consists of 99 items,[9] each on a separate card,
representing five object relations dimensions of the SCORS. (The scale
Capacity for Emotional Investment in Relationships and Moral Standards
was divided into two dimensions, one concerned with Investment in
Relationships and the other with Investment in Values and Moral Standards.) A sixth dimension, Dominant Interpersonal Concerns, focuses on
dominant interpersonal themes in the stories, such as concerns about
protection, dependency, competition, achievement, abandonment, and
rejection.

Each dimension is represented by at least eight items,[10] representing
the five developmental levels for that dimension, as previously designated
on the SCORS. Each item is coded to indicate the dimension and level
represented. For example, the code a21 or a22 indicates an item on the
affect-tone dimension from developmental level 2; an item coded s11 or
s12 indicates an item on the cognitive-structure dimension from level 1,
whereas s51 indicates an item on that dimension from level 5. Examples
of the Q-sort items are given below.

After reading and rating each story individually, the rater then
considers the total set of stories from one individual and sorts the

Q-items into a fixed distribution of nine piles[11] scored 1 to 9. The items scored 9 are considered highly representative of the storyteller; those scored 1 do not describe the person at all, with the remaining cards sorted as appropriate into the piles between 1 and 9. Once the items have been sorted into these nine piles and the score of 1 to 9 has been recorded for each item, they are redistributed into the six dimensions being assessed. It is then possible to compute a score for each of the five object relations dimensions, indicating the story-teller's developmental level on that dimension. This score may be determined simply by using the level of the Q-item with the highest rank (1–9) for each dimension, as the score for that dimension. Alternatively, it is possible to weigh the level of the items for each dimension by their position in the sort (level 2 by pile 7; level 1 by pile 5, etc.) and then obtain an average score for the dimension.

Examples: Assessment of TAT Stories Using the SCORS-Q. To indicate how this interpretive perspective for assessing object relations is used, consider the following story told about TAT Card 15 (graveyard scene). This same story was discussed earlier in the chapter, using an alternative perspective for assessing features of the BPD. The storyteller was diagnosed as a borderline personality disorder.

> "May I comment on the picture? The mood of the picture is almost too imposing or extreme to stimulate very much. Very ghoulish picture, and melodramatic. This man is a Charles Addams character in a German graveyard. Graveyard in East Berlin, also in West Berlin. It was in both at one time. Now the wall is here but the ghouls underneath are all the same. Charles Addams placed this man here, and the man is too shy to die, so he is simply standing there. The way Charles Addams drew him made it impossible for him to associate with life except through the death he is too shy to experience. So he stands there thinking in German, repeating the German word for cold over and over to himself."

This story, scored by an expert in the SCORS-Q approach,[12] yields the following assessment for developmental level on each of the five object relations dimensions. For each dimension, the most characteristic Q-sort item is given.

1. Cognitive structure of representations of people: *s01* "descriptions of people show psychotic disturbance" (the "level" 0 indicates psychotic disturbance).
2. Affect-tone of relationship schemas: *a22* "tends to ward off upsetting or anxiety-provoking views of people or relationships."

3. Emotional investment in *r*elationships: *r11* "tends to depict relationships as interchangeable, unimportant in themselves, or useful primarily for self-soothing." Also characteristic is *r91* "tends to describe loners and not to be disturbed by their aloneness" (the "level" 9 indicates nonpsychotic processes that do not fall on a developmental continuum).

4. Emotional investment in *v*alues and moral standards: *v27* "tends not to think about moral issues, and to show little interest in ethical concerns."

5. Understanding of social *c*ausality: *c01* "narrative concerns of interpersonal events or explanations of people's behavior show psychotic disturbances in thought that render them difficult to follow."

Overall, on the five object relations dimensions, this story is assessed as being at a psychotic level on the dimensions of Cognitive Structure of Representations of People and Understanding of Social Causality. Capacity for Emotional Investment in Relationships is at level 1, whereas the Capacity for Investment in Values is at level 2, as is the Affect-Tone of Relationship Schemas.

Finally, the story is scored for two Dominant Interpersonal Concerns (Westen, 1993) (these are coded consecutively; the code numbers do not indicate developmental level): *d16* "tends to depict themes of diffuse negative affect, psychic pain, internally 'falling apart' or global sense of 'upset' that cannot easily be labelled as any single emotion," and *d21* "tends to depict stories indicative of fears about safety, survival, or protection."

Here is a second TAT story, told about the same Card 15, by another patient with a diagnosis of BPD. This story was also discussed earlier in the chapter.

"This is an elderly man come to his wife's grave. Sort of a sneer on his lips now, looking down and remembering the fact that he did her in. No remorse, sort of a cold narrow person, presume possibly that he killed her because she was the opposite. Sort of like *My Last Duchess*. Do you know the poem *My Last Duchess*? She was greater in spirit than he and he envied this. She could be free in love and spirit and he could not, drew him to poison her or something. Now he has grown older. He does look unhappy. Sneer but maybe regret. Maybe he needs her now. His own miserliness made him poor indeed. But not a great wealth of feeling there. A thin brooding, sneering still and not much future for him. . . . Face seems, see the cheeks, face drawn narrow, narrow chin, flat, selfishness of flesh, as if he had none to spare. Thin in feelings, nothing underneath, derisive feeling but little else."

This story was also scored by the expert who evaluated the previous story. For each of the object relations dimensions, the most characteristic Q-sort item is given.

1. Cognitive structure of representations of people: s01 "descriptions of people show psychotic disturbance," based on a suggestion in the story of psychotic boundary confusion. Also scored on this dimension is: s22 "sees people at times as all good or all bad"; while the description of the characters is very complex, the cognitive structure is scored at level 2 based on the splitting involved.

2. Affect-tone of relationship schemas: a11 "tends to describe people and relationships as grossly malevolent, with little hope of comfort or kindness between people."

3. Emotional investment in relationships: r11 (see above). Also characteristic is: r92 "tends to describe tumultuous, highly ambivalent, or highly conflictual relationships."

4. Emotional investment in values and moral standards: v21 "moral concerns tend to center on reward or punishment rather than guilt"; he is only sad because he needs her now. Also scored is: v32 "appears invested in moral values or social norms and to experience guilt when transgressing"; the storyteller recognizes that the character should feel remorse.

5. Understanding of social causality: c11 "tends to offer highly unlikely, illogical, or distorted explanations of people's behavior or narrative accounts of interpersonal events."

Overall, on the five object relations dimensions, this story is assessed as being at level 1 on Affect-Tone of Relationship Schemas, Capacity for Emotional Investment in Relationships, and Understanding of Social Causality. The average of the two scores (0, 2) for Cognitive Structure of Representations of People would also be level 1. The average developmental level for Capacity for Emotional Investment in Values and Moral Standards is between 2 and 3.

Finally, the story is scored for four Dominant Interpersonal Concerns: d12 "tends to depict themes of victimization," d14 "tends to depict themes of conflictual dependence," d22 "tends to depict competitive themes," and d27 "tends to depict themes indicative of conflicts about self-control."

Further examples of scored protocols with the complete Q-sort are provided by Westen (1993).

Research Studies. The majority of published research studies using Westen's object relationship approach to the TAT have been based on the rating scales of the SCORS. The findings from many of these studies have been summarized by Westen (1993). As an example, the utility of this approach for clinical diagnosis was demonstrated by Westen, Lohr et al. (1990) in a study of patients diagnosed either as BPD or major depressive disorder (MDD). Along with 30 "normal" individuals,[13] patients told stories about seven TAT cards; these were coded by two raters on the four object relations scales. The results indicated that BPD patients could be significantly differentiated from normals by their lower scores (more primitive level of functioning) on all four scales and were frequently lower than the MDD patients. The groups were further compared for the occurrence of very low-level scores (level 1, most pathological) on each of the scales. Again, the BPD patients had a significantly greater percentage of level 1 responses on all four scales than did the normal subjects, and were significantly lower than the MDD patients on all scales except Complexity of Representation, which was nearly significant. Thus, the BPD patients had a large number of stories that centered on need–gratification, that were grossly illogical, in which the characters were viewed as malevolent, and that tended to provide representations of people that were poorly differentiated. Interestingly, at the same time, 46% of the BPD patients produced two or more stories that were scored at level 4 or 5 on this latter scale, a result comparable to normals and higher than the depressive patients, reflecting, presumably, the variability in level of functioning found in persons with a borderline personality disorder.

Westen's SCORS measures were also used to study hospitalized adolescent girls (Westen, Ludolph, Lerner, Ruffins, & Wiss, 1990). Thirty-three of the girls were diagnosed as BPD; 21 were psychiatric comparison subjects, with a diagnosis of affective disorder, anorexia, and other (non-BPD) personality disorders. In addition, 31 normal girls from a comparable socioeconomic background were studied through the local school system. When contrasted with the psychiatric comparison group, the BPD patients differed on two scales: They had lower scores on the Affect-Tone of Relationship Schemas (i.e., had more malevolent object representations) but higher scores on the Complexity of Representations of People scale. When compared to the normal girls, stories of the BPD patients were rated as being at lower levels on three of the scales: Affect-Tone of Relationships Paradigms, Capacity for Emotional Investment in Relationships and Moral Standards, and Understanding of Social Causality. Also, the BPD patients had a significantly greater percentage of level 1 (most pathological) responses on all four scales than did either of the other two groups. A discriminant function analysis based on the object relations scores correctly classified 76% of the hospitalized patients as belonging to either the BPD or the psychiatric comparison group. A similar analysis of the borderline and normal adolescents correctly classified 80% of the BPD patients. A further study with the hospitalized girls revealed significant relationships between developmental history variables and level of object relations on the SCORS (Westen, Ludolph, Block, Wixom, & Wiss, 1990).

Westen's approach has also been used to differentiate between adult BPD and adolescent BPD hospitalized patients (Westen, Ludolph, Silk, Dellam, Gold, & Lohr, 1990). Consistent with the hypothesis that the capacity for object relationships continues to develop beyond the pre-oedipal period of life, the adult BPD patients scored significantly higher than the adolescent patients on Complexity of Representations of People, Capacity for Emotional Investment in Relationships and Moral Standards, and Understanding of Social Causality. Further differences were found when the "neutral" TAT cards (1, 2, and 4) were analyzed separately from the "negative affect" cards (3BM, 13MF, and 15). The developmental differences for Complexity of Representations of People appeared on both neutral and negative cards; for Capacity for Emotional Investment in Relationships in Moral Standards, the difference occurred only on the neutral cards; and for Understanding of Social Causality, only on the negative cards. A discriminant function analysis using all four scale scores from all six TAT cards correctly classified 93% of the subjects as either adult or adolescent BPD patients.

These studies demonstrate that Westen's object relations approach with the TAT is useful in identifying borderline pathology. In addition, they provide important information for understanding the nature of the borderline personality disorder. Typically, the theory has held that borderline adults and adolescents share the same pre-oedipal developmental arrest. If this were so, the two BPD ages should show the same (low) level of object relations development. However, because the results indicate "that object relations in borderlines continue to develop beyond adolescence" (Westen, Ludolph, Silk, et al., 1990, p. 379), the theory of BPD might well be revised to account for the ways in which this development occurs.

THE NARCISSISTIC PERSONALITY DISORDER

Three different interpretive perspectives for assessing the presence of narcissism on the TAT have been suggested. These approaches are all based on clinical descriptions of the narcissistic personality disorder (NPD).

Sugarman (1980), whose approach to studying the BPD with the TAT was discussed earlier in the chapter, considers the NPD to be a subtype of the BPD. In addition to those features of TAT stories that are characteristic of the BPD, Sugarman points to identifying characteristics of stories of the NPD. The main characters in the stories of NPD individuals often *fluctuate between feelings of uncertainty and feelings of wished for perfection and power*, including a sense of inadequacy related to the impossibility of meeting the unrealistically high goals these individuals set for themselves.

This theme is seen in the following story, which was told about TAT Card 14 by a female patient. The story also demonstrates cognitive confusion, along with circumstantial and illogical reasoning.

"This is a young poet. He has just awakened and he is putting himself to the window. That is the way he would do it. I describe his action in those words because he is a poet. He looks out on the rooftops of Paris, his room is very high, it is a garret, and visualizes in the clouds the statue he will later build. Because he is a young poet. If he were older, he would be through building statues. And he will leave his window open all day. He will build the statue with materials he has in his room. Then he will fall in love with it and look for what he put into his statue in the people outside the window. And this will go on and on and on. This looking for, in people, what he has put into his statue and fallen in love with. But he does not find it until he gets out of his room and walks the streets and sees what it is like to look up at the window."

The story line alternates between the young, inexperienced man who strives to create a perfect love object and his difficulty in attaining this goal. Although he creates this idealized perfection, he is unable to find its counterpart in reality. There is an uncertainty as to whether he ever will find it, although he keeps searching.

Narcissism in the Stories of College Populations

The other two approaches to studying narcissism with the TAT have been conducted within normal college student populations. Whether the methods would identify persons with a narcissistic disorder is not known.

Shulman's (Shulman & Ferguson, 1988; Shulman, McCarthy, & Ferguson, 1988) approach has been used successfully to identify strong components of narcissism in the personality of college students. Stories written about TAT Cards 1 and 13MF, along with two early memories, were obtained from 75 college students in an introductory psychology class (sex unspecified) and were scored for narcissism using criteria adapted from the DSM-III (American Psychiatric Association, 1987) description of the narcissistic personality disorder. These criteria included the portrayal of grandiosity, idealization, entitlement and interpersonal exploitativeness, lack of empathy, oversensitivity to criticism, and the need for attention and admiration. Subjects who scored in the top and bottom 12% of the narcissism distribution were subsequently interviewed by an experienced clinical psychologist, who had no knowledge of their projective test scores. On the basis of the clinical interview, the subjects were rated by the clinician as high or low on narcissism. There was significant agreement between the narcissism scores based on the projective tests and the interviewer's judgment: 11 of 13 subjects were correctly classified by the tests. Although not tested statistically, there were clear differences in the scores on each TAT card for the high and low narcissistic groups. There was also evidence that the TAT-based narcissism score correlated with the self-absorption/self-admiration factor of the Narcissistic Personality Inventory.[14]

A similar study was carried out by Harder (1979) with 40 male college upperclassmen who were given 10 TAT pictures along with an Early Memories test and the Rorschach. Based on Reich's (1933) description of the phallic–narcissistic character type, the TAT was scored according to five components which constituted the Ambitious/Narcissistic Style Scale. These included references to (1) intrusiveness/thrusting, (2) exhibitionism/voyeurism, (3) urethral excitation, (4) mastery/competence/power, and (5) "self-potency." Each subject was also rated on an "ambitious/narcissism" scale by the investigator (who was unaware of the projective responses but had considerable interaction with the subject) and, separately, by two other experienced clinicians who rated the subject's self-description. Scores based on the TAT scales were found to relate significantly to the ratings of the clinicians and the investigator.[15]

SUMMARY

This chapter has considered several different interpreters' perspectives for assessing the presence of pathology in TAT stories. These perspectives are based both on theoretical expectations regarding the dynamic factors assumed to underlie the pathology, as well as on clinical observations of the pathology in psychiatric patients. It is assumed that the identifying features that underlie and constitute the pathology (i.e., the narrative features of the pathology) will be expressed in the stories that are told.

Although many of the critical features to be identified in the stories are of a qualitative nature, research studies show that it is possible to state these characteristics with sufficient specificity that reliable ratings may be obtained. In this case, the story interpreter can describe the pathology of a single patient, can address the question of differential diagnosis within groups of patients, and can contribute to an enhanced theoretical understanding of the disorder.

• SECTION IV •

CHANGING
NARRATIVES:
STUDIES
OF NORMAL
DEVELOPMENT

ELEVEN

Developmental Differences in TAT Stories: Children and Adolescents

T his chapter looks in detail at a number of stories told by children to see how they may be used to understand the process of development. In particular, I will focus on the development of gender identity, defense mechanisms, object relations, achievement motivation, and emotional stance as these have been investigated through the study of TAT stories. But first I consider the general question of the use of the TAT with children.

THE USE OF THE TAT WITH CHILDREN

Some psychologists have raised a question as to whether the TAT is appropriate for use with children (e.g., Klein, 1986). Certainly, the large part of both the research and the clinical literature regarding the TAT has focused on adult responses. Kagan (1959) expressed pessimism regarding the use, in general, of projective thematic techniques with children, and Bellak (1975), stating that the TAT is not well suited for use with children, proposed that the CAT be used instead for children ages 3 to 10 years.

The CAT differs from the TAT in at least two important ways: First, the figures in the pictures are animals rather than humans. Second, the situations depicted are relevant to early stages of development: oral conflicts, sibling rivalry, attitudes toward parents and oedipal concerns. The assumption underlying the CAT is that children identify more readily with animals than with persons; there is some research (e.g., Budoff, 1960; Weisskopf-Joelson & Foster, 1962) that suggests that this in fact is true, at least for some children. On the other hand, Bellak hypothesized that some children do better when the scenes of the CAT are redrawn using humans, especially when the children are older and/or brighter.[1] However, a series of studies failed to support this hypothesis (Armstrong, 1954; Biersdorf & Marcuse, 1953; Boyd & Mandler, 1955; Budoff, 1960, 1963; Lawton, 1966; Levitt & French, 1992).

In a further discussion of the issue, Schwartz and Eagle (1986), in their book on the psychological assessment of children, concluded from their years of clinical experience that the CAT does not provide as much information as does the TAT for interpretation of interpersonal interaction. Further, these authors felt that the use of animals as subjects in the pictures "pulls" for regressive interpersonal interaction and also leads to an inhibition of imagination, with the result that the child's "stories" are limited to picture description. Only with the very youngest children (ages 3 or 4) do they suggest using the CAT rather than the TAT.

As discussed in this chapter, there is considerable empirical evidence that the TAT may be used successfully with children, and that the same coding measures that have been developed to study adult personality may be applied to the stories of children.

DEVELOPMENTAL DIFFERENCES: PRESCHOOL THROUGH ADOLESCENCE

Schwartz and Eagle (1986) have provided normative guidelines for the kinds of TAT responses to be expected from children of different ages.[2] They describe the 3- to 5-year-old child as capable of providing only a limited story in which there is a description of the character(s) in the picture and perhaps some description of what they appear to be doing, along with some identification of the objects in the picture. At the upper end of this age group (i.e., age 5), there may be more of a story or elaborated fantasy. Between ages 5 and 7, more details are included in the picture description, but the productions are still largely unelaborated, although occasionally a child may provide a fanciful theme. There tends to be considerable variability among children in this age group, with some giving brief statements, some obsessively repeating a particular theme, and some compulsively accounting for everything in the picture, while others ignore or deny important aspects of the picture. Children in the

7- to 9-year-old group may find the task of storytelling quite absorbing, and their TAT stories begin to have real plots. The stories now have a beginning, a middle, and an end, with complex themes in which motives and feelings are attributed to the characters. Stories from children in the 9- to 12-year-old group tend to be of two types; on the one hand, the story may be rather perfunctory, told in a way that meets all the requirements of the instructions but communicates little else. Alternatively, children in this age group may tell stories that are quite elaborate, and they embark on the process of storytelling enthusiastically and with pleasure.

THE USE OF THE TAT
TO STUDY CHILDHOOD DEVELOPMENT

In addition to these general guidelines, it is possible to use more systematic methods to analyze the TAT stories of children. The different interpretive approaches that have been described in previous chapters, focusing on gender identity, defense mechanisms, and object relations, have also been used in studies with children. In these investigations, the measures have revealed important developmental differences.

Gender Identity

Several investigators have shown that May's (1966) D/E measure may be used with children to reliably assess gender identity. It may be recalled that the D/E measure calculates scores in such a way that the typical feminine pattern (deprivation followed by enhancement) yields a positive score, whereas the typical male pattern (enhancement followed by deprivation) yields a negative score (see Chapter 6). Among children already in school (third-, fourth-, and fifth-graders), May (1971) found the same sex-related differences in fantasy patterns that he had noted with adults. When the stories of these children were coded for the D/E measure, the results showed that the girls had the typically feminine pattern whereas the boys had a significantly more masculine pattern.

Two examples of stories from children of this age group, given to the picture of trapeze artists and scored for D/E, are shown below. The first comes from an 8-year-old girl who is in the third grade. Recall that the scoring scheme allots a positive value to deprivation (D) units that occur prior to the pivotal incident (PI) and to enhancement (E) units that occur following the PI.

"These people were <u>very unhappy</u>. They knew how to do tricks but <u>they couldn't get into a circus</u>. They <u>wanted to</u>. [But one day a circus

master who didn't have anybody to do tricks like this took them in.]
Everybody liked it. They were happy in the end, they were very, very
happy. They really did want to be in the circus."

Score: +5

This story shows a typical feminine pattern, with three deprivation
units before the PI and two enhancement units following. There is a clear
shift in theme and mood from negative to positive, with a total score of
+5.

Compare this story with the next, which comes from an 11-year-old
boy who is in the fifth grade.

"It's a man and a lady in the circus and they're very famous because
they are great trapeze. But the lady and the man are swinging, [and
the man by mistake lets go of the lady], and the lady falls down to the
net. The man's swinging, suddenly the net falls and he falls down
and hits the ground. (HE?)[3] He has to go to the doctor, and he has
lost an arm, and quits the circus."

Score: −7

Here, the story begins on a very positive note, with two enhancement
units. Following the PI, however, everything goes wrong. The story is
filled with negative events, reflected in the six deprivation units scored.
With one enhancement unit ("to the net"), the total score is −7.

Cross-Sectional Studies

In May's (1971) study, the children wrote out their stories. In order to use
the approach to study gender identity in even younger children, it is
necessary to ask the children to tell their stories out loud and to record
these productions, eventually transcribing the narratives. This method
was used by Cramer and Bryson (1973), who compared a group of 48
children just entering school (mean age = 5,7) with a group of 41
elementary schoolers (mean age = 9,7) for stories told about four different
pictures.[4]

The results revealed important developmental differences. On the
basis of scores combined from the four pictures, the younger boys and
girls did not differ on the D/E measure of gender identity. However, the
older girls had significantly more feminine scores than did the older boys
and the younger girls (see Table 11.1). Furthermore, the same pattern of
results was generally found for each of the four individual pictures.

In a second study (Cramer & Hogan, 1975; Cramer, 1975), a
group of young children (mean age = 5,6) was compared with another
group of children who were somewhat older than those of the

previous study (mean age = 11,5). Stories were told about two pictures.[5] As before, the younger boys and girls did not differ on the D/E measure for either picture. However, the older girls showed a significantly more feminine pattern than did the older boys and were more feminine than the younger girls. In addition, the boys in the older group of this study, who were, on average, 2 years older than those in the previous study, showed a stronger masculine pattern than did the younger boys.[6] These results suggest that an increase in the masculinity of boys' sex-related fantasy pattern occurs about 2 years later than the increase in the feminine pattern of girls—a finding that corresponds well with the fact that most girls reach physical maturity about 2 years earlier than do boys (McCandless, 1967, p. 395).

Similar results have been reported by Fakouri (1979) and Saunders (cited in May, 1971; see also May, 1980), who found that the predicted sex differences in D/E fantasy patterns appeared from ages 8 to 9 and older. Saunders also found that this sex-related difference in fantasy patterns was due primarily to the girls, whose D/E scores became significantly more feminine from grades 3 through 8, while the scores for the boys, which were masculine, showed little difference over this age range, findings consistent with those of Cramer and Bryson (1973).

To examine these developmental differences in more detail, Cramer (1980) conducted a large-scale study with 686 individuals varying in age from 3 years to the senior year of college. In all, eight age groups, with approximately equal numbers of males and females in each, were studied: 3–5 years, 6–7 years, 8–9 years, 10–12 years, high school grades 9–10, high school grades 11–12, college freshmen, and college juniors and seniors. All subjects either told or wrote stories about two stimulus pictures. Each of the resulting 1,372 stories was scored by two independent raters who were blind to the age and sex of the storyteller. Interrater reliability (Pearson r's) were determined for each of the eight age groups, and varied from .65 to .92 (trapeze card) and from .76 to .91 (TAT Card 17BM).

TABLE 11.1. Mean D/E Scores, Four Pictures Combined, Boys and Girls

Group	N^a	Mean	Standard deviation
Younger girls	93	0.25	3.00
Younger boys	83	−0.15	2.34
Older girls	82	2.43	5.47
Older boys	74	0.03	3.95

Note. From Cramer and Bryson (1973). Copyright 1973 by the American Psychological Association. Reprinted by permission.
[a]N varies throughout according to the number of scorable stories.

As illustrated in Figures 11.1 and 11.2, there is little difference between males and females at the youngest age level. However, by middle childhood, stories about both pictures reveal a significant difference between boys' and girls' fantasy patterns, and this difference is maximized as the subjects begin to reach puberty. The differentiation is maintained during early adolescence but disappears by the freshman year of college, where, for both cards, gender identity based on narrative stories shows no difference between males and females. However, during the last two college years, a clear differentiation between males and females reemerges.

The lack of differentiation in the narrative measure of sexual identity found in the youngest children is consistent with developmental theories that point to this period of life as a time in which children first begin to establish a clear sense of their sexual identity (Freud, 1933/1964; Slaby

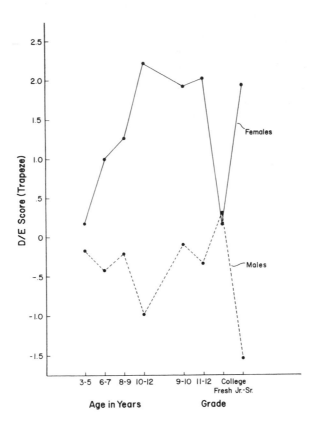

FIGURE 11.1. Deprivation/enhancement scores for trapeze picture: age 3 to college seniors, males and females. From Cramer (1980). Copyright 1980 by Lawrence Erlbaum Associates. Reprinted by permission.

& Frey, 1975). Not until a child psychologically identifies him- or herself as male or female would one expect for this identification to be expressed in thought patterns. The recurrence of a lack of differentiation in sex-related narrative pattern found among the college freshmen is open to at least two different interpretations. On the one hand, it may reflect a regression to the emotional attachments and identifications with both parents that existed during the preschool years, as Blos (1967) has suggested. On the other hand, it may represent a shift in identification, from a same-sex chum during earlier adolescence to an interest in and temporary identification with the opposite sex, a phenomenon described by Sullivan (1953). In any case, the data are remarkably consistent from the two pictures in showing developmental differences across the age span in the scores derived from the stories.

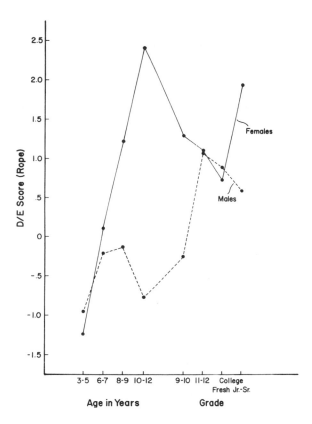

FIGURE 11.2. Deprivation/enhancement scores for TAT Card 17BM: age 3 to college seniors, males and females. From Cramer (1980). Copyright 1980 by Lawrence Erlbaum Associates. Reprinted by permission.

Longitudinal Studies

The striking developmental differences discussed earlier and shown in Figures 11.1 and 11.2 are based on cross-sectional data. From several smaller samples, there are longitudinal data available to support the cross-sectional findings. Ireys (1975) carried out a longitudinal study of younger children from ages 6 to 8, who told stories on four occasions. The results showed that the D/E scores of the girls in the group changed to being more feminine over this period, whereas the boys showed very little change, consistent with the results of the cross-sectional studies reported earlier.

In another study, 29 of the boys and girls who participated in an earlier investigation (Cramer & Bryson, 1973) were retested a year later in a second study (Cramer & Hogan, 1975), and their TAT stories were again scored for the D/E fantasy pattern. Among the 14 younger boys and girls, there was little change in scores from the previous year: Some scores were slightly more negative, some slightly more positive, but the overall changes averaged out to around zero. Among the 15 older boys and girls, however, stories told about the trapeze picture showed clearly that the sex-related narrative patterns were becoming stronger as the children approached puberty. The scores of the girls in this group had become much more positive (mean change = +3.25), while those of the boys had become much more negative (mean change = –3.07)[7] (Cramer, 1975).

In a third longitudinal study, a group of 31 boys and girls who were about to enter adolescence wrote TAT stories on two occasions, separated by 1 year. The stories from 28 of these subjects showed a shift in D/E scores over the year interval; of these, 20 of the shifts were in the direction that would be predicted for the subjects (i.e., females becoming more feminine and males becoming more masculine).[8] Examples of stories from a preadolescent boy who was tested on two occasions 1 year apart illustrate this shift. On the first occasion, he was 11,7 years old. In providing a story about the trapeze picture, he actually told two stories, linked together, as follows:

> "This is a man and a lady that worked in the circus for a long time. They practice a lot and they get a lot of money. There was this one day, they put on the circus and there was millions of people there. It was their turn and they did this cannon act, where they get shot out of the cannon. [They get shot out of the cannon] and everybody claps."
>
> **Score:** 0

(This is the end of the first story. The boy continues . . .)

"There were these other people who <u>asked if they could play</u> at their park; put the circus on at their park. They go to the park and they get up on the stage and they start to practice for the circus. They practice getting shot out of the cannon. There are two cannons that they get shot out of like that. [The girl got shot out of the cannon first and then the boy]. The <u>girl fell down</u> first <u>on the net</u> and then the <u>boy fell down</u> right on top of her. <u>She got her neck broken</u> so <u>she couldn't play in the circus</u>. <u>She went to the hospital</u> and they <u>didn't know if she was going to survive or not</u>. The <u>guy was really worried</u>. They had to figure out some sort of way to cure the neck so they can make it feel better. They sew her neck together and <u>she's all right</u>."

Score: −4

When, as occasionally happens, there are actually two stories provided by a storyteller, each is scored separately and an average is taken. This average yields an overall score of −2.

Looking at this protocol in more detail, the first story told by this 11-year-old boy has an equal number of positive and negative units, resulting in a score of 0. Although there are units prior to the PI, the positive conclusion ("everybody claps") does not follow the male pattern. The score of 0 reflects the ambivalent position of the storyteller.

In the second story from this first occasion, there is a weak score for deprivation prior to the PI (the need to ask if they can play holds the possibility that they will be deprived of the opportunity). Following the PI, we see the occurrence of multiple deprivation units; the ending of this story is full of calamities. Nevertheless, at the very end, the storyteller attempts to reverse course ("she's all right"), as he did in the first story. However, the accumulation of negative units in the second story now outweighs this attempt, and a score of −4 results.

One year later, when this boy was 12,7 years old, he told the following story about the trapeze picture.

"Well, this is a brother and a sister and they work for a circus, Barnum and Bailey Circus, and <u>they like acrobatting</u> for the circus and <u>they like it a lot</u>. And they had a cannon act too where they got shot out of a cannon and so they liked acrobatting and getting shot out of a cannon a lot. [One time in an act, they were getting shot out of a cannon], and <u>they hit each other</u>, and <u>fell on the net</u> and <u>the lady broke her neck</u> and <u>the guy broke his arm</u> so <u>they couldn't acrobat</u> for a long time, 2 years. The <u>girl had to stay in a wheelchair</u> and the <u>guy had to stay in bed</u>. So <u>they stayed there for 2 years in the hospital</u>. After that when they go though, they asked if they could work in the circus again and the <u>doctor said no</u> they wouldn't be able to because of the <u>muscle spasms in</u>

the guy's arm and the neck conditions in the lady's neck so they couldn't be in anymore circus acts and that's all. (HF?) They felt bad because that was their living."

Score: –13

On this second occasion, the story follows a full-blown masculine pattern. Prior to the PI, there are two Enhancement units. Following the PI, with the exception of one positive unit ("fell on the net") the story continues with deprivation after deprivation—broken neck, broken arm, could not acrobat, staying in a wheelchair, staying in bed, staying for 2 years in a hospital, doctor forbidding work, muscle spasms, neck conditions, no more circus acts, and feeling bad—creating even more tragedies than in the previous year. This time, there is no attempt to make it turn out all right in the end, as occurred the previous year, and the resulting score of –13 is strongly negative (i.e, this boy's fantasy story has moved strongly in the masculine direction).

Compare this change with that which occurred in the stories from a preadolescent girl in the longitudinal study. At the time of the first testing, she was 10,4 years old. Her story about the trapeze picture was as follows:

"There was this man and wife and they had a trapeze act. So late at night when they weren't supposed to go into the tent and practice, they wanted to practice. And they were practicing, and practicing and practicing, and they were doing flips and somersaults, and holding on to the trapeze with one hand, and hanging by the heels. [And then the man caught her] and she slipped out of his hands and fell on to the net and bounced right back up and the man caught her up and she got on to the other trapeze and she slipped again, she fell on the net again, and she bounced and she caught hold of the man and she went on over to the tightrope and she walked across and then she went on the trapeze again and she swung over to the platform. The next day was the circus. She fell and she missed the net but nothing happened to her, she didn't have one bruise or anything. But her husband thought the trapeze was too dangerous and they started on clown."

Score: +1

On this first occasion, the story begins with an equal number of D/E units prior to the PI; the pattern in the beginning is thus neither masculine nor feminine. A similar situation continues after the PI. The story vacillates between D and E units, first one, then the other (–D, +E; +E, –D; +E, +E; +E, –D; –D, +E; –D) until the end of the story. The overall score of this 10-year-old girl (+1) is just slightly positive.

A year later, at age 11,4 years, she told the following story about the trapeze picture.

"It's the nighttime and they're practicing on the trapeze but <u>no audience is there</u>, but they're practicing and the man when he's hanging by one of his knees, <u>one of his legs comes undone</u> from the rope and <u>there's no net underneath</u>, and they're still practicing and <u>his leg's still slipping out</u> but <u>he doesn't know it</u> and then <u>his leg comes out</u> all of a sudden. [And the girl she doesn't want him to die because he's important to the circus, so she waits until the next trapeze comes and she gets on the trapeze and she swings over and helps him get his leg back under the trapeze.] But <u>she can't do it</u> so she slides down the rope and <u>she lowers the trapeze thing so he can get out of there</u>. So <u>they were all happy</u> and <u>they were a little afraid</u> to practice again but they waited until somebody else was with them just in case they needed some help so they didn't go up there again until they had somebody else with them. <u>Their act went pretty good</u> 'cause <u>they had a whole bunch of people there</u>. (HF?) They're a little scared maybe because what happened to the boy when his leg came out of the rope. After <u>they feel pretty good</u> because they're not too afraid because they did it pretty good, really good."

Score: +9

This time, a very clear feminine pattern is displayed. Prior to the PI, there are only D units, describing a series of mishaps. Following the PI, there is still evidence of the mix of D and E units (−D, +E; +E, −D), as seen on the first testing occasion, but this time there is a strong positive ending (+E, +E, +E), which, when combined with the typically feminine opening of the story, results in an overall score of +9, which is strongly feminine.

These longitudinal studies all provide clear demonstrations from the TAT of *change* in the sex-related narrative fantasy of preadolescents, showing the value of TAT stories for understanding children's development.

Defense Mechanisms

As discussed in Chapter 7, stories told about the TAT also provide information about the use of defense mechanisms. Starting from the position that defense mechanisms are part of normal development, a theory of defense mechanism development from dual viewpoints has been proposed (Cramer, 1991a). One view focuses on the emergence of different defenses over the course of development. In this approach, different defenses are hypothesized to become salient at different periods of development, such that there is a chronological ordering in the emergence of defenses. The second view focuses on the developmental history of each individual defense as it unfolds from birth to maturity. Here, the concept of defense mechanism development refers to the "life history" of each individual defense; that is, the idea that each defense has its own course of development from birth onward. To test this theory, three defenses were chosen for study: denial, projection, and identification. For reasons explained in the theory (see Cramer, 1991a), it was hypothesized that denial would be predominant during early childhood, projection would be characteristic of later childhood and preadolescence, and identification would become prominent during later adolescence. The various manifestations of each defense as it develops—referred to as the "components" of the defense—were used to develop a scoring system to assess the three defenses in TAT stories (see Chapter 7; Cramer, 1991a).

Several examples of the use of defenses in children's stories follow. The first story was told by a 5½-year-old kindergarten pupil about the trapeze picture. Her story illustrates the use of denial as it is typically found among young children.

> "Acrobats. The lady jumped up. The man might hold her hand. He is! He might slip. But he won't, because his legs are hooked on and he is a good acrobat. The lady won't either, but her hands, they look like they will but they won't. She has shoes on. She is jumping, up right into the sky. She has glasses on top of her head. Their hair is flying up, so her hair won't go down until the man lets her down. (WF?) The man is feeling her arms and the lady is feeling his arms."

In this story, the threat of falling keeps appearing in the story, but each time the storyteller denies that it will happen—"he won't," "the lady won't either," and "they won't." The story also provides an excellent example of the very concrete response often found at this age; to the examiner's inquiry, "What are the people feeling?" the child responds, "The man is feeling her arms. . . . " In addition, the story shows the typical feminine D/E pattern, which is unusual in such a young girl.

In the second example, also from a 5½-year-old girl, we see denial used on a more primitive level, where the defense creates a perceptual distortion and a disruption in reality testing. Again, the story was tape-recorded as the child responded to TAT Card 17BM.[9]

> "This is a statue, climbing down a rope. (WH?) He falls and then breaks. And then somebody builds him back up and he does the same thing over again."

Although nearly all children, regardless of age, see the figure clinging to the rope as a live man, this little girl turns the figure into a statue.

Given the subsequent course of the story, it appears that she is concerned about the possibility that the figure will fall. In order to quell her anxiety about injury or death, she denies that the figure is alive; if it is not alive, it cannot be hurt and cannot die. This denial is carried out through a misperception; the human being is misperceived as a statue. However, the denial is not completely successful. It leads to a disruption in reality testing, where the statue exhibits animate behavior by "climbing down a rope." When the concern about falling and its consequences is expressed ("He falls and then he breaks"), we see how the perceptual denial allows the child to avoid and undo the anxiety-laden fear of death: Because it is a statue, the pieces can be put back together again, and so there is no harm, nothing to be feared. But the issue is not put to rest completely, for the whole process is then repeated.

The use of projection, which becomes stronger in middle childhood and preadolescence, is illustrated in the following story told by an 11-year-old boy about the same TAT card.[10]

> "Once there was a story about a man and he was building a house and then some warriors came along and broke down the house and were trying to kill him. Luckily he escaped and went away on his horse. Trying to get into the government building, he climbed up a rope and got in and killed the emperor."

This story, although short, is striking in its demonstration of projection. Although the TAT picture depicts a single man clinging to a rope, the storyteller adds a band of murderous warriors, an escape horse, and a murdered emperor. As there is nothing in the picture to suggest these characters, they are clearly derived from the storyteller's own aggressive fantasies, projected onto the benign stimulus card. The story also illustrates the two sides of projection. In the beginning, a man, apparently minding his own business, is benignly building a house. Along come some men described as "warriors," to whom is attributed both the intent to destroy the man's work and the wish to kill him. The story concludes, however, with the hero himself carrying out the intentions that had previously been attributed to the warriors—namely, killing someone.

Identification, as manifest in projective stories, may occur at all ages but is more frequent during adolescence and adulthood.[11] In fact, it is not uncommon that the entire plot of an adolescent's story may revolve around issues of identity and identification. When identification occurs in the stories of young children, we sometimes see examples of its more primitive components.

In the following three stories, the entire plot is taken up with various aspects of the identification process. The first story was written about

TAT Card 1 by a 17-year-old girl, a student in the twelfth grade. The picture on the card shows a young boy sitting at a table, on top of which rests a violin.

> "A little boy facing a violin. His parents have forced him to play the violin, when he'd rather be outside playing baseball. He is sitting looking at his violin and thinking. He is wondering why his parents are making him do something he doesn't want to do. He is frustrated because he is too young to be able to express his own view on things, but he isn't too young to think of them. Bigger people than he are always telling him to do things that don't make sense. Why do his parents want him to sit inside on a beautiful day and play a violin?—As he gets older he will either realize that his parents were trying to help him. He will see that what they were doing was for his own good. He will practice his violin diligently and become quite interested and good at it. Or, because his parents made him play the violin, he decides that he hates it, and shuts out any interest of the violin or music. It was his parents' interest, and not his to begin with, so he figures it's stupid."

This story nicely portrays a number of themes involving identification and, in a sense, illustrates the course of its development. Almost immediately, the storyteller goes to a central conflict between the child's wish for pleasure and the parents' imposition of rules and restrictions. It is, of course, in the mind of the storyteller that this conflict between unrestricted gratification and adult demands is taking place. As such, it indicates that the parents' mores have been internalized; the internalization of adult standards is one aspect of identification. In the way the demands are portrayed in the story, they have not yet been fully integrated into the self ("he is wondering why his parents are making him do something he doesn't want to do"). Rather, they appear as an introjected other who is engaged in a struggle with the pleasure-seeking self. Despite the noticeable differentiation of self and other at this point, it soon becomes clear that the boy is not yet ready to separate from the other ("he is too young to be able to express his own view"); the focus stays on what the "bigger people" tell him to do. These controls, however, which govern his behavior, continue to be experienced as alien to his own self (they "don't make sense"). Secondary identification, which involves a change in the ego whereby the values and sanctions of the identified-with figure become one's own, has not yet occurred in the young boy of the story.

The story continues and raises the point that in order for secondary identification to occur, the boy must grow older. Then, he adopts the parents' point of view; he sees that "what they were doing was for his own good." His behavior now is governed by this identification; he gives up his pleasure-seeking orientation and acquires the capacity for work (he practices "diligently").

The storyteller then takes us one step further in the ongoing process of identification. Not content to leave the boy in a state of secondary identification, the issues of separation and individuation are raised once more. Whereas when he was younger he was only able to *think* about being different, now the boy is able to *act* on rejecting the parents' views. He "shuts out any interest of the violin" and works to differentiate himself from his parents through devaluing their interests ("he figures it's stupid"). Taken as a whole, the story can be interpreted as representing the developmental stages of identification—from introjection through adolescent individuation.

A rather different outcome occurs in a second story written about the same TAT picture by a 17-year-old girl in the eleventh grade.

"This boy, John, is a very talented young musician. Constantly on the road, performing. He has played at such renowned places as Carnegie Hall and Denver Athenaeum. Even though he's only 4. John was practicing one day when he stopped, looked at his violin, and started to think. 'Why do I practice 6 hours a day? I am always on the road and never get a chance to make friends my own age.' He begins to wonder if he wants more from life than just music, music, music. John goes and starts to talk to his mother. They have a long talk. And when John leaves the room he feels as his mother does. Now John is concert master of the Vienna orchestra."

This story again focuses on several aspects of identification. It begins with a boy who already shows evidence of having modified his own ego to include adult concerns: He has adopted an orientation toward a profession ("musician"), the work ethic ("constantly on the road, performing"), and status as judged by adult standards ("Carnegie Hall and Denver Athenaeum"). There is no suggestion here that these activities are ego alien, imposed by (introjected) adults. Rather, they seem to represent what he, the musician, feels himself to be. The first hint of possible tension comes when we learn that this working professional is but 4 years old. There is a sense of dissynchrony here; 4-year-olds are not expected to have identified so strongly with the adult world. We have, then, a case of premature, precocious secondary identification. As the story progresses, the boy begins to move into the next phase in the identification process—namely, to question the values acquired through secondary identification ("Why do I practice . . . ?") and to begin the second individuation process. To do this, he expresses the need to turn to persons outside his family and his own generation ("a chance to make friends my own age"). As the disengagement from the earlier identification proceeds, he experiences the sense of insufficiency that accompanies the loosening of old ties; he "wonders if he wants more from life than just music."

It is at this point, however, that the forward progress in the course of identification comes to a halt, for the boy goes back to his mother rather than continuing to separate from her. That this regressive path might be followed has been foreshadowed for us by the earlier recognition that this boy's attainment of secondary identification was precocious. Attained prematurely, it suggests that the creation of ego structures needed to support further development may have been bypassed. Lacking the necessary inner strength for progression to the next phase of identification and to disengagement from the parents, the boy instead falls back onto the earlier attachment to his mother. As they talk, the regression continues, until, when he leaves the room, "he feels as his mother does." Although he had been on the brink of the second individuation process of adolescence, he regresses back to the point of a nondifferentiated merging with her; their feelings are indistinguishable. The story ends by indicating that John continues in his life to be fixated at this early level of primary identification.

Yet another way in which issues involving identification may be expressed in projective stories occurs in a third story—an example from an adolescent boy. On first reading, the story may be understood as symbolic of a growing boy's concerns about his sexuality. In a broader sense, the story reflects concerns about the process of identification, including the discovery of masculine sexual identity, as it is passed down from one generation to the next.

> "At the age of 12 John lives with his mother. His father has died many years ago and all he has left him is this violin. John sits and looks at it, puzzled by its strange shape. From time to time he plucks at its strings with his fingers. As time passes, he becomes fascinated with it. He soon discovers that it is not an ordinary violin. By picking it up and bracing it to his neck and just by resting the bow on its strings his hand seems to move by itself and make beautiful sounds. He does not reveal his discovery to anyone. The more John played the better things began to sound, until one day he picked up an ordinary violin and found that he could play it also. His mind and body had coordinated themselves after having played so much that they were now at home with any violin. So John found peace with his instrument and had a good life making and playing violins."

This story begins with a boy who is on the verge of puberty. He has been without a male identification figure for many years. However, his deceased father has left him a (male) legacy. This is problematic for the boy, who, without a (male) model, is puzzled over how he is to use it. As the boy gets older, he increasingly focuses his interest on the enigmatic masculine object. Then, as though his inheritance from his father guides him, he is able to use his hand to produce pleasure from this male legacy. Initially, this activity is carried on in secret.

With time and more experience, the boy is able to reveal his masculinity in public. At this time, his masculine psychological identification is established and is coordinated with his masculine physiology and masculine drives. The development of this stable identification allows him to continue his life in a happy and productive manner.

These three stories illustrate some different ways in which the issue of identification is expressed in the TAT stories of adolescents. Although identification is more likely to appear in the stories of this age group, the following story, told by a 4-year-old boy to TAT Card 17BM, illustrates the use of a primitive precursor of identification—namely, incorporation.

> "He's climbing on a rope. He's trying to get up onto a beanstalk. He saw a mean, big, old giant. The giant gets his muscles to make his bread. He said, fe, fi, fo, fum, I smell the blood of the Englishman. I'll grind your muscles to make my bread. And he does. Then, he gets the giant's muscles, and now he's a giant."

This story, which includes elements from a well-known childhood folktale, is constructed around the conflict between the young, growing boy and the big, powerful adult. The youth wants to succeed; he is trying to get ahead in life. But the old giant is mean and tries to destroy him by robbing him of his strength. It is in the storyteller's idea of how this conflict between young and old is resolved that we see the primitive use of incorporation. First, it appears that the giant will win by taking the boy's muscles, grinding them into bread and then, presumably, eating the bread. Through oral incorporation, the giant will have destroyed the boy's strength and will have added to his own. This latter possibility—that through incorporation one acquires the characteristics belonging to the object to be incorporated—is made most clear in the turnabout that occurs at the end of the story. For, in the end, the boy gets the giant's muscles and thus becomes a giant. Although there is some confusion in this story about who is incorporating whom, the message is clear: It is through eating, or incorporating the other, that one acquires the strength of the other.

Cross-Sectional Studies

As illustrated through the previous stories, children's TAT productions are rich with evidence of defense use. Systematic research with the TAT has also shown that there are reliable differences across the developmental spectrum in children's use of defense mechanisms (Cramer, 1987, 1991a). Beginning with stories from 42 children ages 5 to 12 years old, and subsequently with stories from 320 additional children, the method of TAT analysis for the use of the three defense mechanisms was applied (Cramer, 1987). The subjects represented four age groups (mean ages = 5,8; 9,10; 14,6; and 16,0), with an equal number of boys and girls in each age group. It was hypothesized that the use of defenses by children could be characterized by a developmental hierarchy such that denial, the most primitive and least complex of the three defenses, would be strongest in the youngest group of children. Projection, a defense of greater complexity, was predicted to be relatively stronger among children in middle childhood and preadolescence. Identification, the most complex of the three defenses, was expected to be relatively stronger among late adolescents.

The results of the study confirmed these predictions. Children in the youngest age group used significantly more denial than any other age group. Projection was used significantly more often by the middle two age groups, and identification was used significantly more often by the oldest three age groups, with a steady increase in the use of identification across these three age groups (see Figure 11.3). A subsequent study of the TAT stories of 28 adolescents (Brody & Layton, 1989, cited in Cramer, 1991a, p. 262) again found that identification was used more in this group than projection, which was used more than denial.

Using this approach, a further study by Avery (1985) supported the conception of a developmental hierarchy of defense use in children, as determined from TAT stories, and demonstrated predictable relationships with other personality variables. In this study of fourth-, fifth- and sixth-graders from diverse socioeconomic backgrounds, there were consistent findings showing that use of the lower level defense of denial was negatively related to level of ego development, independence, and self-determination, whereas use of the higher level defense of identification was positively related to higher levels of functioning in these areas. Projection, developmentally between denial and identification, was neither positively nor negatively related to these personality variables.

Two other studies have demonstrated the validity of the use of TAT stories to assess defense mechanisms in children by showing that the measure is sensitive to changes in defenses that would be predicted to occur as a result of changes in environmentally produced stress.[12] In an experimental study (Cramer & Gaul, 1988), second- and sixth-grade children told TAT stories both prior to and following a game-playing intervention in which the children were led to believe that they either had

or had not been successful at the game. It was predicted that the
experience of failure would increase the use of defenses in stories told
following the failure experience. The results supported the prediction:
The children who experienced failure were more likely to use the lower-
level defenses of denial and projection. On the other hand, the experience
of success was followed by greater use of identification.

A second study demonstrated that stress from real-life trauma was
related to defense use (Dollinger & Cramer, 1990). A group of boys, ages
10 to 13 years, who had experienced a lightning strike during a soccer
game in which one boy died were subsequently asked to tell stories to two
pictures that depicted lightning-related scenes. From the defense scores
of these stories and from clinical ratings of the boys' psychological status,
it was determined that the boys who made the greatest use of defenses,
and especially the defense of projection, showed the least degree of
clinical upset. In this case, the use of an age- and sex-characteristic defense
was successful in staving off anxiety about the traumatic event.

The cumulation of this evidence, which consistently supports a
developmental model of a hierarchy of defenses, and which is consistent

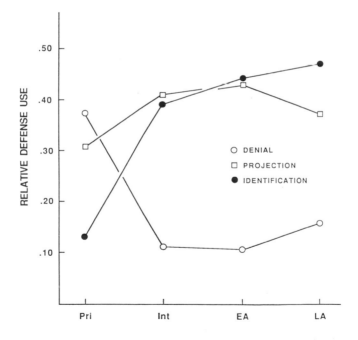

FIGURE 11.3. Defense mechanism scores: primary, intermediate, early adolescent, and late adolescent groups, boys and girls. From Cramer (1987). Copyright
1987 by Duke University Press. Reprinted by permission.

with the theoretical conception that the use of defenses will increase under conditions of stress or anxiety, provides ample support for the utility of using children's TAT stories to assess the use of defense mechanisms.

Longitudinal Studies

There is also some longitudinal evidence using this TAT measure that demonstrates the development of defense mechanisms. Twenty children from two age groups were followed over a period of 1 to 2 years. The younger group, with an average age of 6 years at the beginning of the study, told stories on four occasions over a 2-year time span; the older group, who were 8 years old at the beginning of the study, told stories on three occasions over a 15-month time span. The same pictures were presented on all occasions, and the stories were scored for the use of the three defenses of denial, projection, and identification (see Figure 11.4). The results showed clearly that across the age range of 6 to 9 years old, the use of denial decreased, with the sharpest decrease occurring during the first 9 months.

Projection, on the other hand, markedly and steadily increased across the age groups studied; by late childhood, the use of projection remained at a high and steady level. Identification was used minimally by the children when they were at the preschool and early childhood ages but began to slowly increase as the children reached middle childhood; by the end of middle childhood, the use of identification surpassed the use of denial. These longitudinal findings confirm the idea that defenses develop gradually, each with its own pattern of increasing and decreasing use over the developmental life span.

To illustrate this change, the stories given by three children—Adam, Beth, and Carol—over the course of 1 or 2 years are presented below. In each, a shift in the predominant defense may be noted.

Adam. The following set of stories to TAT card 17BM were told by Adam, who was 6, 8 years old at the time of the first testing. At the time of the fourth testing, he was 2 years older.

Time 1 (Age 6,8)

"I know he's climbing a rope. Looks like he's climbing up some sort of a wall . . . up a castle wall or out of a castle wall. (WH?) I think he's actually climbing out of a castle and there's a wall next to him. (WH?) Maybe he's escaping. (WH?) He runs. I think he escapes. Lots of men are chasing him. (HF?) Sad."

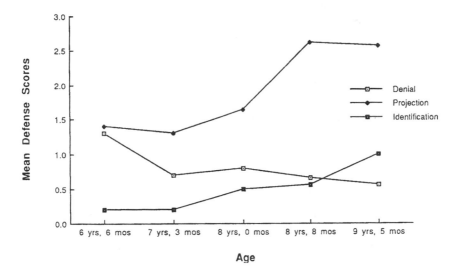

FIGURE 11.4. Defense mechanism scores, longitudinal study: ages 6 to 9 years, boys and girls combined.

Here we see the common story of the hero escaping from and being chased by others. This projection of hostility and the need to flee from it yields a projection score of 2; neither denial nor identification is scored in the story.

Time 2 (Age 7,5)

"Oh, I've seen this one before. Well, he's climbing up a wall and I think he's thinking if he falls what's going to happen. He's climbing up the wall to get out of a prison. And he's climbing up to get to the tower where the princess is and capture her. But he's actually sort of swinging on the ropes, it looks like. (HE?) He captures the princess."

On this second occasion, we see the same theme of escape as before. However, this time the escape is from prison. Further, rather than being chased (i.e., being the victim) the hero now assumes a more active role and pursues his own victim, by capturing the princess. The use of projection (score: 2) continues as the predominant defense; no other defenses are manifest.

Time 3 (Age 8,0)

"Well, it looks like a man escaping from prison—you know how they have those big walls. And he's got a big fence on the other side—tries to get over that, too. And he's trying to get out. The expression on his face is sort of happy. It looks like a strong guy (I'd hate to run into him). His feet are trying to go up and his nose looks happy, too, But his eyebrows sort of go down. (HE?) He gets caught."

The escape theme continues. At this third occasion, a new element of projection appears—the hyperattention to facial nuances in an attempt to justify projected emotions. Again, projection is the predominant and only defense used in the story. (score: projection = 3).

Time 4 (Age 8,8)

"Well, he looks like he's pretty strong. He's climbing up a wall. Maybe he's climbing up a wall to get away from lions—or maybe he's just climbing out of the prison. Looks like he's been somewhere that isn't very pleasant because he doesn't have anything on. He looks sort of happy. Maybe he's climbing up to get somewhere—inside somewhere. And he wants to get inside so he can see the King. But the guards don't let him. They gave him a beating cause he tried to break in. And he climbed up the wall and he finally got into the King. Then the King called the guard and he grabbed his sword from the shelf and then when the guards caught him he had to fight them. And he fought. And then they looked at each other, they turned around, threw their swords away—the guards tried to stop them but they just ran away. And they got home and had some soup."

At the age of 8½, Adam shows a continued use of projection, now with even greater intensity. There is also the beginning of evidence for the use of identification in the introduction of the figure of the king, and in the justified punishment given him for his wrongdoing. The increase in projection comes about in part through the addition of ominous characters and objects to the story—additions not justified on the basis of the picture itself. Thus lions, hostile guards, and a sword are added to the situation, along with the projected hostile actions of beating and fighting. In addition, we see the use of circumstantial reasoning to defend against the anxiety created by the nakedness of the central figure: "Looks like he's been somewhere that isn't very pleasant because he doesn't have anything on" (score: denial = 0, projection = 7, identification = 2).

Beth. The following stories were told about the trapeze picture by Beth, who was 6,3 years old at the time of the first testing and 7,8 years old at the third testing occasion.[13]

Time 1 (Age 6,3)

"Swinging on a rope . . . and the man's hanging onto a woman and he's on something that is swinging and he's in a tent, a big tent. The lady fell down. (WH?) She lands on a mattress. And the man falls down, he landed on a pillow. (HE?) Good. They went up again. They started again. (HE?) Good. (HF?) Fairly good."

Although much of this story is taken up by describing the picture, as is common for children of this age, there is one dramatic happening introduced by the storyteller—namely, the fall. It is at this point that we see the use of the defense of denial to ward off the anxiety about the possible ensuing disaster. Although it is conceivable that a mattress could cushion the impact of such a fall, the thought that a pillow could ensure a safe landing is highly unrealistic (i.e., indicates the denial of reality). This story thus demonstrates the use of the defense of denial, which is typical of this age group (score: denial = 1, projection = 0, identification = 0).

Time 2 (Age 7,1)

"They're swinging. The man is a little strange. (WF?) They're thinking that they're not going to fall, but they do. They're dead."

On the second occasion, the anxiety around the possibility of falling is also present, as is the use of denial to alleviate the anxiety ("thinking that they're not going to fall"); however, the defense is not successful ("they do [fall]"). This time, however, the unease of the storyteller is defended against through the use of a new defense—projection; the uneasiness is placed onto the hero ("the man is a little strange"). Aggression is also projected ("they're dead"); on the previous occasion, aggression had been defended against through the use of denial (score: denial = 1, projection = 2, identification = 0).

Time 3 (Age 7,8)

"Yeech! I saw that picture. They're swinging. The lady falls. The man is still up there. And then the man falls and they both died. (HF?) They're thinking they are the greatest acrobats but they're the awfulest."

On the third occasion, the use of denial has disappeared. Projection is the only defense shown ("they both died"). There is also evidence for the beginning of self-reflection, an aspect of identification, in the comment "they're thinking they are the greatest acrobats but they're the awfulest." Because this evaluation is directed toward another (the characters) rather than the self, it is not given a formal score for identification (score: denial = 0, projection = 1, identification = 0).

Carol. The following stories were told about TAT Card 17BM by Carol, who was 8 years old on the first testing occasion. In them, we see greater use of projection initially, with the beginning use of identification as she gets older. At the last test date, she was 9,4 years old.

Time 1 (Age 8)

"Well, he's trying to escape from some battle or something. He's trying to do it pretty fast. And he's trying to get down to the bottom of the building and he's not feeling so good because he doesn't like the fight that's going on. And he's trying to get down to the bottom and he's in a real rush. And he wants to get down really bad. (HE?) And so he gets down to the bottom and he goes back up again because he's a real weirdo. And when he goes up he finds that he was only dreaming and he found himself just laying in bed."

This first story has the common "escape" theme, trying to get away from some projected danger—in this case, "the fight." We see the projection of personal discomfort onto the hero in the comment "he's a real weirdo." Demonstrating the transition stage this girl is in, the end of the story illustrates the effort to deny the whole event by turning it into something unreal—a dream (score: denial = 1, projection = 3, identification = 0).

Time 2 (Age 8,9)

"This is a man that was climbing up a rope and he's kind of like Tarzan, but he's a different man, though. And he fights crime and he was climbing up a rope to watch a parade. Then he saw somebody kidnapping a lady. And now he's climbing down a rope and going down to stop the man. Then he got down and he found some witnesses and they said he went off into a cave. And the man went down to the cave and found the man and brought him to the police. (HF?) He's very proud because he fought one of his first crimes."

This story presents a rather different plot, and a reversal from being the victim who is being acted upon to being the actor who is involved in bringing about justice. While there is still the projection of danger ("somebody kidnapping a lady"), the use of identification has emerged as an important defense. The central figure is clearly described as being *like* (identified with) a popular hero, and he behaves in a way that shows a clear identification with the laws and principles of society (score: denial = 0, projection = 1, identification = 2).

> Time 3 (Age 9,4)
>
> "This man is going to be in a movie. He's practicing for a movie because he's going to star in a movie and he's going to be Tarzan. And he doesn't know it but he's being chased by criminals. And the criminals are trying to get him but he thinks he's getting away from what's going to be in the movie, an ape or something. And the criminals can't catch him and he was going to set a trap for the ape but he trapped the criminals instead. And he didn't know that he had trapped them and he said, 'Hey, I've trapped something.' And he went down there and said, 'I'm sorry.' Then he let them go. Then the police said to him, 'There've been some criminals around here—have you seen them?' And he said, 'Oh no, I've only seen a couple of guys.' The police said, 'Where'd they go?' and he says, 'They went into that store over there.' And so the police go over there and they were in the store. And they get them. (WF?) Wow, I don't know that."

In the last story of this sequence, the use of identification has become stronger. Now the hero is not only "like" Tarzan, as in the previous story; here he is "going to be" Tarzan (i.e., assume the identification completely). Again, the moral forces of society are made victorious in the end. Projection continues to be manifest in this story, both in the "chase" and "trapping," and in the addition of "criminals" to the situation. Also, there is an attempt to defend against the projected hostility through the use of denial: "The criminals can't catch him" (score: denial = 1, projection = 3, identification = 2).

Object Relations

The method for using TAT stories to assess the nature and level of object relations, which was developed by Westen (1991a, 1991b) and described in Chapter 10, has been employed successfully to demonstrate developmental differences in subjects ranging in age from early childhood to late adolescence. This measure, based on the theoretical and research literature from psychoanalytic and social cognition approaches, is designed to reflect the quality of the individual's interpersonal behavior and the processes that mediate the capacity for relatedness to others. The original interpretive method (the SCORS) consisted of four scales, each of which was scored at five levels. The four scales assess the complexity of representations of people, the capacity for emotional investment in relationships and moral standards, the understanding of social causality, and the affect-tone of relationship paradigms. Underlying this approach, and the development of the scales, is the assumption that there is a developmental progression in the quality of object relations, with lower levels on the first three scales representing developmentally earlier periods and higher levels characterizing later periods of development. The fourth scale, affect-tone, is assumed to be independent of level of development.

Two empirical investigations supported these assumptions. In the first (Westen et al., 1991), second-graders (mean age = 7,9) and fifth-graders (mean age = 10,8) told stories about TAT Cards 1 and 17BM. The stories were transcribed and coded by two raters who did not know the age or sex of the subjects. Interrater reliability was high for the four scales, ranging from .91 to .96.[14] The results showed the predicted developmental differences: Fifth-graders had significantly higher scores for complexity of representations, emotional investment, and social causality. As predicted, there were no developmental differences on the affect-tone dimension. Further, an inspection of the percentage of subjects in each grade who were rated at each level of the object relations scales showed a clear developmental pattern: More second- than fifth-graders were rated at the lower scale levels, and more fifth- than second-grades were rated at the higher levels.

In a second investigation (Westen et al., 1991), ninth-graders and twelfth-graders told stories about six TAT cards.[15] Each story was coded on each scale by two raters, with interrater reliabilities ranging from .86 to .95.[16] The majority of subjects in this adolescent sample were female (62% of the ninth-graders and 84% of the twelfth-graders), a factor that may be important because, in the first investigation, the fifth-grade girls had higher scores than the boys on all four scales.[17]

The results again indicated that the older subjects (twelfth-graders) had higher scores on the three predicted object relations scales (complexity of representations, emotional investment, and social causality) but not on the affect-tone dimension. Further, inspection of the results from the two investigations indicated that the ninth-graders in the second study had higher mean scores on the three critical object relations scales than did the fifth-graders of the first study, as would be expected. However, a comparison of these means is not completely justified. In addition to the gender imbalance, different stimulus cards were used in the two studies; further, it does not appear that any correction was made for story length, which was probably greater in the older subjects, with the ensuing possibility of higher scores. However, Westen et al. (1991) have considered the possible relationship between the scale scores and the issue of verbal fluency, and concluded that verbosity, per se, does not lead to higher scores. Rather, they concluded that subjects at higher levels of development may use more words to describe their more complex object representations.

Achievement Motivation

Children's stories have also been used to assess age differences in the presence of achievement motivation (McClelland et al., 1953; see Chapter 15). In a large-scale study of 3,000 boys and girls (Veroff, 1969), children were asked to make up a story in response to a series of questions asked about two pictures—a man in a white shirt seated at a desk and two men at a machine.[18] The questions were similar to those used in a nationwide study with adults (Veroff, 1961; discussed in Chapter 12). For each picture, the child was asked, "What are the men doing?" "What are the men thinking?" "What do they want?" and, "What will happen?" For each picture, the story was coded achievement imagery = 2, task imagery (executing a task, doing something) = 1, imagery unrelated to achievement = 0. Scores were summed over the two pictures; each child could thus have a score of 0 to 4.

The results for boys and girls indicated that there was a steady increase in achievement motivation scores from first grade to sixth grade, with no reversals (see Table 11.2). Statistical tests indicated highly significant age differences.[19] There was also a significant effect attributable to sex, with boys scoring higher than girls. Veroff believed that some of the sex differences in the TAT motivation scores, at least among the older children, might be related to girls having more of a social comparison orientation about achievement, whereas boys had more of an orientation to achievement that involved autonomy.

Many additional studies using the TAT approach to measuring achievement motivation have been carried out with children. Summaries of this work may be found in Atkinson (1958), McClelland (1961), Smith (1969), and Rosen and D'Andrade (1959), among others.

Emotional Stance

Another systematic approach to studying children's TAT stories has been developed by Stewart and her colleagues (Stewart & Healy, 1985; Stewart, Sokol, Healy, Chester, & Weinstock-Savoy, 1982; Stewart, Sokol, Healy, & Chester, 1986; for a discussion of this approach, see Chapter 15). The "inner emotional stance" TAT measure has been used to assess the reactions of children to life changes, and to test the hypothesis that the emotional stances of receptivity, autonomy, assertion, and integration represent a sequence of reactions that occur within an individual over time in response to a changed environment. This sequence is understood as an internal process of adaptation rather than development, although the stances may be linked theoretically to the four stages of psychosexual development (oral, anal, phallic, and genital).

Several investigations chose school transitions as the life change to be studied. Two research designs were used: Some studies compared the TAT stories of subjects who were pretransitional with those who were posttransitional; other studies compared subjects who had just experienced the transition with those who had experienced it in the past (e.g., 1 or 2 years earlier). Initially, a cross-sectional design was used; most of the findings from these studies were subsequently replicated using a longitudinal design.

Using a cross-sectional design, the reaction to various transitions in school was studied. A comparison of children who were just entering school (kindergarten and first grade) with those who had been in school for 2 years (second grade) indicated that the stories of the transition group showed an almost exclusive preoccupation with issues of receptivity and autonomy, whereas the stories of the posttransitional group reflected almost entirely issues of assertion and integration (Stewart et al., 1982). That these results were not simply due to cohort differences was demonstrated in a subsequent longitudinal study in which the same children were retested 1 or 2 years later. Those children who had just experienced the transition at the first testing occasion, showing lower-level emotional stances, by the time of the second testing had shifted toward a higher-level emotional stance, becoming like the posttransitional group of the first study. This latter group, who were not experiencing a transition at the time

TABLE 11.2. Mean Achievement Motivation Scores, Grades 1–6, by Sex

Grade	Boys[a]	Girls[b]
1	1.89	1.78
2	2.02	1.87
3	2.29	2.09
4	2.34	2.13
5	2.56	2.23
6	2.65	2.41

Note. Adapted from Veroff (1969). Copyright 1969 by Russell Sage. Adapted by permission.
[a]Total $N = 1,025$.
[b]Total $N = 1,051$.

of the first testing, when retested 1 to 2 years later, did not show a change in level of emotional stance (Stewart et al., 1986).

These results, of course, could be explained as reflecting changes due to development rather than to environmental changes, because the older children showed a developmentally higher-level emotional stance. That this is not a sufficient explanation of the findings is demonstrated by subsequent investigations that found the same shifts to occur among older subjects. Further, when pretransitional subjects were compared with older subjects who were experiencing a transition, there was a stance shift in the opposite direction (i.e., from a higher level to a lower level of functioning).

A second and third transition period in school occurs when students move from elementary to junior high school, and again from junior to senior high school. An initial cross sectional study compared the TAT stories of pretransitional students (sixth- and ninth-graders) with those of students who had experienced the transition (seventh- and tenth-graders). As a whole, the transitional subjects did not show the expected lower-level emotional stance scores. However, social class was discovered to be an important factor in determining the students' reaction to the transition: Middle-class students did show the expected drop in emotional stance scores, whereas working-class students showed a slight increase (Stewart et al., 1982).

A subsequent longitudinal study of this transition (Healy & Stewart, 1984), which retested the pretransitional subjects a year later, immediately following their entry into junior or senior high school, found that after the transition, they were more preoccupied with lower-level affective stances. Again, there was an interaction with social class and also with sex: Middle-class girls were strongly affected by the school transition and showed a marked drop in level of emotional stance, whereas working class girls were unaffected. Boys from both socioeconomic groups were equally and strongly affected by the transition.

Another educational transition occurs when students enter college. In developing the measure of emotional stances (Stewart, 1982b), students who had just experienced this transition (i.e., freshmen) were compared with those who had presumably adapted to it (seniors). A comparison of their TAT stories indicated that the freshmen were more preoccupied with earlier issues of receptivity and autonomy, whereas the seniors expressed more concern for issues involving assertion and integration. These differences between freshmen and seniors, which were found in three different colleges, were assumed to be due to, and to reflect, the nature of the process of adaptation to the new college environment. The alternative explanation—that the differences are due simply to development, or maturation—is less acceptable in this sample when one considers that the level of scores of the freshmen—their preoccupation with issues of receptivity and autonomy—are comparable to those of the children who were just entering elementary school (Stewart et al., 1982). Stewart suggests that the preoccupation of the freshmen with earlier emotional levels reflects a *"re*experiencing of issues first experienced at far younger ages" (Stewart, 1982b, p. 1110) and reflects their current process of adaptation.

A further cross-sectional study of the transition to college (Stewart et al., 1982) found that freshmen had lower scores on the measure of emotional stance than did sophomores. The effects of this period of adaptation to college—the first year—were confirmed in a subsequent longitudinal study (Stewart et al., 1986). College students who were tested as freshmen and again as sophomores showed the expected increase in level of emotional stance but did not change after the sophomore year. In this longitudinal study, however, it was the men students who showed a significant increase in stance score from the freshman to the sophomore years; the women did not change. No sex differences were found in the cross-sectional study.

SUMMARY

This chapter demonstrates how the TAT has been used to discover important developmental changes in the personality of children and adolescents. Developmental differences and changes have been found with the D/E measure of gender identity and with the measure of defense mechanisms, as well as with the measures of object relations, achievement motivation, and emotional stance.

The seven studies of gender identity all yielded consistent results. Boys and girls did not differ in gender-related fantasy patterns in early childhood (ages 3 to 6 years); by ages 8 to 9, differences appeared and continued until late adolescence, when lack of differentiation occurred again. By the end of the college years, both males and females showed the typical sex-related pattern.

The six studies of defense mechanisms were also all consistent in supporting a developmental model of defense use. Denial was found to be characteristic in the stories of young, preschool children. Projection was characteristic of the stories from middle childhood. Identification became more prominent in late adolescence. Further, each of these defenses was found to have a developmental history of its own, gradually increasing and/or decreasing across childhood and adolescence.

Developmental differences in level of object relations was investigated in two studies using the TAT. In one, it was found that fifth-graders manifest a higher level and quality of object relations than do second-graders. In a second study, twelfth-graders were found to be at a higher level than ninth-graders. Although the two data sets are not strictly comparable, the combined results show a steady increase in level and quality of object relations from early elementary school to the end of high school.

In one very large-scale study of achievement motivation in children, the results showed a clear and steady increase in the strength of the achievement motive from first to sixth grade.

Finally, the TAT has been used to document changes in children's and adolescents' level of emotional stance and adaptation as related to transitions in educational placement (beginning school, moving to junior high school, to senior high school, and to college) in both cross-sectional and longitudinal studies.

Overall, the same interpretive perspectives that have been found to be useful in the interpretation of adult TAT stories have been found to be equally informative when used with the stories of children.

• TWELVE •

Developmental Differences in Adult TAT Stories

T
he TAT was designed for use with adults in both clinical and research settings. The majority of studies with the TAT have been carried out with young adults (often college students) as the subjects. Descriptions of normative stories for each TAT card are generally based on the themes occurring in the stories of this young adult population. Interestingly, despite the fact of an increasingly large elder population, and the fact that the TAT is one of the 10 tests most frequently used by practicing clinicians,[1] a survey carried out by Lezak (1987) revealed that there are no American or European old-age norms for the TAT. Although Bellak (1975) has created a special test for senior citizens (the SAT),[2] the majority of investigations continue to use the TAT with both young and older adults. In this chapter, I review studies that have used the TAT to study adult development.

DEVELOPMENTAL DIFFERENCES AMONG OLDER INDIVIDUALS

Studies of Achievement, Affiliation, Power, and Intimacy Motivation

Two extensive studies of American adults, ages 21 to 80+ years, were conducted by Veroff and his colleagues, who collected a large number of stories, once in 1957 and again in 1976 (Veroff, 1961, 1982; Veroff, Atkinson, Feld, & Gurin, 1960; Veroff, Depner, Kulka, & Douvan, 1980; Veroff, Reuman, & Feld, 1984). Each of these studies allows cross-sectional comparisons of adults at different developmental periods over the life span. Together, they provide the opportunity for comparisons of cohort differences (i.e., the comparison of same-age adults from different generations). The TAT stories of these adults,[3] corrected for length of protocol, were scored for the presence of various motives, or needs, including nAchievement, nAffiliation, and nPower (including fear of weakness [Veroff (1957) method] and hope of power [Winter (1973) method]; see Chapter 15). Considerable attention was given to controlling for possible interviewer differences, to training the coders for consistency, to assessing interrater reliability, and to reassessing reliability at three different points during the coding procedure.

The 1957 sample, described as a "cross-section of Americans living in private households, selected by means of probability sampling" (Veroff et al., 1960, p. 2), consisted of 1,619 men and women ages 21 to 65 and older. Subjects were grouped into 5-year age intervals (21 to 24 years, 25 to 34 years, and so on) making possible a comparison of the motive scores across the several age groups. For men, the results suggested that nAchievement remains fairly constant from early adulthood (ages 21 to 34) to middle adulthood (ages 35 to 49), although there was some increase with age among middle-level[4] and lower-level occupations.[5] In the older age group (50+), men in middle-level occupations showed a decrease in nAchievement. For nAffiliation, men showed virtually no change across the age span. Power motivation (fear of weakness) showed a peaking at middle age (35 to 54 years) for men who did not go beyond a grade-school education; this result was not found with men who had more education. On the other hand, nPower (hope for power) showed a peaking at midlife (ages 40 to 54) for all men, regardless of level of education.

For women, there was a decline in both achievement and affiliation motivation across the life cycle. Differences in power motivation were more closely related to educational level. Fear of weakness decreased across the age span for women with only a grade school education but increased for women with high school or college backgrounds. On the other hand, hope of power increased among the oldest women (55+) of grade-school or college background, with less change among the high-school-educated women.

This same analysis of motive scores was repeated with the stories gathered 20 years later from the 1,498 subjects in the 1976 sample. Of particular interest were parallel age trends in the data from the two testing periods; consistent effects across the two generations tested would provide more reliable evidence for attributing developmental meaning to age differences found. For men, the new results were consistent with the earlier findings regarding nAchievement; there was little change from early to middle adulthood, with a slight decrease in the 55+ age group.

No consistent age effects across the two samples were found for nAffiliation. Power motivation (fear of weakness) was found to remain relatively unchanged across the age span[6] whereas hope for power was consistently higher during middle age, especially the period from 40 to 49 years (Veroff, 1982), or 50 to 54 years (Veroff et al., 1984), followed by a decrease in older years (Veroff et al., 1984).

The most consistent results for the two subject samples were found for women. Both achievement motivation and affiliation motivation showed a clear decline across the life cycle. The decrease in affiliation motivation was found both for women who worked outside the home and for those who did not. It also was found for women who were married or divorced as well as for those who were mothers or who had been married but had no children. The only women who did not show this decline in nAffiliation were those who held high-prestige jobs (Veroff et al, 1984). Although there was also a consistent decline in nAchievement with age, this decrease reflected primarily less story imagery referring to career aspirations or social comparison with peers. However, imagery referring to competition with standards of excellence did not decrease.[7] From this, Veroff et al. (1984) concluded that older women in our society show a decline in the career orientation component of achievement motivation but not in the more general competence orientation. The results for the two samples of women were also consistent in showing that neither of the measures of power motivation showed any reliable change with age. The relationship between educational level and changes in the two power measures found in the earlier sample did not appear in the second group of women.

Age and/or developmental effects were also investigated by looking for cohort effects—that is, determining whether the age differences that were found might be due to differential historical/social factors which would affect one cohort differently than another, thus leading to apparent age effects that were really due to cohort differences. In this case, a cohort that was relatively high on a particular motive in 1957 would continue to be high in 1976. To examine this question, the data from the two testing occasions (1957 and 1976) were combined, and five cohorts, based on the year of birth of the subjects, were formed. Cohort 1 included all individuals who were born between 1927 and 1936 and who were thus 21 to 30 years old in 1957 or 40 to 49 years old in 1976. Cohort 2 included all individuals born between 1917 and 1926, and so on (Veroff, 1982; Veroff et al., 1984).

The results of this analysis were clear in showing that there were no cohort effects for men on the achievement, affiliation, or power motives. Rather, the results indicate that "adult motivation shifts as men proceed through the life cycle" (Veroff, 1982, p. 108). For women, although there was no evidence for cohort effects regarding power motivation, cohorts did appear to make a difference for achievement motivation.[8] Women in cohort 1 who were 21 to 30 years old in 1957 (thus forming the youngest age group at that time) had high nAchievement scores; women from this cohort had even higher levels of achievement motivation in 1976, when they were 40 to 49 years old, and this level of achievement motivation was considerably higher than that of women of comparable age (40 to 49) in 1957. Women in cohort 5, who were 60 to 69 years old in 1957 were very low in nAchievement at that time; women from this cohort also had low achievement scores in 1976, when they were over 80 years of age.[9]

These results may be interpreted to reflect the influence of the historical/social circumstances of the society in which these women were living. The 1950s introduced the idea of the "feminine mystique" and changing social roles for women, followed by consciousness-raising and affirmative action programs which supported possibilities for women's achievement. All this occurred during the time the achievement motivation of cohort 1 was high and presumably helped to sustain it. Because cohort 5 did not receive this social support during their young adult years, there was an ensuing decline in their achievement motivation.

A comparison of the results from the two periods provides further information about changes in American motives over the 20-year period from 1957 to 1976. This comparison is made more meaningful by the fact that the same storytelling format and the same pictures were used in both studies, and the raters who coded motive scores in 1976 were trained to be consistent with the scoring conventions used by the raters in 1957.[10]

In order to determine the effect of time of testing, the scores from both testing dates were combined into one distribution for each motive. The scores from each date were then compared to the median score for the total distribution, and the percentage of men and women at each date who were above the median score was determined (see Table 12.1). These comparisons revealed several differences between the 2 years that were independent of age and education effects. In 1976, men had much weaker affiliation motivation scores than in 1957, and they had stronger power motivation scores; both the fear of weakness and the hope of power components were stronger in 1976. Women, in 1976, had higher achievement motivation, consistent with the historical/social analysis suggested above; this was true for women at all educational levels. Women also had stronger power motivation (fear of weakness) in 1976 than in 1957 (see Table 12.1).

In order to interpret these findings, the authors examined changes in responses to individual pictures, as well as considering the overall scores. From these analyses, they concluded that the higher level of achievement motivation in women in 1976 represented a general increase in women seeking achievement not only in the workplace but also in other realms of life. In addition, it reflected women responding to increased opportunities "for self-definition through achievement" (Veroff et al., 1980, p. 1259). Men, however, did not show clear-cut changes in achievement motivation. This seemed to be related to two factors: The first, beginning in the 1960s, was the disillusionment of the counterculture with the idea that achievement provides a basis for self-definition; the second

TABLE 12.1. Comparison of American Motives: 1957 versus 1976; Percentage of Scores above Median

	Men		Women	
	1957	1976	1957	1976
Achievement				
21–24	58	41	42	61
25–34	48	56	44	67
35–44	50	60	43	59
45–54	48	46	40	63
55–64	40	60	38	56
65+	42	44	32	46
Affiliation				
21–24	58	41	53	56
25–34	57	40	51	61
35–44	57	42	52	48
45–54	54	41	52	48
55–64	66	37	35	42
65+	58	33	36	37
Power (Veroff)				
21–24	29	71	45	65
25–34	33	68	48	56
35–44	41	64	42	55
45–54	41	67	45	48
55–64	27	63	39	61
65+	42	60	41	51
Power (Winter)				
21–24	33	62	46	57
25–34	41	53	54	51
35–44	44	59	40	48
45–54	59	57	42	49
55–64	45	39	55	45
65+	50	47	50	46

Note. From Veroff et al. (1980). Copyright 1980 by the American Psychological Association. Reprinted by permission.

was the factor of a tightening job market over this period. The authors further suggest that a cultural shift occurred—away from the importance of achievement toward the influence of power—as a means for success in the marketplace.

In fact, over this 20-year period, both men and women showed an increase in the "fear of weakness" aspect of power motivation, especially in the interpersonal world. The authors suggested that this may reflect the changes in sex roles that occurred over this time span, for these had previously defined power relations between men and women. It is suggested that men reacted to this loss of interpersonal power by shifting to a need for power in relation to other men, as is seen in an increased "hope for power" theme in the workplace. As mentioned earlier, for men, power seemed to have displaced the importance of achievement in the workplace. In turn, this focus on power is generally incompatible with affiliative goals, which, as noted earlier, had declined in men over this time span. The decrease in affiliation motivation was especially true in stories about the workplace but was also found regarding family relationships, consistent with the changes in power relations discussed above. It is further suggested that women's reaction to increased "fear of weakness" has been to focus on achievement goals in the workplace rather than "hope for power" goals, and that this focus on achievement among women has not interfered with maintaining their affiliation motivation.

The TAT stories from the 1976 sample were also evaluated for nIntimacy (McAdams & Bryant, 1987). Stories told by 1,208 adults to the six TAT cards used for scoring the other motives (nAchievement, nAffiliation, nPower: [Veroff] and nPower [Winter]) were scored for nIntimacy by a highly trained rater, with scores adjusted for length of story. As was found for nAffiliation, older women obtained lower nIntimacy scores than did younger women; in fact, the decrease was consistent and linear across the adult years. Men, on the other hand, remained relatively stable in nIntimacy across age, again consistent with the findings for nAffiliation. For both men and women, nIntimacy showed a substantial correlation with nAffiliation, although, as discussed in Chapter 15, there are good empirical and theoretical reasons for considering these as measures of two separate dispositions.

There were also sex differences in the relationship between nIntimacy and other personality variables. For women, there was a weak positive relationship between nIntimacy and nPower (Winter's hope for power) and weak, positive relationships between nIntimacy and a sense of happiness and of gratification. For men, there was a negative relationship between nIntimacy and nPower (Veroff's fear of weakness), and a positive relationship with uncertainty.

Attribution of Male and Female Personality Traits

A second large-scale study of older adults was carried out by Neugarten and her colleagues, studying older individuals residing in Kansas City during the 1950s (Neugarten, 1964; Neugarten & Gutmann, 1968). Subjects ranging in age from 40 to 70 years told stories to a number of TAT and TAT-like cards, in order to study age-related differences in the attribution of personality traits to males and females. The TAT was also used to study ego-mastery style and ego energy as a function of age.

As part of this larger study, Neugarten and Gutmann (1968) asked male and female subjects from two age groups (40–54, n = 73; and 55–70, n = 58) to tell a story about and describe the four characters depicted in a single TAT-like card; the characters varied in age and sex. Focusing on the descriptions of the older man and older woman, there were very interesting differences between the younger and older subjects. These differences could best be characterized along a continuum of dominance and submission; a six-category scale was devised to define this continuum. For perceptions of the older man, the six categories reflected the impact of the man on the situation and the extent to which others deferred to him; the categories ranged from "altruistic authority" (most dominant) to "passive cerebral" (most submissive). For perceptions of the older woman, two themes were intermingled with the dominance–submissiveness continuum: The first theme—"control over others"—reflected whether the older woman was seen as dominant and controlling or as submissive and controlled. The second theme—"the nature of impulsivity"—indicated whether the older woman was viewed as benign and nurturant or self-assertive and aggressive.

The results showed that the age of the storyteller was a significant factor in the attribution of dominance–submissiveness to the stimulus figures; further, this relationship was reversed as a function of the sex of the stimulus figure. Middle-aged subjects (ages 40 to 54) perceived the male figure as being dominant and powerful in the family whereas the female figure was perceived as subordinate, submissive, benign, and nurturant. Among the older subjects (55 to 70), however, the male figure was described as submissive whereas the female figure was seen as dominant, authoritative, self-assertive, and aggressive. Thus there was an age-related shift occurring in the perception of the personality of older males and females.[11] Statistical analyses indicated that only age was a significant factor in determining these results; neither sex of subject nor occupational class was related to the shift.

A cross-sectional study of the effect of social status on the shift in perceived female power raises questions about the importance of age, per se, in determining the shift (Todd, Friedman, & Kariuki, 1990). In this investigation, older women (mean age approximately 50 years) and younger women (mean age approximately 26 years), of higher and lower social and economic status, from two countries (United States and Kenya) gave stories to TAT Card 4, which shows a man, who appears upset, looking away from a woman, who is holding on to him. The female and male characters of the stories were scored blindly by two raters on several dimensions involving interpersonal power, theme, and outcome. The results showed a significant interaction between age and status, such that the higher status, older women produced higher power scores for the female character, whereas the lower-status older women did not. Consistent with this finding, the higher-status women's stories ended optimistically with the female character getting her way, whereas the lower-status women's stories had negative outcomes. The authors interpreted these results to mean that only women of higher-status show a positive shift in power with age. However, they caution that because this is a cross-sectional rather than longitudinal study, it is not possible to know whether the women in the older groups had in fact been equivalent in power perception when they were younger. It is possible that women in both status groups had increased in power perception with age but that the baseline scores differed when they were younger, as a function of status.

One additional study (Pasewark, Fitzgerald, Dexter, & Cangemi, 1976) compared the themes of stories to TAT cards given by females from three age groups, matched for occupational level: adolescents (ages 14 to 16), middle-aged (ages 30 to 44), and older (ages 60 to 89). The older women provided the most themes expressing dependency but the fewest story outcomes with a pessimistic outlook. Themes of loneliness were greatest among the adolescent and the older women, as were stories with a general tenor of unhappiness.[12]

Ego Mastery Styles and Ego Energy

Gutmann (1964) continued this investigation of age-related personality changes in adulthood. The focus in this study was to identify styles of ego mastery which were used to manage both inner stress and external concerns. TAT stories from subjects in three age groups were evaluated: 40 to 49, 50 to 59, and 60 to 69.

Gutmann found three major styles of ego mastery to appear in these stories, representing a continuum of ego strength. The most vigorous, effective style of ego functioning was termed "active mastery"; the most stress-laden, maladaptive style was termed "magical mastery." Between these two, in terms of ego strength, was the style termed "passive mastery."

Although all three styles of ego mastery occurred in the stories of men and women subjects, they were expressed via different themes and content by the two sexes. For men, under the category of *active mastery*, some stories portrayed a hero who could be described as a "self-asserter," moving directly and aggressively toward the goal, not deterred by resistance or challenge from others. For other stories in this category, the hero was described as an "achievement doubter" who, although moving vigorously into the world, had inner reservations about doing so and tended to alternate between assertion and deference. For women, the category of active mastery included two different themes. Stories of "rebellious daughters" involved assertion against a restrictive (usually maternal) authority, whereas themes of "moralistic matriarchs" revolved around the idea that morally lax young people must be guided and disciplined by an older woman. In general, men who manifest either of the active mastery subtypes had in common an assertive orientation, whereas the two subgroups of women were alike in maintaining active mastery by externalizing guilt. For men, the struggle expressed was with an impersonal environment or with passive aspects of themselves that interfere with achievement. For women, the conflict expressed was with people.

The second category, *passive mastery*, was expressed by men in two subthemes. The "adaptive conformer" style described heroes who were deferent, in whom the direct expression of aggression or self-interest was ego alien and who disavowed competitiveness. The "depersonalized conformer" style was characterized by a focus on the impersonal aspects of the environment, with a disengagement from feelings; the disavowed motivations were projected onto the distant world. In both cases, there was a withdrawal from active engagement in the external world.

For women, passive mastery was expressed in two different subthemes. The "maternal altruist" style reflected a discomfort with aggression; an intropunitive stance was characteristic, with a reliance on reaction formation. In the other subtheme, "passive aggressor," the woman lacked the external supports to allow the intropunitive stance to be effective. Constriction and an apathetic conformity to convention characterized the ego functioning of this substyle.

Finally, the category of *magical mastery*, as it occurred in men, involved marked misinterpretations and distortions of stimuli. When faced with difficulty, the reaction was to "alter the world by perceptual fiat, not by realistic, instrumental action" (Gutmann, 1964, p. 126). For women, also, the use of this style of ego mastery involved distortions and misperceptions of reality, often with the inappropriate attribution of aggressive and sexual feelings to the stimulus figure.

Table 12.2 shows that there are clear age-related shifts in the expression of these styles of ego mastery, and that these shifts differ somewhat in men and women subjects. The ego mastery style of younger men is characterized by a central theme of activity. Their engagement is with the external world, not within themselves. Older men, on the other hand, do not see themselves moving outward in an assertive fashion. Rather than express their own aggression, "they ascribe power and determination to impersonal, external forces, to whose mandate they must adapt themselves" (p. 128). Mastery is now achieved by passive "circuitous routes" (p. 128). For women also, active mastery shows a clear decline with age whereas magical mastery shows a decided increase. In contrast to men, women show little change with age in the passive mastery style.

In the process of interpreting these results, it is important to note that the seven TAT cards used in the study are heavily loaded with male pictures. TAT Cards 1 and 17BM both depict a single male; 6BM is the "mother–son" card; 7BM is the "father–son" card; 4 and 10 show a male and female in a heterosexual relationship, with the male in a physically dominant position. Only Card 2, with a female in the foreground and a man and woman in the background, is not male dominated. Thus, it is difficult to know whether the finding that older women subjects show declining evidence of active mastery is a reflection of their feelings about themselves (i.e., older women), which would be in disagreement with the findings of Neugarten and Gutmann (1968), or whether this is their perception of older men, which would agree with Neugarten and Gutmann's findings. If this is so—that the responses of women in this study reflect their attitudes about men, not women, then the increase in the magical mystery style is less a reflection of changes with age in the personality of women than it is a change in women's perception of men. From this point of view, the findings would also be interpreted to mean that both men and women, as they age, perceive men as being less active, but only men perceive themselves as being more passive whereas women perceive them as being more irrational.

This same approach, using TAT stories to determine adult developmental differences in styles of ego mastery, has continued to be used by

TABLE 12.2. Relationship between Ego Mastery Styles, Age, and Sex

	Age 40–49		Age 50–59		Age 60–70	
	Men	Women	Men	Women	Men	Women
Active mastery	59%	53%	39%	40%	24%	21%
Passive mastery	27%	22%	39%	33%	47%	29%
Magical mastery	14%	25%	22%	27%	29%	50%

Note. Adapted from Gutmann (1964). Copyright 1964 by Henry Holt Publishers. Adapted by permission.

Gutmann in cross-cultural studies (Gutmann, 1985). Stories from younger and older men in Navajo, Lowland Maya, and Highland Maya societies have consistently shown that the younger men had the highest proportion of active mastery responses, which markedly declined among the older men, who were more likely to show passive or magical mastery styles. These cross-sectional findings were replicated in longitudinal TAT studies from both Navajo and Druse societies. Although there was some variation across societies in the rate and degree of change in the mastery styles, the general developmental sequence—active, then passive, then magical mastery—was maintained.

Ego mastery styles, as assessed from TAT stories, were also found to differ in women as a function of differences in life-span developmental level (pre- or postempty nest). Cooper and Gutmann (1987) studied the ego mastery styles of middle-aged women who either did or did not have at least one child under age 18 still living at home. All the women, ages 43 to 51, were currently employed as teachers and had been continuously employed for 6 to 29 years. Stories were told about five TAT cards (1, 2, 4, 7GF, and 17BM). For all except Card 1, the stories of the "pre-empty nest" women made greater use of the passive mastery style, whereas those of the "post-empty nest" women showed greater use of active mastery. The authors related these findings to the "parental imperative perspective," which suggests that during the developmental period of parenthood "the female's masculine traits, such as aggression, must be repressed in order to preserve the harmonious atmosphere which is optimal for the successful raising of the children" (p. 347). However, once the active parenting period is concluded, this repression is no longer necessary, and these assertive traits can now be manifest.[13]

The empty nest syndrome was also studied, using the TAT, by Bedford (1989). In this study, Bedford was interested in how the presence or absence of children might affect the parents' attitudes or feelings about their own siblings. Sixty adults between the ages of 30 and 69 were assigned to either the child-rearing group, meaning that at least one child was still a minor and had not left home, or the empty nest group, meaning that all the subject's children were grown and no longer lived at home. There were an equal number of men and women in each group. Each subject also had a living sibling who was within a 3-year age span of the subject. TAT cards were adapted to show pairs of same-sex characters of about the same age; these figures were described to the subjects as being "sisters" or "brothers." Written stories to these six pictures were coded for the occurrence of themes of affiliation, conflict, and separation. The results indicated that the two adult groups (children present vs. empty nest) did not differ in the frequency of affiliative or conflict themes, but those adults—both women and men—who were still raising their own children showed more concern about sibling separation. Although not discussed by the author, it may be assumed that this group was also younger and thus closer in time to their own childhood and their shared experiences with siblings. The study also found that women expressed more sibling conflict in their stories than did men, regardless of their child-rearing status.

In a further study of adult developmental differences, Rosen and Neugarten (1964) used the TAT to focus on the "ego energy" of men and women from three age groups (40 to 49, 50 to 59, and 64 to 71), representing three socioeconomic classes. Available ego energy was measured along four dimensions: ability to integrate wide ranges of stimuli, readiness to perceive or deal with conflictful situations, tendency to perceive vigorous and assertive activity, and tendency to perceive or be concerned with feelings and affects. The results indicated a steady and significant decrease with age on each of the four measures. There were no differences attributable to sex or social class. The authors concluded:

> The differences among the age groups lend support to the hypothesis that with increased age there is less energy available to the ego for responding to, or maintaining former levels of involvement in, the outside world. The implication is that the older person tends to respond to inner rather than to outer stimuli, to withdraw emotional investments, to give up self-assertiveness, and to avoid rather than to embrace challenge. (p. 99)

Again, it should be noted that all but one of the five TAT cards came from the "masculine" set.

This cross-sectional study was followed up with an investigation by Lubin (cited in Neugarten, 1964), who retested 93 of Rosen and Neugarten's subjects 5 years later 14 and compared their ego energy scores from the two occasions. Of the four age groups studied, three (ages 55 to 59, 60 to 64, and 65 to 69 at the second testing occasion) showed a significant decrease in ego energy from time 1 to time 2. The failure to find this change among the very oldest subjects (ages 70 to 76) was explained by the author in terms of the unusual health and robustness of this group of individuals who had successfully survived into the seventh decade of life.

Emotional Stance

The TAT "emotional stance" measure of Stewart, discussed in Chapter 15, has been used for studies of change or transition in adults, generally showing a lower emotional stance level during the transitional period. Important life transitions for adults occur around the experiences of marriage and parenthood. A cross-sectional study (Stewart et al., 1982) compared the emotional stance level of individuals planning to be married (currently engaged) with those who were recently married. Both the recently married women and men had lower stance scores than did the engaged women.[15]

A longitudinal study (Stewart et al., 1986) added to these findings. A comparison of the emotional stance of men and women who were just beginning marriage with that found a year or two later indicated a shift to a higher emotional stance at the later date.

In studying the effects of the significant life changes of parenthood, it appeared that the process of adaptation differed for men and women, and that the effect of other experiences during this time of life made it difficult to establish clear patterns of change in emotional stance. A cross-sectional study of couples who were either expecting or had given birth to a first child (Stewart et al., 1982) revealed an interaction between transitional group and sex: Men showed the transitional effect (lower emotional stance) prior to the birth of the child, with a higher score after the birth, whereas women showed the opposite results, with a lower stance score following the birth of the child. A longitudinal follow-up of these expectant and new parents 2 years later (Stewart, Sokol, Healy, & Chester, 1986) failed to show any simple overall pattern of change in emotional stance.

THE RELATIONSHIP BETWEEN TAT MOTIVATIONAL MEASURES AND SUBSEQUENT BEHAVIOR: LONGITUDINAL STUDIES

Several longitudinal studies have demonstrated that TAT measures of nAchievement, nAffiliation, nPower, and other motivational measures are successful predictors of subsequent behavior. In an investigation carried out at the American Telephone and Telegraph Company, McClelland and Boyatzis (1982) administered six TAT cards to 311 male entry-level managers. These stories were then scored for nAchievement, nAffiliation, nPower (Winter's system), Activity Inhibition, and Stewart's emotional stances (also termed "stages of adaptation"). Scores were corrected for protocol length and transformed to standard scores,[16] allowing direct comparisons across the various measures. Of particular interest in this study was the assessment of the leadership motive pattern (LMP), defined as (1) nPower standard score equal to or greater than 45 and equal to or greater than the nAffiliation standard score, (2) activity inhibition standard score greater than the median, and (3) a raw score of activity inhibition greater than or equal to 2.

The job performance of these men was followed up 8 years later (n = 262) and again 16 years later (n = 246) in order to determine the level of management they had attained and the type of managerial position held. "Technical" managers were in positions involving the construction, installation, and maintenance or repair of telephone equipment; "non-technical" managers were in positions involving customer services, accounting, marketing, administration, and personnel-related functions. The results of the study indicated that those men who had shown the leadership motive pattern on entry into the company had reached higher levels of management at both the 8- and 16-year follow-up than had men not showing this pattern. However, this finding occurred only for men who were in nontechnical managerial positions. Stewart's measure of emotional stance was also found to be related to level of management attained after 8 years, for nontechnical managers; those individuals who had earlier scored at stages III and IV had attained higher levels of management that those who had scored at stages I and II. Interestingly, nAchievement was not related to management level either 8 or 16 years later, although the highest nAchievement scores were found within the nontechnical managers who were at a low management level (level 3, on a 7-point scale) 16 years later. Overall, the results were interpreted to mean that managerial success in these positions was associated with (1) concern about influencing others, (2) less concern about being liked, and (3) a moderate to high degree of self-control. However, for men in technical managerial positions, the TAT measures of motivation had little predictive power.

In a second longitudinal study of men (Winter, Stewart, & McClelland, 1977), nPower was found to be significantly, although negatively, related to the career level of the men's wives. The TAT stories given by 51 men when they were freshmen at a prestigious New England college were scored for nAchievement, nAffiliation, nPower, and self-definition (Stewart & Winter, 1974; see Chapter 15). Seventeen years later, a follow-up questionnaire was given to these men which asked for details of their present life, including their career and their wife's career. The wife's career was coded on a 4-point scale, ranging from no work outside home (scored 1) to lifetime career in a field traditionally male (scored 4). The husbands' TAT scores from their freshman year were then related to the wives' later career levels. The results indicated that the wife's career level was negatively related to the husband's nPower score (Winter's system), positively related to the husband's nAffiliation score, and unrelated to the husband's nAchievement score. In addition, there was a positive but insignificant relationship between the husband's scores on self-definition and the wife's career level.[17]

The authors offered three possible explanations for the negative relationship between the husband's freshman nPower score and the subsequent career level of his wife. It is possible that the husband's nPower motive influenced the kind of wife he chose. It is also possible that the wife's choice of a husband was affected by her perception of his motives and suitability for her career plans. Finally, the husband's motives could have led him, after marriage, either to encourage or discourage his wife's choice and striving in a career.

In a third longitudinal study, McAdams and Vaillant (1982) investigated the relationship between TAT measures of motivation and subsequent psychological adjustment. The study involved 57 Harvard men who had been part of the large-scale Grant Study of Adult Development. These men, drawn from Harvard classes of 1942–1944, had been selected on the basis of being psychologically "sound." At age 30, they were given the TAT; stories from five of the cards were used to score nAchievement, nAffiliation, nPower (Winter's system), and nIntimacy. Over the next 17 years, the psychological adjustment of the men was determined from information about income level, occupational promotion and enjoyment, days of sick leave, marital enjoyment, regular vacations, pastimes with friends, drug or alcohol misuse, and psychiatric visits. To determine the relationship between motive score and adjustment, a mean split was used to divide the subjects into high- and low-motive groups; the adjustment scores of the two groups were then compared. The results indicated that higher adjustment scores were obtained by subjects who were high in nAchievement, nAffiliation, and nIntimacy, but only the last comparison was statistically significant. Within this group of men selected for psychological soundness, nIntimacy as determined from the TAT at age 30 was a significant predictor of psychological adjustment nearly 20 years later.

Finally, in a study that included both women and men, Skolnick (1966a, 1966b) examined the TAT stories of subjects who had participated in the Oakland Growth Study. Stories were told once when the subjects were ages 17 to 18, and again 20 years later.[18] However, different pictures were used on the two occasions, making longitudinal comparisons somewhat difficult. The stories were scored for nAchievement, nAffiliation, and nPower.[19] Several categories of aggression were also scored. The TAT scores from late adolescence and middle adulthood were correlated with a large number of behavioral and personality measures from both time periods, for males and females separately. Many correlations among the variables were calculated, and the question whether the significant results exceed chance expectation—not tested by the author—must be kept in mind while discussing the findings.[20]

The results of this study are numerous and complex. Although the focus in this section of the book is on longitudinal relationships, there were also a number of interesting findings from this investigation showing relationships between TAT motivational measures and personality/behavioral variables during adolescence, and again during adulthood. These findings are presented first, followed by the longitudinal results.

During adolescence, boys' scores for nPower were positively related to drive for control, overt aggression, leadership, being social, having an effect on the group, prestige, and self-assertiveness. Boys' scores for nAchievement were not related to personality or behavioral variables. For girls, however, nAchievement was positively related to IQ and nPower was related to leadership in high school. Scores on nAffiliation in adolescence were not related to the personality or behavioral variables for either boys or girls.

In adulthood, *nPower* scores for the males showed a similar pattern of positive correlations with personality and behavioral variables to that seen in adolescence: leadership, being social, having an effect on the group, prestige, and self-assertiveness in senior high school were all found to be related to adult nPower scores. For the females in adulthood, as was true for the adolescents, there were few significant correlations with nPower. In adulthood, *nAchievement* was correlated with adolescent and adult IQ and with adolescent strictness of superego, for both men and women. For adult men, nAchievement was correlated with the California Psychological Inventory (CPI) measure of achievement via conformity, whereas for women nAchievement correlated with the CPI measure of achievement via independence. This latter finding suggested to the author an interesting sex difference in the meaning of nAchievement: Women who are high in nAchievement appear to be more individualistic, different, and expressive than high nAchievement men, who are more conforming (Skolnick, 1966a).

For adult men, *nAffiliation* was negatively related to the adult CPI measure of sociability. For women, there was a negative relationship between nAffiliation and adolescent drive ratings of succorance.[21] Skolnick suggests that the nAffiliation measure in adulthood may thus be seen as compensatory, reflecting deprivation or lack of affiliation but not lack of striving in this area.

This study also demonstrated longitudinal consistency in TAT-based motivational dispositions over a period of 20 years. For men, a significant correlation was found between adolescent and adult TAT scores for both nPower and for the general category of aggression; for women there were significant correlations across the years for nAchievement, nAffiliation, and the aggression subcategories of verbal aggression and victimization (Skolnick, 1966b). In addition, for the women, adolescent scores on nAchievement correlated with aggression as observed in adult interviews.

Overall, the findings of this study showed longitudinal consistencies in motivational scores derived from the TAT, although these consistencies over time differed for males and females. There were also meaningful and direct relationships between the TAT measures and related behaviors, as measured by ratings or situational observations, both in adolescence and adulthood. Again, these differed according to age and sex. In general, adolescent behavioral scores predicted adult TAT scores better than adolescent TAT scores predicted adult behaviors. This finding has been interpreted to mean that the TAT motivational imagery is more a result than a cause of action (McClelland, 1966).

The findings of Skolnick (1966a, 1966b) were refined in a study by Elder and MacInnis (1983), who focused on the relationship between nAchievement in adolescent females and subsequent adult behavior. The database consisted of nAchievement scores, as coded by Skolnick (1966a, 1966b), of adolescent girls ages 17 and 18 years, information obtained from the Strong Vocational Interest Blank (SVIB) at that time, and information about the lives of these women as young adults.[22] The primary question behind this study was whether nAchievement in women might have different manifestations in those who were oriented toward educational advancement and a career, as compared to women whose orientation was family-centered and domestic. In order to determine the career or family orientation of the adolescent girls, a counselor highly experienced with interpreting the SVIB used its results to establish two groups of girls. One group was considered to have a wholly domestic interest pattern; the other group had a partly career focus and partly domestic interest pattern. These two vocational groups might be expected to follow different life trajectories in the expression of nAchievement. For the first, domestic group, achievement might be expressed through mate selection, marriage, and building a family. For partly career-focused women, nAchievement might be expressed through personal accomplishments in work and community.

When adolescent nAchievement scores were correlated with these later-life events, it was found, as predicted, that the career-oriented women with high nAchievement married later and had their first child at a later age as compared to those with lower nAchievement and as compared to those women who had a domestic orientation. Among the domestically oriented women, those with high nAchievement reported having a greater number of children and greater marital satisfaction than did those with lower nAchievement. These factors were not related to nAchievement for the women with career interests.[23] Overall, adolescent nAchievement was significantly related to later-life events, but the pattern of these correlations was quite different for the two groups of women.

One other longitudinal study has investigated the relationship between a single TAT measure and behavior of the subjects at a later point in time. Stewart (1978) studied the relationship between women's TAT scores on a measure of self-definition/social definition (see Chapter 15) and their subsequent life responses to stressful situations. TAT stories were obtained from 57 female first-year students attending a prestigious New England college and were scored for the self/social definition. Seventeen years later, when these women were 31 years old, they were interviewed about stress and their response to stress. The results confirmed the hypotheses that self-defining women tend to see a *problem*, regardless of its content, as located in the environment, rather than within the self. However, they tend to see the *solution* to the problem as located within themselves, and thus they may reasonably plan to initiate action to solve the problem. Self-defining women were thus more likely to make instrumental responses to their problems, whereas socially defined women made noninstrumental responses or no active responses at all. The results also confirmed the hypotheses that self-defining women are better able to clearly articulate the nature of their problems and their solution, to identify more causes of these problems, and to present their problems in a broad social context.

SUMMARY

This chapter has focused on the ways in which the TAT has been used to study developmental differences in adults. The results of these investigations have yielded consistent findings.[24] In two large-scale studies, the TAT was used to investigate motivational differences as a function of age. The two studies produced quite similar findings, although they were conducted 20 years apart. In both 1957 and 1976, for men, nAchievement was found to remain relatively constant from early to middle adulthood, with some decrease found after the ages 50 to 55. Likewise, both studies found the nAffiliation of men to remain unchanged across the adult life span, while nPower (hope for power) was found to be higher during middle age, especially ages 40 to 49.

The results were also largely consistent for women. Both nAchievement and nAffiliation were found to decrease across the adult life span, and there were no consistent changes with age found for nPower. However, although there were no cohort effects for men (i.e., age, rather than birthdate, was the primary factor determining the results of the two studies) for women, cohorts did appear to make a difference for achievement motivation. Women who began their adulthood in the 1950s did not show the drop in nAchievement over the ensuing 20 years that would have been predicted from the cross-sectional data obtained from the first study. Presumably, changing social conditions for women during that period contributed to their maintaining a higher level of achievement motivation. Social status has also been found to interact with age in relation to women's scores on power motivation.

Longitudinal studies, comparing the TAT scores of the same individuals from late adolescence with those obtained 20 years later found significant consistencies in the nPower and aggression scores of men, and in the nAchievement and nAffiliation scores of women. Although these results are somewhat different than those obtained from the cross-sectional data discussed earlier, there are several possible reasons for this. First, although the *mean* level of any dimension may increase or decrease from one time to another, if the ranking of subjects on that dimension remains the same, the correlation between the two sets of scores will be significant, indicating that there is consistency across time. Second, the longitudinal results reviewed here cover only the beginning years of adulthood; it is not known whether the consistencies would continue after age 38 (the age at second testing).

Further TAT studies of developmental differences across the later years of life were consistent in showing that, during the ages from 40 to 70, men and women increasingly perceive the male personality as less active, more submissive, and having less ego energy available. Men also increasingly perceive the male personality as being more passive and somewhat more irrational, whereas women perceive the male personality as being strikingly more irrational. It is less clear how the perception of the female personality changes with age, owing to the biased selection of TAT cards in the majority of the studies. In the single study to present cards with both male and female figures and to ask explicitly for a description of each gender, there was a clear age-related shift in the perception of the (older) female figure, from an attitude of being submissive, subordinate, benign, and nurturant to one of being dominant, authoritative, self-assertive, and aggressive.

Longitudinal studies with adults have found that TAT measures do, in some cases, successfully predict future behavior. For example, scores on leadership motive pattern obtained from men entering the work force significantly predicted the type of managerial position obtained by the men up to 16 years later. A measure of emotional stance was successful in predicting, 8 years later, the management level reached by these men.

Another longitudinal study demonstrated a relationship between college men's power motivation scores and the career level of their wives, as determined 17 years later. A further study demonstrated that the TAT scores for intimacy motivation derived at age 30 were a significant predictor of psychological adjustment some 20 years later. A longitudinal study of college women found that those who scored high on the "self-definition" dimension of the TAT (as compared to "social definition"), when interviewed 17 years later about their responses to stress, were more likely to perceive solutions to problems as located within themselves and to make instrumental responses to those problems. Those women who had earlier scored high on the "social definition" dimension made noninstrumental or no responses to problems.

On the other hand, adolescent TAT measures of nAchievement, nPower, and nAffiliation, although showing some consistency with similar measures taken 20 years later, were relatively unsuccessful for predicting to selected *ratings* of adult drives and demographic status. However, a refinement of the research strategy taking into account different vocational interest patterns of the women in the study demonstrated a relationship between strength of adolescent nAchievement and subsequent adult behavior.

Considering the broad range of subjects, ages, personality variables, and TAT measures discussed in this chapter, it is clear that a systematic approach to storytelling has proven to be a successful research strategy in the study of adult development.

• SECTION V •
RESEARCH ISSUES WITH THE TAT

• THIRTEEN •

General Issues
in TAT Research

To carry out research in which the TAT is used as a means for studying personality, the researcher should be aware of a number of important issues—issues that emerge repeatedly in critical analyses of the TAT. Although these issues are often debated on a semiphilosophical level, there is in fact a body of research that has attempted to provide empirical knowledge relevant to the debated concerns. In this chapter, these issues and the relevant research are presented.

One issue that arises in both research and clinical contexts revolves around the choice of TAT cards to be used. The issue here is whether the particular selection of cards serves to bias or skew the results. Certain cards, it appears, are more likely to elicit story themes of one type, whereas other cards seem to "pull" for different types of stories. To assess card pull, knowledge about normative stories is helpful. However, it is also important to consider what is known about gender differences in reaction to TAT pictures, as well as information regarding independent evaluations of the pictures themselves. The first section of this chapter considers those issues related to card pull.

Another issue is whether the original TAT cards, which depict white, middle-class characters, are appropriate for use with minority subjects. An extensive series of studies contrasting the TAT with a storytelling measure developed for use with minorities are presented in this chapter.

A third issue of importance is how, or whether, the length of story a subject tells is relevant to the evaluation of that story, when standard coding procedures are used. It has been proposed, for example, that evidence for validity of the TAT measure of achievement motivation—namely, the correlation between the TAT measure and a criterion measure of achievement—was entirely spurious, due only to differences in story

233

length across subjects (Entwisle, 1972). Several correction methods that have been proposed to adjust scores for story length are discussed in this chapter.

CARD PULL

From early on, it was recognized that the different TAT cards tended to elicit different types of stories, needs, motives, and affects. Card pull refers to this phenomena. A summary of some early research in this area appears in Bellak (1975, pp. 153–154, 161) and in Murstein (1961, pp. 234–268). A theoretical discussion of the issue is provided by Peterson and Schilling (1983).

The issue of card pull has been addressed in two different ways. In the more frequent approach, a description of themes commonly elicited by each card is provided; that is, card pull is assessed in terms of the types of stories told about the picture. In the second approach, the stimulus picture itself is evaluated, independent of any story that might be told. Each of these approaches is discussed here.

Normative Stories

Several authors have provided extensive discussions of the typical story themes generated by the various TAT cards (e.g., Bellak, 1954, 1975; Henry, 1956; Holt, 1978; Rapaport et al., 1946; Stein, 1955). A most comprehensive discussion of common themes is provided by Holt (1978), who reviews and distills the findings of some 20 different studies of "norms" for the TAT. Holt integrates and summarizes this material for each card, indicating, for example, the percentage of subjects in various studies who described the pictures in a particular way (e.g., the characters' sex, status, illness, and defects) as well as typical themes and omissions. This source is probably the most complete set of "norms" (largely qualitative) available for the TAT on a picture-by-picture basis.[1]

Generally, it has been noted that some cards pull for stories about parent–child or family relations (e.g., Cards 1, 2, 6BM, 6GF, 7BM, and 7GF), whereas others pull for stories about heterosexual relationships (Cards 4, 10, and 13MF). Additional pictures will pull for stories with themes of aggression (Cards 3BM, 8BM, 11, 12M, 13MF, and 18GF), or will be prone to elicit depressive ideation (Cards 3BM, 3GF, 9GF, 12BG, 14, 15, and 17GF). Finally, some cards are more likely to pull for thematic material expressing a concern about being controlled by others, sometimes with homosexual overtones (e.g., Cards 5, 12M, 17BM, and 18BM). Generally, the clinician selects a set of pictures that samples each type of card pull in order to tap into the storyteller's functioning in these important areas of personality. That is, the selection of different stimulus cards is purposely used to pull for different types of information about the storyteller's personality.

This strategy is often very helpful for clinical purposes, both in revealing the individual's way of responding to significant psychological areas and by indicating areas that are either avoided or overly stressed. For example, if Card 13MF fails to elicit a story involving heterosexuality, or if Card 1 prompts a story filled with aggression, these are deviations from the typical card pull, and thus are significant.

Murstein (1961) noted that the first 10 cards are more likely to elicit material that is emotionally relevant to the storyteller. Thus clinicians tend to use these cards more than the second 10, which tend to elicit stories of a more impersonal, symbolic nature. However, "the meaningfulness of stories for personality evaluation seems to follow a curvilinear relationship with ambiguity, with the medium-ambiguous pictures facilitating the expression of the most revealing stories" (Murstein, 1961, p. 242).

In a systematic study of card pull, Ehrenreich (1990) compared the stories given by 70 female college students about five frequently used TAT cards (Cards 1, 2, 3BM, 12M, and 13MF). Each story was scored on four dimensions: drive expression, defensive pattern, dependency pattern, and locus of control[2]; the results showed that their occurrence was statistically different across cards. Higher drive expression was elicited on Cards 3BM, 12, and 13MF than on Cards 1 and 2. Lower-level defenses were more frequent on Cards 3BM and 13MF; higher-level defenses were more frequent on Card 2. Internal locus of control was more frequent on Card 2, whereas external locus of control was more frequent on the other cards. Likewise, independence of characters was more frequent on Card 2, whereas dependence was more frequent on Cards 1, 3BM, and 12M.[3] Unfortunately, the generalizability of these findings are limited by the subject sample being entirely female.

One further study of card pull investigated the direction of the climber on Card 17BM, in connection with the hypothesis that climbing *up* would be associated with an optimistic personality and climbing *down* with a pessimistic personality (George & Waehler, 1994). The results failed to find an association between optimism–pessimism and direction of climbing. However, differences in climbing direction were associated with sex, with women more likely (64%) to see the character as climbing up than men (35%).[4]

Related to the issue of card pull, some TAT cards have been found to elicit a wider variety of themes than others. For example, in a study by Newmark and Flouranzano (1973), 20 TAT cards were given to 30 white male hospitalized psychiatric patients, ages 26 to 49. The top 10 cards, in terms of number of themes elicited, were, in rank order: 4, 1, 3BM, 13MF, 12M, 18BM, 8BM, 2, 6BM, and 7BM. A similar study by Cooper (1981), with 75 adolescent males, ages 11, 14, and 17, found seven of the same cards to be among the top 10 in terms of number of themes elicited.[5] Haynes and Peltier (1985), studying adolescent male delinquents, interestingly, found that nine of the cards identified by Neumark and Flouranzano (1973) were identified by clinicians as those used most often. These studies show considerable agreement regarding usefulness of the different cards, although determined in quite different ways.[6]

Gender Differences

As in the above study, it has also been found that different TAT cards pull for different types of stories as a function of the storyteller's sex, a finding that provides a confounding condition with Murray's original idea that there should be separate male and female cards. In a well-designed study to investigate this issue (Worchel, Aaron, & Yates, 1990), it was found that the "female" TAT cards (i.e., those labeled "GF"), in comparison to the "male" ("BM") TAT cards, elicited more "general concern" themes from *both* men and women storytellers. These general concern themes included issues of separation, effort, conflict, ambivalence, acceptance, fear, escape, verbal hostility, and sexuality—issues I would characterize as being concerns about relationships with other people.[7] However, themes of withdrawal and anxiety occurred as a function of an interaction between stimulus card sex and subject sex: The female TAT cards elicited more withdrawal themes and more anxiety from men subjects, whereas the male TAT cards elicited more withdrawal themes and more anxiety from women subjects.

The findings of this study, based on a factorial design (men and women storytellers responded to male and female TAT cards) are important for understanding both the question of card pull and that of sex differences in TAT stories. As pointed out by Worchel et al. (1990), previous research designs often confounded subject sex with TAT card sex (see the review of 25 years of research on the question of sex differences in TAT stories by Stewart & Chester, 1982). Although these studies used both male and female TAT cards, very often only female subjects were studied. For example, in studying achievement motivation, and using the standard male arousal procedure prior to the TAT storytelling, six of the eight studies reviewed used women subjects only. The majority of these studies showed that male TAT cards elicited higher achievement scores. Further, a review of studies that used a gender-relevant arousal procedure (Stewart & Chester, 1982) showed that five of the six studies used women subjects only; two of these studies found an interaction between arousal condition and sex of TAT card. In reviewing the research on affiliation motivation, only one study was found in which both male and female TAT cards were used, and this study included only women subjects. The results indicated that women had higher affiliation scores, following arousal, on the female TAT cards. However, the need for a full factorial design before interpreting this finding is clear once one reconsiders the finding of Worchel et al. (1990) that female TAT cards elicited more material dealing with interpersonal relationships for both men and women.

Further information on the interaction between sex of TAT card and sex of subject comes from a study by Chusmir (1983, 1985). Using a population of men and women working managers in their early 30s who were studying in a graduate program of business administration, half the group was given McClelland's standard six pictures for measuring achievement, affiliation, and power motivation. The other half of the subjects were given a "balanced for sex" set of six pictures in which half the pictures depicted females and half males. The results indicated that the sex of the TAT pictures had no significant main or interaction effects for scores on achievement or power motivation. However, the balanced-sex pictures produced higher *affiliation* scores than did the male-only pictures, and this effect was stronger in the women subjects than in the men. These findings confirm and extend those reported by Stewart and Chester (1982). However, it should be noted that the subject sample is rather atypical.

A further study (Katz, Russ, & Overholser, 1993) investigated the hypothesis that storytellers would identify more with stimulus characters of the same sex as themselves, which was the original rationale for having "male" and "female" TAT cards. However, examining the stories of college students told to three male and three female cards, there were no gender-based differences in the amount of fantasy, affect, or length of stories for the two types of cards.

An additional study by Pollak and Gilligan (1982) found that the production of violent imagery in stories differed as a function of the interaction of gender and thematic context. Using two TAT-like pictures which pulled for themes of affiliation (a man looking at a picture of his family; a couple sitting on a bench by a river) and two which pulled for themes of achievement (two women in lab coats; two acrobats on a trapeze), they found that college men gave more violent images to situations involving affiliation, whereas college women gave more violent imagery to situations involving achievement. Subsequent studies, however, did not replicate these results (Benton et al., 1983; McAdams, Lester, Brand, & Lensky, 1988; Weiner et al., 1983).[8]

Cue Value of Picture

A different approach to assessing card pull has been to obtain an evaluation of the content of the TAT cards independently from the types of stories they might elicit. Indeed, the original selection of cards was based on the idea that pictures with males as the main characters would elicit better stories from men, whereas pictures with females would elicit better stories from women.

A systematic study of the cue value of pictures, independent of the stories written about the pictures, was carried out by Jacobs (1958), who asked subjects to rank order 12 TAT and TAT-like pictures for the "concerns" being expressed by the person(s) in the picture. The concerns included descriptions of achievement, affiliation, power, avoidance of failure, hunger and thirst, sex, safety, and guilt, among others. Results giving the mean rank value for each concern, for each picture, are provided. Differences in the cue value of pictures for affiliation were noted to be helpful in explaining discrepancies in earlier studies of affiliation in that some of these studies used stimulus pictures with a high cue value for affiliation, whereas others used (different) pictures in which the cue value was lower.

A similar procedure was used by Birney (1958) who determined college students' ratings of magazine pictures for the presence of various achievement themes. The overall achievement score rating for each picture was then compared with achievement motivation scores obtained from stories written about those pictures by a different group of college men. The results indicated a reasonably strong correlation between the rating of picture "pull" for achievement themes and the actual presence of those themes in the stories written.

Yet another study by Haber and Alpert (1958) used the rating procedure described above, as well as a picture paired-comparison technique to determine the achievement pull for a set of pictures. Subsequently, the achievement motivation scores for stories written to these pictures by a different group of subjects were found to be highly correlated with the subjects' achievement ratings. However, when the story writers themselves were asked to rate the pictures for achievement themes, the correlation between their own ratings for individual pictures and the achievement imagery in their individual stories to those pictures was close to zero.[9]

In another approach to assessing the characteristics of the TAT cards themselves, subjects were asked to select, from a group of three cards, the one that was most different (Alvarado, 1994). Each card was regrouped with other cards and judged a number of times. Degree of similarity was found to correspond more to the affective tone of the relationship depicted in the pictures rather than to the normative themes that appear in subjects' stories.

A different approach to assess card pull was used by Campus (1976). Using a separate set of cards for men and women, subjects were asked to write a story for each card, imagining that they themselves were a person in the picture. Then, they were asked to rate this person on a list of adjectives, chosen to represent 17 of Murray's (1938) needs.[10] Campus (1976) provides a list of cards with high and low ratings on each need for men and women separately, and the stimulus ambiguity (i.e., variability in ratings across subjects) of each card is given. This is an interesting approach to measuring card pull, although the results may be more descriptive of the subjects than of the TAT cards.

There are many other examples of card pull that are apparent from observation of the results reported in the research literature. Typically, researchers will selectively use those TAT cards that pull best for the psychological trait or motive being studied.[11] Thus, both from the research literature and from clinical description, it is clear that the results obtained from any investigation using the TAT will be significantly determined by the choice of TAT cards used and, more complicated, by the interaction of storyteller sex with the cards chosen. As shown later, the interaction with subject ethnicity may also be an important factor.

These findings regarding card pull have implications for certain kinds of research with the TAT. As discussed by Veroff et al. (1960), if the investigator wants to contrast the relative strength of several different TAT motive scores within the same sample of subjects, attention must be given to card pull. Because we know that some TAT cards "pull" for the expression of one motive and others pull for different motives, the relative strength of each motive will vary according to the selection of TAT cards used. Thus, the mean score for motive X may be consistently higher than that for motive Y, and Y higher than Z, not because of "true" differences in motive strength but because of differential card pull. In this case, the absolute score indicating a very strong expression of motive Z may not approach the average score obtained for motive X. In order to make the distribution of scores for each motive equivalent (have equivalent meaning), Veroff et al. (1960) suggest using the separate score distributions to assign percentile ranks to the scores for each motive. These percentile rank scores then provide a common "scale" whereby the strengths of the several motive scores may be compared. However, because percentile scores do not represent an interval scale and may not be further manipulated algebraically, an additional transformation of the percentile scores through normalizing the distribution of percentile ranks (assigning a mean score of 50 and a standard deviation of 10; that is, creating standard T scores) is suggested. In the Veroff et al. (1960) study, these T scores

removed the differences among mean scores across the different measures of motivation and across sex. However, the correlations between
story length and T scores were nearly identical as those between story
length and raw scores, so that a correction for story length was still
necessary.[12]

Research Cards

In addition to these standard TAT cards, other pictures have been
developed for use in research studies and with special populations. For
example, May (1980) found in his studies of sexual identity that a picture
of a man and woman swinging on a trapeze is most successful in eliciting
relevant stories, and McAdams (1982a), studying intimacy motivation,
successfully used a picture of two persons sitting on a park bench. Pictures
of these and other research cards, and the areas of personality investigation in which they have been used, are provided in Atkinson (1958), in
McClelland and Steele (1972), and, recently, in Smith (1992).

Other sets of pictures have been developed for use with such special
subject groups as children (see Chapter 11), senior adults (see Chapter
12), and minority groups including Native Americans, African-Americans, and Hispanics (see Costantino, Malgady, Rogler, & Tsui, 1988).
Indeed, of 66 research studies reviewed between 1978 and 1988 which
were reported as using the TAT,[13] only 29 clearly used Murray's cards; 17
studies clearly did not use TAT cards although "TAT" was included in the
title of the research paper. For the remaining 20 studies it was not possible
to determine which cards were used (Keiser & Prather, 1990).

SPECIAL CARDS FOR MINORITY GROUPS

A second general issue to be considered when using the TAT for research
or clinical purposes is that of "match" between the figures portrayed on
the stimulus cards and the racial/ethnic background of the storyteller.
For example, it has been noted that minority children often given minimal
responses to such projective tests as the TAT and suggested that this might
be due to a difficulty in identifying with the white characters shown in
the TAT pictures. For this reason, a number of investigators have attempted to develop alternate sets of pictures in which the characteristics
of the people depicted are similar to those of the minority group being
tested.[14] Various attempts to develop sets of cards appropriate for Native
Americans and for separate Indian tribes have been discussed by Dana
(1986). For African-Americans, Thompson (1949) changed the white
figures of 10 of the TAT cards into black figures and found that African-

American male college students' story length was increased, as compared to the length of stories given to the standard pictures of Murray's TAT.

However, as pointed out by Costantino, Malgady, and Vazquez (1981), subsequent studies failed to confirm Thompson's results.[15] Bailey and Green (1977) suggested that this failure might be due to the way in which the black TAT cards were constructed—namely, simply by putting dark skin on white characters. For this reason, Bailey and Green (1977) constructed an experimental set of TAT cards in which the characters were drawn to show African-American facial features, hair texture, and style of dress. The responses of African-American male high school and college students, and adult noncollege students (ages 25 to 45) to these experimental TAT cards were compared with responses to Murray's original TAT and to Thompson's modified TAT. The results of this study were interesting in that they showed that while the African-American subjects rated the tests with black characters as facilitating their story production (as compared to Murray's test with white characters), in fact there was no difference, across tests in the actual expression of four of Murray's needs—nAchievement, nAggression, nSex, and nSuccorance. The subjects also made ratings of their ability to relate personal feelings to each test; the three tests did not differ. The results of this study thus indicate that the use of racially congruent stimulus cards may elicit some more positive ratings about the test material (and thus, perhaps, enhance test rapport), but that response content is unaffected. Contrary to the assertions of Costantino et al. (1981) and Lefkowitz and Fraser (1980), Bailey and Green (1977) did *not* report that the black TAT pictures elicited longer protocols than the white TAT cards.

In another study of possible content differences in responses to Murray's TAT and to Thompson's TAT, the stories of African-American and white low socioeconomic status (SES) high school students were evaluated for "future-time perspective" (Sheikh & Twerski, 1974). The results indicated that white students showed a constricted time perspective on the black TAT but for African-American students there was no difference between the two tests.

The question of differences in story content and story length by African-American subjects to white and black TATs has also been investigated using the Themes Concerning Blacks (TCB) pictures developed by Weaver (described in Triplett & Brunson, 1982). One study compared the stories of 5- to 8-year-old African-American boys and girls to TCB and TAT pictures; an attempt to match for similarity of content and character situation in the two tests was made (Triplett & Brunson, 1982). As in Weaver's original study, although the race of the characters depicted was identified correctly, there was no difference in story length between the TCB and the TAT. However, judges' ratings of the feeling tone of the stories to the two sets of cards differed:[16] The majority of the TCB stories were positive, whereas the majority of the TAT responses were negative.

A similar study of feeling-tone differences, using the TCB and TAT, was reported by Dlepu and Kimbrough (1982). The stories of African-American boys and girls ages 5 to 11 were rated for positive or negative feeling tone, and the children's picture card preferences were determined. Again, there was an attempt to match the TCB and TAT cards for common themes. Of the six "matched" pairs, for three the feeling tone was more positive for the TCB cards[17]; for one pair, the TAT card was more positive[18]; and for two pairs the differences were not great.[19] In general, the children preferred the TCB cards to the TAT cards, although the preferences were far from unanimous (boys, 70% to 30%; girls, 60% to 40%).

In the above studies, racial influences on the TAT responses generally have been evaluated by varying only one critical factor—the race of the stimulus figure. Only one study varied both race of stimulus figure and race of subject. To these two important factors, a third—race of test administrator—was added by Lefkowitz and Fraser (1980). African-American and white male college students either were given four of the standard Murray TAT cards or were given these cards redrawn so as to change skin tone, physiognomy, and hair texture to produce African-American figures. Stories were told individually to African-American or white male clinical psychologists and were subsequently scored for nAchievement and nPower,[20] corrected for protocol length. The results indicated that the two motive scores were not related to race of stimulus figure, to race of test administrator, or to race of subjects. Nor were any of the two-way interactions significant. However, white administrators elicited longer stories from both African-American and white subjects. In addition, length of story was *negatively* correlated with motive scores for African-Americans but showed a low positive correlation for whites, as is generally reported.

The issue of racial "pull" of stimulus pictures has also been investigated with Hispanic subjects, a group for whom there is relatively little information available regarding the appropriateness or validity of available personality tests (cf. Costantino, Malgady, & Rogler, 1988; Costantino, Malgady, Rogler, & Tsui, 1988). To remedy this situation, the Tell-Me-A-Story (TEMAS) test was constructed as a storytelling procedure for Hispanic students (Malgady, Costantino, & Rogler, 1984). The test consists of 23 chromatic pictures: 12 pictures are given to both sexes and 11 more are specific to one sex. The pictures portray Hispanic characters interacting in familiar urban settings and depict situations that require the resolution of a psychological conflict (e.g., complying with parents vs. playing with peers). The pictures were structured to pull for nine personality variables, described below; the authors report that experts judging the pictures reached 71–100% agreement regarding the "pull" of each picture.

The pictures are presented in random order, and subjects are asked to tell a 2- to 4-minute story that will answer three questions: What is happening in the picture now? What happened before? What is going to happen in the future? The examiner may conduct an additional inquiry if needed to elicit further information.

Each story is scored for nine personality variables, six structural variables, and five affective states. The personality variables are rated on a 4-point scale, with a score of 1 indicating a highly maladaptive solution and a score of 4 indicating a highly adaptive resolution in the story. The personality variables are: interpersonal relations, aggression, anxiety/depression, achievement motivation, delay of gratification, self-concept, sexual identity, moral judgment, and reality testing. The structural variables include verbal fluency (number of words), reaction time, total time, unanswered inquiries, omissions, and transformations. The affective states consist of happy, sad, angry, fearful, and neutral.

The psychometric properties of TEMAS were investigated with low SES Puerto Rican children (Malgady et al., 1984). A clinical group of 210 children (grades K–3) was selected on the basis of teacher referrals for maladaptive behavior; a nonclinical group consisted of 73 children from the same public schools (grades K–6) who were not undergoing psychotherapy and did not show personality disturbance or behavior problems. A comparison of the responses of the two subject groups (using only nine pictures) indicated that the public school group had more adaptive scores than did the clinical group on all of the nine personality variables; they also had higher scores on all affects, including anger and fearfulness, possibly indicating less defensiveness in this nonclinical group. On the other hand, the clinical group had higher scores on the structural variables of omissions, transformations, reaction time, and unanswered inquiries and a lower score (nonsignificant) for word fluency. These latter findings affirm the importance of formal as well as content variables in the use of storytelling techniques.

Although the authors report that age was not correlated with scores in the public school sample, in the clinical sample age was positively correlated with scores on word fluency, anxiety, and reality testing and negatively correlated with stimulus omissions and stimulus transformations. Given these findings, it is thus possible that age, rather than pathology, was responsible for the difference between the clinical and public school subjects on these variables, for there were relatively more young children in the clinical sample (grades K–3, $n = 210$), as compared to the nonclinical sample (grades K–6, $n = 73$). Estimates of reliability for the 20 variables—both interrater reliability and internal consistency—varied, being high for some dimensions and low for others.[21]

Estimates of concurrent validity were carried out with the clinical group, correlating the scores on all TEMAS variables (nine pictures) with eight criterion measures, including ego development, teacher behavior ratings, mother behavior ratings, delay of gratification, self-concept, disruptiveness, and aggression. All the TEMAS variables correlated with more than one of the criterion variables, with the exception of TEMAS aggression, which was unrelated to any criterion variable including the criterion measure of aggression. Likewise, TEMAS scores on "delay of gratification" were unrelated to the criterion measure of delay of gratification. Of the 160 possible correlations between 20 TEMAS and 8 criterion variables, 63 were significant. However, there is a lack of specificity or rationale for this host of obtained relationships. Instead, there is evidence that maladaptive scores on a variety of TEMAS variables are correlated with maladaptive scores on a variety of criterion variables, and that a total maladaptive TEMAS score might be expected to correlate with other measures of maladaptation. The meaning of the individual TEMAS variables, however, is less clear.

In an early study with the TEMAS (Costantino et al., 1981), urban Hispanic boys and girls ages 9 to 12 years old were given six pictures from the TEMAS test and six pictures from Murray's TAT. The results indicated greater verbal productivity (i.e., longer stories) to the TEMAS,[22] supporting the hypothesis that the typically shorter responses of minority children on projective tests is not due to some cognitive or verbal deficit but rather is a function of the ethnicity of the stimulus materials.

However, the authors did not consider the possibility that the greater verbal productivity to the TEMAS pictures by Hispanic students was due to the greater number of characters presented in the TEMAS pictures (27+ characters) than in the TAT pictures (8 characters). Even if the stories were limited to simple picture description, there are more characters to be described in TEMAS. To address this confound, one needs to know whether the same differences in verbal productivity would be found when non-Hispanics take the TAT and TEMAS and/or when the TEMAS pictures are redrawn with the characters having non-Hispanic features.

The above study was in fact carried out (Costantino & Malgady, 1983), although not for the reason indicated above. The stated purposes for this second study were to increase the number of TAT (17) and TEMAS (31) pictures used, with the intent of enhancing estimates of internal consistency for verbal fluency; to broaden the age range sampled (grades K–6); to add both African-American and white comparison groups; and to provide a parallel nonminority TEMAS for the purpose of assessing the effect of ethnicity of characters on verbal fluency. The presence of the last two conditions allows us to determine, in addition, the effect of multiple characters on the TEMAS as a possible critical variable in determining verbal fluency.

In this study, three groups of children (Hispanic, African-American, and white) were given all three versions of the storytelling task. The results indicated a significant interaction between subject group and test version. Both Hispanic and African-American children gave longer responses (greater verbal productivity) to the minority *and* nonminority TEMAS than to the standard TAT pictures; for white children, verbal productivity did not differ across tests. Because the depiction of minority characters (vs. nonminority characters) on the TEMAS did not influence story length for minority students, the authors concluded that it is the presentation of familiar environmental scenes (which were the same in both versions of TEMAS), rather than the depiction of congruent racial characteristics, that is responsible for increased verbal productivity. However, it is equally true that because both the minority and nonminority versions of TEMAS depicted a larger number of characters than did the TAT, it may be that the presence of more characters is responsible for the longer stories from the minority children, whereas the white children were unaffected by number of characters and/or urban minority middle-class scenes. Furthermore, the authors' conclusion, which focuses on the factor of familiar environment, does not explain why the white children did not show greater verbal productivity on the TAT (more familiar environment) than on TEMAS, nor does it explain why the productivity of African-American and white children was equivalent on the TAT. An adequate explanation for the interaction between stimulus card characteristics and verbal response is still awaited.

A study in which TEMAS successfully discriminated between public school and clinical outpatient Hispanic and African-American children was reported by Costantino, Malgady, Rogler, and Tsui (1988). Using 23 cards from the minority version of TEMAS, bilingual Hispanic and African-American examiners elicited stories from 100 clinic children (mean ages = 10,5 and 12,1, respectively; sex unstated) diagnosed as adjustment disorder (about 50%), conduct disorder (22%), developmental disorder (14%), or anxiety disorder (remainder of group) and 373 children who were students in New York City public elementary and intermediate schools (mean age = 9,4 for both schools; sex unstated). Stories were rated on nine personality variables for degree of adaptation/pathology. After group differences in age, SES, and score differences related to ethnicity, were controlled for, a discriminant function analysis indicated that the TEMAS scores significantly differentiated between the clinical and nonclinical groups. Further, 89% of the children were accurately assigned to clinical or nonclinical groups on the basis of their TEMAS scores. In addition, TEMAS was somewhat more successful with Hispanic than with African-American children in differentiating clinical from nonclinical subjects; however, the results also were statistically significant within each ethnic group.

In yet a further study, Costantino, Malgady, Colon-Malgady, and Bailey (1992) studied the validity of the *non*minority version of the TEMAS with white, inner-city children. The results of a discriminant analysis indicated that the TEMAS profiles successfully differentiated between a group of normal-functioning public school children ($n = 49$) and a second group of children who were outpatients at community mental health clinics ($n = 36$).

STORY LENGTH

Another issue that becomes apparent in the interpretation of the TAT stems from the fact that people tell stories of varying lengths. This is sometimes an interindividual variable—some people characteristically tell long stories while other people are more brief—and as such provides a source of information about individual differences. Differences in story length may also appear as an intraindividual variable, where presumably the shift from long to short stories within the same storyteller is related to differential reactions evoked by the different cards or to other variations in the psychological state of the storyteller. For the clinician, these variations are grist for the mill; they constitute part of the formal determinants, discussed earlier, for interpreting the psychological processes of the storyteller. For the researcher, however, variations in story length may pose a problem, possibly producing spurious results.[23] Clearly, there is greater opportunity for higher scores in a longer protocol. Should, then, a higher score resulting from a long protocol be assumed to reflect a greater intensity of the trait being measured, or should that score be adjusted in some way to acknowledge the length of the protocol? For example, should the intensity of the trait be inferred from the *relative* strength of a score—relative to the total fantasy output or relative to scores on other traits derived from the same story? Especially when one is comparing subject groups which differ in age, intelligence, or verbal ability, the possibility that differences in story length have a direct effect on scores obtained becomes very important. The problem of differences in story length affecting the scores obtained has been dealt with in several ways. In the following sections, several different approaches to this issue are discussed.[24]

Adjustment Tables

In the manual accompanying the TAT (Murray, 1943), it is suggested that whenever story length diverges very much from the standard of 300 words, a correction factor should be used to adjust the scores. The manual provides a table with the adjustment factor to be applied to stories of varying lengths, with scores from short stories being adjusted upwards and scores from long stories being adjusted downwards.

This approach was adopted by Walker and Atkinson (1958). Using TAT-like pictures to assess fear in soldiers who had been exposed to the explosion of an atomic bomb, the experimenters found considerable variation in the length of stories written (0 to 344 words). Because fear scores correlated significantly with story length, an adjustment was needed. The correction procedure involved establishing several story length intervals, each with a range of 30 words[25]; each subject within that interval was assigned a standardized z score for fear, based on the mean and standard deviation of the fear scores for control subjects with stories of that length. In this way, subjects whose fear score was at the mean for stories of a given length would have an adjusted standard score of 50, regardless of the absolute magnitude of their fear score. This adjustment reduced the correlation between story length and fear score from .41 to .02.

Percentage Scores

Another approach used to adjust for differences in story length is to express the TAT scores as a percentage of words in the story. In this case, the score for each variable is expressed in terms of its incidence, per 100 or per 1,000 words, or whatever other word unit seems reasonable. The percentages obtained for the variable scores may then be transformed into standard scores, with a common mean (e.g., 50) and a common standard deviation (e.g., 10).[26]

Relative Scores

A different approach, which may be used when more than one variable is being scored in each story, is to calculate relative scores. For example, if one is scoring several types of motives (X, Y, Z), the relative strength of each separate motive (e.g., X) is determined for each subject as a proportion of the total motive strength $(X + Y + Z)$ expressed in the story. Thus the relative strength of motive X is calculated as: X divided by $(X + Y + Z)$. The use of such ratio scores, however, results in certain limitations for performing statistical analyses.[27]

Regression Analysis

A commonly used approach in contemporary research is to count the number of words in each subject's story and then correlate total words with the scores obtained from that story. If the correlation is statistically significant, it is used as a basis to adjust the raw scores, through regression analysis, to account for differences in story length.[28] An example of this approach and an extensive discussion of the comparability of scores obtained from story protocols of varying lengths are provided by Veroff et al. (1960). In this large-scale study of more than 1,600 adults, the authors found that story length correlated between .21 and .28 with TAT scores of achievement, affiliation, and power motivation. They noted that even higher correlations (.41 to .51) between motivation scores and story length have been found in other populations (e.g., high school students and soldiers), especially when the time allotted for storytelling is short (less than 4 minutes) or uncontrolled. When such a correlation exists, a person who tells a longer story has a greater chance of obtaining a high TAT score.

Veroff et al. (1960) suggested that the best correction for story length would be one based on the average correlation obtained for several different TAT scores and story length.[29] For example, if three different motive scores are obtained from the same protocols, the average of the three correlations between motive score and story length (number of words) is the best estimate of the degree to which story length influences the opportunity to obtain a high score. In this study, the average correlation was used to establish a regression line of motivation scores on length of protocol, and for each interval of story length, the "expected" motivation score was determined. This average expected score (obtained for each motive separately) was subtracted from the average obtained score, and this difference score was used as a correction factor for each subject's individual scores, based on the length of the subject's story. Thus, if the subjects told short stories, a correction factor was added to their TAT scores; if stories were long, a correction factor was subtracted from the TAT scores. In this way, the resulting residual scores can be used to make comparisons within and across groups without concern that differences in story length are unduly influencing the findings.[30]

This method to adjust motive scores for story length has been described succinctly by Gurin, Veroff, and Feld (1960), referring to their large-scale study of TAT-derived motives in American adults (see Chapter

12): "All motive scores used in the analyses were residualized scores based on the regressions of each motive on story length" (McAdams & Bryant, 1987, p. 400).

SUMMARY

In this chapter, a number of the important issues pertaining to the TAT, around which there has been controversy, have been discussed. One of these issues—that different TAT pictures tend to "pull" for different themes—is approached in two different ways. In the first, the stories told to different pictures have been studied and categorized as to prevalent themes. Source references that may be consulted to identify the normative themes are provided in the chapter. The influence of card pull for scores obtained from a set of TAT cards is considered, as is the interaction between storyteller sex and card pull. A second method used to identify card pull has been to obtain ratings of the pictures, per se, separate from the types of stories that are actually written to the pictures.

The chapter also reviews a number of studies devoted to the question of the appropriateness of the TAT for minority subjects, along with a discussion of alternative sets of pictures. The results of these investigations of the interaction between stimulus card characteristics and subject ethnicity are found, at this point, to be inconclusive.

The third section of the chapter focuses on the issue of differences in story length and how this may affect scores obtained. Several different methods that have been used to adjust scores to account for differences in length are explained.

The next chapter addresses issues of reliability and validity.

• FOURTEEN •

Questions
of Reliability
and Validity

P roblems regarding the reliability and validity of projective tests have plagued projective tests from the beginning. Although it is undoubtedly true that for the use of the TAT in clinical practice, "The interpreter is inseparable from the test when the validity of a technique like the TAT is in question" (Holt, 1951, p. 222), it is also true that, for the researcher, the question of stability and repeatability of measurement (i.e., reliability) is an important one.

In this chapter, the recurring questions of the reliability and validity of the TAT are examined. Then, questions regarding the appropriateness of conventional psychometric methods for studying the reliability and validity of the TAT are considered. New approaches to understanding reliability with measures of human motivation are discussed, and supporting evidence for validity is provided.

TRADITIONAL PSYCHOMETRIC APPROACHES

Reliability

Traditionally, there are four approaches to the measurement of reliability. The first is *interrater* reliability—the degree of agreement between two individuals who are rating or scoring the same sample of behavior. This approach to the study of reliability is conceptually quite different from the remaining three. Interrater reliability is concerned with the question whether the measure under question yields the same results when used by rater A as when used by rater B. It does not imply that the behaviors being studied must be absolutely consistent from moment to moment or, in the case of the TAT, from story to story. It asks only that regardless of whether the behavior is consistent or changing, both raters agree on the kind of consistency or change that occurs.

The other three approaches to reliability rest on the a priori premise that the behavior (trait, motive, attitude) being measured is fixed, stable, and unchanging. This supposition underlies the well-known theoretical definition of a test score: The obtained test score (X) equals the subject's "true" score (T) plus an "error" score (E); any variability in the obtained score is attributed measurement error or chance factors because the "true" score is defined, a priori, as unchanging. Reliability, in this case, depends on the magnitude of "chance error" in measurement. It is important to keep in mind that this untested assumption of complete immutability in the trait being measured underlies the *test–retest, split-half or equivalent forms*, and *internal consistency* approaches to measuring reliability.

Interrater Reliability

The earliest studies with the TAT (Morgan & Murray, 1935; Murray, 1938) did not seem to be concerned with the question of reliability—interrater or otherwise. However, a detailed scoring scheme of needs and press was worked out (e.g., Murray, 1938), and raters who were trained through practice and group discussions at the Harvard Psychological Clinic were reported to have achieved high levels of interrater reliability (Tomkins, 1947). A review of the early reports on interrater reliability (Tomkins, 1947) indicated considerable variability in the obtained coefficients, ranging from +.30 to +.96, depending on what kind of TAT protocol was being interpreted, the experience of the interpreter, and the scoring scheme employed.

In contemporary psychological research the problem of interrater reliability has been dealt with successfully by creating carefully detailed scoring manuals and training raters in the scoring procedure. Through the use of a standard scoring manual, extensive examples, and a set of practice stories, neophyte raters can learn to score TAT stories with a high degree of interrater reliability. Currently, interrater category agreement greater than 85%, or a rank-order correlation coefficient greater than .85 between two raters, or between a rater and practice materials scored by an expert, is considered an adequate level of reliability for research purposes (Fleming, 1982; McAdams, 1982a). Many current research studies with the TAT reach this level (see Chapter 14). It seems clear, then, that once adequately trained, two observers can demonstrate a high degree of consistency in the use of TAT measures over a variety of stories for a variety of different psychological dispositions. The problem of interrater reliability has been solved.

Other Approaches to Reliability

However, there are those who would argue that high interrater reliability is not a sufficient demonstration of test reliability. From this point of view, even though two raters may assign identical scores to each story, if the scores from one story do not correlate with those from the next story, some critics argue that the total score is based on a series of unrelated numbers (e.g., Entwisle, 1972). As discussed earlier, this argument and the remaining three approaches to reliabil-ity are based on the a priori assumption that the psychological disposition under study is unchanging, as though fixed in stone. Although the rationale for this assumption derives from the measure-ment of physical properties in our environment (e.g., the length of a log does not change from the time of its first measurement to that of its second measurement), a moment's reflection indicates its inade-quacy for our purposes. Although the length of a cut log may not change, the length of a *growing* tree does change over time. Would anyone then conclude that if our measuring instrument yields a length of 5 feet on one occasion and 6 feet on a subsequent occasion, the instrument is unreliable? The point is that living organisms do change over time,[1] and any theory of measurement that is based on a premise of fixed rigidity of the characteristic being measured is clearly inappropriate. To measure test–retest reliability with an ap-proach that does not allow for change in the disposition being measured is a futile exercise.[2]

In addition to this unwarranted assumption of psychological rigidity, the traditional approaches to reliability (other than interrater) also assume that the *test* consists of a random sampling of behavior (items) from a larger pool of homogeneous behaviors (items). This assumption is particularly important in considering split-half, equivalent forms, and internal consistency approaches to reliability. The greater the homogene-ity of the test items, the higher the intercorrelations among them, and thus the higher the reliability coefficient obtained.

In the case of the TAT, however, the items (cards) are clearly not homogeneous. On the contrary, heterogeneity was the underlying prin-ciple for the selection of the cards from the original pool. Pictures were purposely included to represent different age and sex groups, and to evoke different "root fantasies" (Morgan & Murray, 1935). In other words, the goal of the test construction was to have minimal item overlap. Although it might still be possible to obtain consistent scores across pictures/stories, it is clear that the test was not designed or based on a rationale that would produce a high reliability coefficient (i.e., the rationale that items be homogeneous).

Thus, the psychometric assumptions of trait immutability and item homogeneity are not relevant for the TAT, and measures of reliability based on these assumptions are equally irrelevant. If the disposition being measured by the TAT happens not to change from one testing occasion to the next, the test–retest reliability may appear to be high; if the disposition does change, the reliability may appear to be low. Likewise, assuming a temporarily unchanging disposition, the selection of more similar pictures may yield a higher internal consistency coefficient, while the selection of dissimilar pictures would yield a low coefficient. In the former case, what is needed is an independent measure that would indicate change or stability in the psychological disposition or, short of this, a demonstration that a planned experimental intervention to change the dispositional strength would increase or decrease the score obtained, thereby reducing the reliability coefficient.

Test–Retest Reliability

The above factors, however, are generally not taken into account in critical reviews of the TAT. One of the most influential of these articles, which cast a long shadow, was published by Entwisle in 1972. Systematically summarizing a selection of published and unpublished data for the achievement motivation measure, Entwisle reported test–retest reliabilities from periods of 1 month to 10 years that varied from .12 to .32. She suggested that the problem of memory from one occasion to the next may be responsible for the low correlations, thinking that subjects may feel they should do something different on the second test occasion.

In response to this often cited critique of test–retest reliability, Smith (1992) has pointed out several problems with Entwisle's (1972) analysis. The main problem is that studies that were well executed were lumped together with those that were poorly conducted (e.g., had poor interrater reliability, used too few cards, or used different, nonequivalent cards on the two occasions) and both adequate and inadequate studies were given equal weight in the analysis. Further problems include, in some of the studies, long time intervals between tests (e.g., up to 10 years) and the failure to consider a study with positive results.[3] Smith estimates that if one considers only those studies that were adequately carried out, the test–retest reliability for nAchievement is around .50.

To test Entwisle's suggestion that low retest reliabilities may reflect the subject's effort to tell a different story the second test occasion, Winter and Stewart (1977) measured power motivation in the TAT with 70

Wesleyan University students. At the time of the retest, approximately 1 week later, the students were given different instructions. Some were asked to write the same story they had on the first testing occasion, some were asked to write a different story, and some were in a "no instruction" condition in which they were told not to worry about whether their stories were similar or different from the first set of stories. The results showed that both the same-story and no-instruction condition yielded relatively high test–retest reliability coefficients (r's = .61 and .58, respectively), whereas the different-story instructions yielded a noticeably lower coefficient (r = .27). The authors concluded from these findings that under ordinary circumstances, subjects instruct themselves to give different stories (i.e., to be original) on the second testing occasion. However, when the self-instruction set to give a different story is broken, as in this study through experimental instructions, the retest reliability will increase.[4]

The no-instruction procedure was repeated by Lundy (1985) with 87 high school students for the TAT measures of affiliation motivation and intimacy motivation. As in the power motivation study above, the test–retest reliabilities over a 1-year interval were reasonably high (r's = .48 for intimacy motivation and .56 for affiliation motivation). Lundy points out that these retest reliabilities are in the same range as those obtained over similar time spans for three highly respected objective personality tests— the MMPI, the CPI, and the 16PF.

Perhaps even more important, from a psychometric standpoint, these retest reliability coefficients were considerably higher than the internal consistency (alpha) coefficients (which ranged from −.18 to .32)— a situation that traditional psychometric theory says is impossible (e.g., Entwisle, 1972; Nunnaly, 1968). Based on the statements of these psychometricians, Lundy (1985) concludes that "the assumptions of classical psychometrics are not met with the TAT, and that alpha is therefore an inappropriate measure for this test" (p. 144).

These studies, in which instructions were varied, demonstrate just one intrapsychic reason why subjects may change from one occasion to the next. Obviously, there are a host of other internal factors that will produce temporal change. Fleming (1982) has suggested three other reasons that test–retest reliability may be lower than desirable. First, she suggests that the retest is a psychologically different experience, and that once the test has been taken, it cannot be repeated. This idea has long been part of the training of clinicians—that is, that test materials should not be publicly displayed because familiarity with the test items may modify test responses. A second point, noted by a number of researchers with the TAT, is that there seems to be a "refractory phase" in which a subject having just given a particular response tends to show resistance to giving the same response again. Winter (1973) has pointed out that this "refractory phase" or "sawtooth effect" may occur not only between test occasions but also within a single test administration, so that motive scores vary with the order of stories told, irrespective of the particular stimulus pictures being presented. McClelland (1980) points out that this sawtooth effect has been known ever since Atkinson's 1950 doctoral dissertation on the TAT and achievement motive scores.

Third, and related to the findings of Winter and Stewart (1977) and Lundy (1985; also in Fleming, 1982), Fleming suggested that the subject's memory for the original response "contaminates" the test, and that the retest is a matter of recall, not reliability. However, Lundy's (1985) subsequent report on memory for previous responses demonstrates that this is not true. Lundy points out that the only way that memory might have an effect is if the subject recalls an earlier story given to a particular picture and then gives the same story to that *same* picture on a subsequent occasion. In his study, he compared the reliability of motive scores for stories written to the same pictures with the reliability of scores for stories written to different pictures. If memory was an important factor, same-picture stories should show higher reliability. However, he found that the reliability for motive scores for the same pictures (the only place that memory for previous stories could play a role) was not greater than reliability for motive scores across different pictures.

Unfortunately, when Kraiger, Hakel, and Cornelius (1984) tried to investigate this same issue, they used summary results, combining estimates of memory from four different stimulus cards, and compared these with estimates of motive stability summed over the four stories. This approach ignores the obvious fact that "memory" can only apply to stories given to the same stimulus card on two occasions. By collapsing the data across stimulus pictures, a subject might obtain a memory score that is similar to the stability score, but the memory score could easily be based on picture A and/or picture B, whereas the stability score is being based on picture C and/or picture D. Such data obviously tell us nothing about the role of memory for a story to a particular picture in producing similar motive scores in stories told to that picture.

Finally, Tomkins (1947) discussed the point that retest reliability depends on the stability of the personality and its fluctuations over time; the longer the period between tests, the greater the possibility for personality change, which in turn would reduce the correlations between the scores of the two testing occasions. It is important to note here that fluctuations in the personality over time are considered to be "error" factors in the definition of reliability in which the "true score = obtained score + error score"; thus these fluctuations detract from reliability. As we will see next, the contemporary approach to the measurement of motivation is based on a model that expects, and thus accounts for, temporal fluctuation in motive expression (Atkinson, 1982; Atkinson, Bongort, & Price, 1977).

Split-Half and Equivalent Forms

The question of reliability as determined from the split-half or equivalent-form approach was also discussed by Entwisle (1972). Reviewing first the published literature on achievement motivation, Entwisle noted that the split-half reliability coefficients vary from .19 to .43, and the equivalent-form coefficients vary from .10 to .64.

One of the problems in using the split-half method is that the number of pictures to which a subject can reasonably respond is low; Entwisle (1972) suggests that six pictures may be a maximum. This means that when one half of the test is being compared with the other half, there are only three items in each half, which is a very small sample on which to determine statistical reliability. In the studies she reviews on split-half reliability, typically either four or eight pictures were used. Statistically, the fewer the number of pictures, the lower the reliability coefficient will be, given the same degree of correlation between the two halves of the test. Entwisle's report demonstrates this: In one study, when the coefficient obtained from eight pictures (.19) was adjusted by the Spearman–Brown formula for a hypothetical test with 20 pictures, the reliability value increased to .54. This increase in split-half reliability attendant upon a hypothetical increase in number of TAT pictures (items) has also been demonstrated by Cramer (1991b).

Although the small number of items (pictures) hampers the split-half approach to reliability, the development of equivalent forms is tedious, if not impossible, with the TAT. At bottom, both the split-half and the equivalent-form approach are based on the assumption that the items in the current test are homogeneous, and that there are more such homogeneous items available to construct a second form of the test. As we have discussed, these are not the assumptions that underlie the TAT. Furthermore, studies using equivalent forms often confound this approach with the test–retest approach, introducing substantial time intervals between the administration of the two forms. This was true in all but one of the studies that Entwisle reviewed.

Internal Consistency

Statistical measures such as Cronbach's alpha and the Kuder Richardson$_{20}$ formula are examples of measures of internal consistency. In this approach to the study of reliability, the basic idea is that the more similar (homogeneous) the scores obtained for each item (i.e., the greater the interitem correlations), the more reliable the test. In this conception, the total variance of a test consists of two parts: The variance specific to the separate items and the covariance between items. The greater the proportion of the total variance that is attributable to interitem covariance, the greater the reliability of the test. Thus, the more similar the items, the more they will correlate with each other, and the greater the interitem covariance.

Again, it is clear that this conception of reliability is based on the assumption that the items (i.e., pictures) should be homogeneous. It does not allow for a test strategy in which items are purposely chosen to represent different areas of personality, nor does it allow for a conception of personality in which the disposition being measured may vary in expression from picture to picture, due either to the different picture pull or to a "refractory phase" in the expression of the disposition.[5] The importance of these two factors for determining the method to be used in assessing reliability and validity with the TAT is considered below in the discussion of the "dynamics of action theory."

A different kind of issue regarding internal consistency is related to the number of items in the test. As is the case with split-half and alternate-form reliability, the statistical measure of internal consistency is importantly influenced by the number of test items. If the individual interitem correlations are low, which would ordinarily lead to a low reliability coefficient, this can be compensated for if there are a large number of items, for an increase in the number of items rapidly increases the number of covariance terms. Increasing the number of these terms increases the total interitem covariance, which in turn increases the reliability coefficient. However, if a test has few items, as is the case with the TAT, then there are fewer interitem correlations, and each one must be higher if the total interitem variance is to reach an acceptable level.

Entwisle (1972) summarized this situation as follows: "Other tests, for instance the Scholastic Aptitude Test, have low interitem correlations, but the number of items is sufficient to compensate. With few items, the items must be highly related for a reliable instrument to emerge" (p. 385). Although this statement is true statistically, one must ask: Does it make sense conceptually? If an item has a low intercorrelation with other items, how does it become a better *item* when it is one of many, than when it stands alone? As a single item, it is no better than a single TAT picture that shows a low correlation with other pictures. Although amassing a group of items with low intercorrelations may raise the numerical value of the statistical coefficient, conceptually, any six of those items may be no more internally consistent than any six TAT pictures. Thus, in fact, the total score of a multi-item test with low interitem correlations is just as equally made up of "a series of unrelated numbers" (Entwisle, 1972, p.

383)—albeit there are more of them—as is the total score of a TAT for which the interitem correlations are low.

In sum, considering the issues and findings discussed earlier, it seems clear that there are serious questions regarding how, or if, traditional psychometric approaches are appropriate for measuring the reliability of TAT scores.[6]

Validity

There are a number of issues to be considered when addressing the question of the validity of the TAT. A primary concern is the criterion to be used to evaluate TAT measures. Should the criterion be observed behavior, or scores from other tests? If the latter, does it matter whether these tests are similar in form and rationale (e.g., projective tests) or dissimilar (e.g., self-report questionnaires). This issue of test and criterion format—conceived more broadly as respondent versus operant measures—is discussed later in the chapter.

A different issue is concerned with the nature of the relationship that might expected between TAT measures and validity criteria; that is, do we expect positive, linear relationships, or might the relationship between fantasy and behavior be inverse or curvilinear? Another issue is whether the criteria for validity should be external to the story itself, or whether one might specify criteria based on material internal to the story. And finally, as is true for the issue of reliability, does it make sense to speak about the "validity of the TAT"?

As mentioned in Chapter 2, Tomkins (1947), more than other early advocates of the TAT, was concerned with questions of reliability and validity. In his thoughtful analysis of how validity might be demonstrated with the TAT, he took the point of view that one cannot meaningfully ask whether the TAT is a valid test, any more than one can ask whether the experimental method is a valid method. Rather, he said, the appropriate question in both cases is whether inferences based on the test, or method, are likely to be true. Thus, we cannot make statements about "the validity of the TAT." Instead, we may ask, to what extent do scores from a particular TAT measure relate to other criteria in a predicted manner.

Tomkins also considered the case in which the correlation between a TAT measure and a criterion variable might not be any greater than the correlation between some other personality measure (e.g., life history information) and that criterion variable. However, unlike Entwisle (discussed later), he did not conclude from this that the TAT measure was thus superfluous. Rather, he demonstrated that when used in combination, the correlation of the two predictive measures with the criterion variable is increased over that obtained for either measure alone. The point, then, is that the existence of a relationship between the TAT measure and some other personality measure, or of each of these measures with the criterion variable, does not, de facto, disqualify the TAT measure from being valid. On the contrary, these types of relationships have formed the background for the traditional psychometric approaches to validity.

To demonstrate concurrent, predictive, and some forms of construct validity, one looks for a theoretically predicted relationship between the TAT measure and some independent measure of personality. In this regard, TAT measures have been criticized by those who note that the correlations obtained are not as high as those obtained, for example, from self-report questionnaires. In reply, TAT researchers have noted that questionnaire scores tend to correlate well with scores from other similar questionnaires, but that they are less successful in predicting real behavior: "the magnitude of prediction obtained with questionnaires is not impressive, hovering around nine percent of the variance" (Fleming, 1982, p. 75). On the other hand, there has been considerable evidence in contemporary research that TAT scores do correlate with independent measures of behavior in meaningful ways. This information is reviewed in other chapters of the book.

Entwisle (1972) used her analysis of the reliability of the TAT achievement motivation measure to suggest why, from her point of view, the measure had low predictive validity: "the lack of predictive validity most likely stem[s] from low reliability of the measure" (p. 389). She went on to say that, when there is evidence for a correlation between the achievement motivation score and some external criterion, such as school grades,[7] this is most likely mediated by differences in the length of stories told. That is, because length of story correlates with motive score (in her sample, r's ranged from .29 to .74, depending on the subject group) and also school grades (in her sample, r's = .17 to .56), she argued that the correlations between motive score and grades (in her sample, r's = −.11 to .47) were mediated by story length.

Unfortunately, the idea of adjusting motive scores for story length and then determining whether any of the remaining grade variance was predicted by (adjusted) motive scores was not considered.[8] As discussed in Chapter 14, contemporary studies that have adjusted for verbal productivity have found that motive or defense scores do relate to criterion variables and do support theoretical predictions. Further, a study by Reuman, Alwin, and Veroff (1984), which related achievement motivation to job satisfaction in adult males, found that although the TAT motivation score and story length were positively correlated, only the TAT score was significantly related to job satisfaction. Clearly, the TAT motivation score was measuring something distinctly different from that reflected in story length.

A somewhat novel approach to the study of validity with the TAT was used in an investigation by Richardson and Partridge (1982). They suggested that the validity criteria for a TAT measure may come either from within the story itself or from some measure external to the story. In this approach, selected TAT variables are related either to different variables measured *within* the story which theoretically would be expected to be related to the selected variables; alternatively, the selected TAT measures are related to variables occurring *outside* the story, such as demographic data. Using as a database the responses of 1,428 subjects from the large-scale national studies by Gurin, Veroff, and Feld (1960) and Veroff, Douvan, and Kulka (1981) (see Chapter 12 for a discussion of these studies), the authors scored the TAT stories for three "family" variables (references to marriage, references to interpersonal conflict, and total number of family stories) and two "peer" variables ("inequities in status" and "peership"). The "family" variables of references to marriage and number of family stories were validated against *external* variables. The first variable correlated with marital status; the second was correlated with living in a family environment but not with other external demographic variables.[9] The variable of reference to interpersonal conflict was validated against an internal (to the TAT story) variable: More conflict occurred in stories with family as compared to nonfamily, themes. The "peer" variables of status and peership were found to be valid when related to such other internal variables as references to age, powerlessness, and shared activity. They did not relate to external criteria. Overall, the adequacy of this approach for demonstrating validity is clearly tied to the theoretical appropriateness of the internal and external variables selected.

A rather different approach to the issue of TAT score validity was presented by Lazarus (1961, 1966). Lazarus proposed that, theoretically, the relationship between TAT motive scores and particular criterion measures of motive behavior might be expected to be either positive *or* negative, depending on the conditions (external and internal) surrounding the expression of the motive. On the one hand, motives may be *directly* expressed in TAT fantasy and in criterion behavior, in which case the relationship will be positive (the "typical" evidence for validity of the measure). However, there are other situations in which the relationship between motivation and behavior may be negative. For example, if the expression of motives is blocked from motoric discharge, the motives may be expressed in TAT fantasy rather than being expressed behaviorally (the *substitutive* principle). Alternatively, the expression of a motive in fantasy may be inhibited when either external sanctions or internal proscriptions against the motive are forceful (the *defensive* principle), even though the underlying motive itself may be strong. In the case of the substitutive principle, the correlation between motive scores derived from fantasy and motive scores derived from other behavior will be negative. In the case of the defensive principle, the relationship between fantasy motive scores and drive strength will be negative.

Lazarus (1966) stressed, however, that both the substitutive–defensive principles and the direct expression conception are needed to understand the relationship of measures of motivation derived from TAT fantasy to other measures of motivated behavior. The problem, as he posed it, was to determine under what conditions the contents of storytelling are directly related to motivated behaviors, and under what conditions they are negatively related. In turn, he suggested that the direct expression of motives—in fantasy as well as in criterion task performance—is likely to occur when the subject perceives the task as requiring reality testing or problem-solving behavior (i.e., instrumental behavior). However, if the subject perceives the task as one involving playfulness, the substitutive principle will more likely apply. Lazarus proposed that TAT story content should thus be differentiated into that reflecting the operation of secondary process, problem-solving activity and that reflecting primary process functioning, as seen in wishful or playful fantasy. Under conditions that foster secondary process thinking, a positive relationship between TAT content and other behavioral evidence of the motivation would be expected; under conditions that foster primary process thinking, a substitutive, or negative, relationship would be expected. This focus on the importance, for the study of validity, of how and for what purposes the subject is giving a response, as this determines the expected relationships between TAT measures and other measures of behavior, appears again in the more recent work of McClelland (1980), discussed later.

The importance of how subjects are instructed to give TAT responses has been demonstrated experimentally by Lundy (1988), who showed that various situational or instructional variables may affect the validity of scores derived from the TAT. Lundy (1988) demonstrated that modifications in the instructions provided subjects prior to story writing may have profound effects on the degree to which the motive scores obtained correlate with validity criterion measures. In his study of some 200 high school students (predominantly seniors), he found that measures of nAchievement, nAffiliation, and nPower correlated significantly with criterion measures when the subjects were given neutral instructions that encouraged relaxed and unstructured responses to the stimulus pictures. However, nonneutral instructions that provided an ego threat, or an indication that the TAT was a personality test, or that stressed that the stories should be structured (i.e., follow rules and instructions carefully) resulted in motive scores that did not correlate with the criterion measures (i.e., failed to support the validity of the TAT motive measures). A similar finding showing the importance of instructions for measures of *reliability* was reported earlier (Winter & Stewart, 1977).

PROBLEMS WITH THE TRADITIONAL PSYCHOMETRIC APPROACH

The determination of test reliability and validity, in classical test theory, is based on the "true score" measurement model discussed above—a model that states that the obtained score (X) consists of the true score (T) plus a quantity due to measurement error or random error (E). Further, this theory posits that the empirical validity of a test, as determined from the correlation of test scores with some criterion measure, cannot exceed the square root of the reliability of the test. Thus, low reliability means that adequate validity is impossible. Recently, the appropriateness of this model for determining the validity of achievement motivation (and, by inference, other TAT-based measures) has been called into question in the context of two different, but related, theoretical orientations discussed here.

One of the strongest, and most persuasive confrontations with the arguments of those who advocate the traditional psychometric approach (e.g., Entwisle, 1972) has been presented by McClelland (1980). Beginning with the observation that the focus on issues of reliability is an attitude peculiar to psychometricians, McClelland reminds us that experimental psychologists do not concern themselves with the question whether, for example, a subject in a memory study would recall the same number of items if retested on another occasion.

To expand on this point, we may note that, in fact, when subjects in a memory experiment are retested, it is generally done to demonstrate a *change* in degree of recall as a result of some intervening experience, including the passage of time. Further, the question whether the subject responds in the same way to *all* of the items within each category to be remembered is not of central importance, that is, "internal consistency" is not an issue.

To illustrate this point, let us consider the "false recognition" paradigm used in experimental studies of memory. In this situation, a list of words is presented to the subject for learning. Subsequently, the subject is tested for memory using a longer list of words, some of which were presented originally (the "target" words) and some of which are new words. Among this latter group of "distractor" words, some are related (either semantically or associatively) to the target words and some are unrelated. The experimenter is primarily interested in responses to the related words. In the typical result, many of the target words are remembered (e.g., 9 out of 10 are responded to in the same way, with the subject saying "yes"), some of the related distractors are "remembered" (4 out of 10 are responded to in the same way), and only a few of the unrelated distractors are "remembered" (i.e., 9 out of 10 are responded to in the same way, with the subject saying "no"). If the responses to these three categories of words were to be used to determine the split-half or internal consistency reliability of the three measures of memory (target words, related distractors, and unrelated distractors), the reliability for the target measure and the unrelated distractors would obviously be higher than that for the related distractor measure, for there is more consistency in responding to the target and unrelated words. However, it is the responses to the distractor items which are of primary interest to the experimenter, and it is these items that are regularly used to test theoretical models of memory.

If experimental psychologists were to make such a reliability determination, which they do not, would they then conclude that the distractor measure was unreliable? Obviously not; responses to any one of these distractors is considered meaningful, and it is not necessary or even expected that all the items in this measure will be responded to in the same way. Further, the whole experimental paradigm is based on the understanding that responses to the distractor items represent "errors," and it is the manifestation of these errors—even if infrequently or irregularly occurring—that is theoretically meaningful.

Considerations such as these raise questions, if not problems, for the traditional psychometric opinion that without adequate reliability, the test cannot have validity (i.e., the position that validity cannot exceed reliability). Further, as we will see next, studies based on computer simulation and experimental test indicate that this opinion is not supported with data derived from TAT stories, that is, it *is* possible to have validity without having internal reliability (Reuman, 1982).

CONTEMPORARY APPROACHES

Operant and Respondent Measures; Implicit and Self-Attributed Motives

McClelland (1980) has discussed and clarified the crucial and intrinsic difference between responses to the TAT and responses to self-report questionnaires and couches this in language that is familiar to "tough-minded" psychologists. The production of a TAT story, he says, is like Skinner's operant response. Although the subject is in a standardized testing situation, the exact stimulus and directing set that eventuate in a response are unknown and likely vary from subject to subject. The response itself is spontaneous and not under the control of the examiner; thus the nature and form of the response will vary from subject to subject.

In contrast, responses to self-report questionnaires are more similar to respondent behaviors. The stimulus is clearly specified (the test question is focused and specific), the response alternatives are fixed (e.g., mark "True" or mark "False"), and subjects are given a directing set: They are to report on how they actually behave, would behave, or have behaved (including thoughts) in the past.

The importance of this distinction between operant and respondent measures lies in the repeated finding that the two types of measures generally do not correlate with each other, even when they are described as measuring the same personality disposition. It is this fact that traditional psychometricians have used to challenge the validity of operant measures like the TAT. According to their reasoning, if the two measures that purport to measure the same disposition do not correlate, one of them must not be valid. Because the respondent measure has higher reliability, the traditional psychometric theory concludes that the validity of the respondent measure is greater, and "therefore" it is the respondent measure that is valid and the operant measure (the TAT) that is invalid. However, if the traditional psychometric approach for determining reliability is not appropriate for the TAT (see above), this reasoning about validity is flawed. Further, both contemporary theory and evidence from research now support the position that the two types of measures are assessing different things (see Weinberger & McClelland, 1990). It is no longer a question of one measure being valid and the other not. Rather, the question is, valid for what?

McClelland (1980) argues that operant and respondent measures relate to different aspects of personality—what clinicians might refer to as different "levels" of functioning. Operant measures, as used by McClelland and his colleagues, assess implicit motives,[10] whereas respondent measures assess values, including self-evaluation. Implicit motives are dispositions that drive, direct, and select behavior. Thus individuals who have a strong implicit motive should manifest greater evidence of these three aspects of behavior than individuals who are weakly motivated. Using two measures of achievement motivation— one operant (the TAT) and one respondent (the Edwards Personal Preference Inventory)—McClelland convincingly demonstrated that it is only the operant measure that accurately identifies individuals whose behavior matches theoretically predicted expectations. The respondent measure produced either chance results or findings in the opposite direction from theoretical expectation. This striking result sets the stage for McClelland's central argument in these papers—namely, that only operant measures are successful in predicting real-life spontaneous behavior over time, whereas respondent measures are most successful in predicting performance involving such immediate choices as other respondent measures.

The strength and importance of this argument has been demonstrated repeatedly by McClelland in recent years. For example, McClelland (1989) reports studies that show that it is operant, fantasy-based measures, rather than respondent, self-report measures, that turn out to be related to criterion physiological changes for the variable under study. Referring to an early food-deprivation study (Atkinson & McClelland, 1948; McClelland, 1951), he notes that while food-related themes in the TAT increased over the course of 1 to 16 hours of food deprivation, self-report ratings of hunger increased from 1 to 4 hours but did not increase further between 4 and 16 hours of deprivation. Clearly, the fantasy measure better reflected the known physiological condition of the subjects. Likewise, in a study of visual-evoked potentials in response to looking at power-related pictures, the TAT-based measure of nPower correlated with the differential evoked potential response to the power pictures, whereas self-reports on being energetic, vigorous, and lively (components of being dominant- or power-oriented) did not correlate with the physiological response. TAT fantasy measures of power motivation also correlated with the physiological measure of stress (increase in norepinephrine) connected to taking an examination, whereas a self-report adjective checklist and a measure of internal locus of control did not. In another experimental study, subjects watched a film on loving relationships and then completed a self-report mood adjective checklist that included feelings of being loved and friendly. The subjects also wrote TAT stories that were scored for the affiliation motive. Only the TAT scores correlated with physiological variables (dopamine concentrations in the blood or saliva) after the film. Further demonstrations of the relationship between TAT measures of motives and physiological variables are discussed in Chapter 15.[11]

More recently, McClelland and his colleagues (McClelland, Koestner, & Weinberger, 1989; Weinberger & McClelland, 1990) have referred to the operant–respondent difference as a distinction between implicit motives and self-attributed motives. Implicit motives are derived from more primitive, biologically based needs, are intrinsically associated with affect, and are most easily expressed in free-response situations. They are best assessed using such fantasy or expressive techniques as the TAT. Self-attributed motives are rooted in self-conceptions, which are largely based on learning, and are best assessed using self-report techniques. McClelland suggests that the best prediction of behavior occurs when both implicit and self-attributed motive measures are used. Implicit motives provide an impulse toward certain types of goals, whereas self-attributed motives define the particular area in which the impulse is expressed (McClelland et al., 1989).

Using this dual approach, TAT measures of implicit motives have also been shown to correlate with real-life behavior in ways that are different from the correlations found with self-attributed motives. For example, in a study examining the relationship of child-rearing variables to implicit and self-attributed motives in adulthood (McClelland et al., 1989), it was found that the TAT-based nAchievement measure was related to developmentally earlier, more biologically connected events, whereas self-attributed achievement scores were related to childhood events involving verbal communication or parental expectations and rules.

An extensive discussion of a wide variety of studies that support the thesis that measures of implicit and self-attributed motives are qualitatively different—in fact, may be orthogonal—is provided by Weinberger and McClelland (1990). Meta-analyses of more than 100 studies of both TAT-based and self-attributed measures of achievement motivation (Spangler, 1992) found that both types of measures related positively to criteria outcome measures, and that the size of the effect was greatest for the implicit measures in the presence of intrinsic incentives, whereas the effect was greatest for the self-attributed motives in the presence of external incentives. Recent studies explicitly designed to compare TAT-based motive scores with those from self-report questionnaires have yielded inconsistent results. For example, Emmons and McAdams (1991) found that TAT measures of achievement, intimacy, and power do correlate significantly with certain self-report measures (the Personality Research Form; PRF) of the same dispositions, and that the results from both types of test were significantly related to a subject-generated list of personal strivings (Emmons & McAdams, 1991). On the other hand, King (1995) found no correlation between implicit and self-attributed motives.

Dynamics-of-Action Theory

The second theoretical orientation that calls into question the appropriateness of traditional true-score test theory is the "dynamics-of-action" approach of Atkinson and Birch (1970, 1978; see also Atkinson, 1982). Central to this theory is the distinction between the strength of an underlying motive (the "genotype") and the variability in the expression of this motive at any point in time (the "phenotype"). The expression of the motive in imaginative thought is expected to be variable from moment to moment, although over longer stretches of time the total amount of emitted motive expression should be constant. The implication of this point of view, for the measurement of motivation via stories told to TAT cards, is that the appropriate unit of measurement is not the story given to one card versus the story given to a second, third, or fourth card but, rather, the expression of the motive over the entire time span of the test (i.e., over the total set of cards combined).

In this conception, the expression of the motive on the first card might be quite different from that on the second, which in turn might be quite different from that of the third. For classical test theory, this would result in very low reliability (low internal consistency). Yet, the total score, summed over all cards, could indeed be an accurate representation of the underlying motive strength, and thus could accurately (validly) predict a relationship between the motive and a criterion variable.

In fact, this possibility—that a test could be valid without being reliable, in the classic sense, has been demonstrated through computer simulation by Atkinson et al. (1977) and through empirical study by Reuman (1982). Based on the idea that there may be many different moment-to-moment patterns of motive expression, each of which, nevertheless, sum to a constant amount over a specified time interval, Atkinson et al. (1977) used a computer to generate cases in which there was considerable interitem variability (i.e., low reliability), but the total scores were still successful in predicting a criterion variable (i.e., adequate validity). In this way, they demonstrated that the total amount of motive expression over a fixed interval of time can provide a valid measure without the test being reliable as traditionally determined.

Reuman (1982) further explored the basic conflict between the dynamics-of-action theory—which expects behavior to vary over time, given a stable personality and a constant environment—and classical test theory, in which the true-score measurement model expects constant behavior over time in a constant environment. Based on computer simulations, Reuman proceeded to show that when there is greater variability in the expression of a motive over a finite time interval, the motivational imagery thus assessed is likely to possess *greater* construct validity than when the phenotypic variability is quite low. In addition to demonstrating this theoretically and through simulation, Reuman also created experimental situations in which the expressed variability was manipulated. Using a procedure similar to that of Winter and Stewart (1977) (see earlier description, pp. 253–254), male subjects wrote stories to eight TAT cards under one of three instructional conditions designed to increase or decrease story variability. For each subject in each condition, the variability of achievement motivation scores across the eight TAT cards was determined, and this variability was related to a standard validity criterion for achievement motivation (number of arithmetic problems attempted). Overall, the results indicated that the validity coefficient was higher for those subjects who had greater story-to-story variability than for those subjects whose stories were less variable. For the same set of data, the internal consistency measure (i.e., reliability) of the highly variable subjects was extremely low. According to classical test theory, it should not have been possible for these highly variable subjects to show evidence for validity. However, the obtained results are in agreement with the dynamics-of-action theory which postulates that greater observed variability will enhance the validity of the measure.

Reuman's (1982) analysis, which asserts that the true-score measurement model is inappropriate for TAT motivational measures, is based on a theoretical position regarding motivation in which random error variance (i.e., variability in observed motivational strength scores) across moments in time is to be expected. Reuman et al. (1984) have used this idea to study the question of the validity of TAT-based measures within the framework of the true-score model, focusing on the idea that a large proportion of the variance in the obtained scores is due to random measurement error (Reuman, Alwin, & Veroff, 1984). This approach to validity hypothesizes that the relationship between the *theoretical* construct being measured (e.g., need Achievement) and a *theoretical* construct it is expected to predict (e.g., work satisfaction) may be significant; that is, that the "true" scores of these two constructs may be significantly related. However, if the random measurement error of either or both constructs is substantial or substantially different, the obtained estimate of the relationship between the two constructs will be biased, producing an underestimation of the validity of the theoretical construct. This is because, as noted before, the empirical validity of a test, when determined by the correlation between the obtained test score and the obtained validity criterion measure, cannot exceed the square root of the measure of test reliability.

To test this hypothesis, Reuman et al. (1984) used a causal modeling approach based on methods of confirmatory factor analysis to assess the validity of the TAT need achievement measure, taking into account and correcting for random measurement error. This approach was successful in demonstrating the validity of the need achievement measure; in addition, it provided evidence that the relationship between the TAT measure and the criterion measure was not due to a spurious mediating variable of story length, as Entwisle (1972) previously claimed.

SUMMARY

This chapter addresses the issues of reliability and validity as they pertain to the TAT. Certain assumptions of traditional psychometric approaches are examined and shown, for a variety of reasons, to be inappropriate or inadequate to evaluate measures such as the TAT. At issue here is the important distinction between operant measures of implicit motives and their appropriate unit of measurement, as compared to respondent measures of self-attributed motives, typically measured by a series of discrete, self-report items. Although the true-score psychometric model may be appropriate for determining the reliability and validity of respondent measures, a theoretically different, dynamics-of-action model has been found to be better suited to demonstrating the validity of operant TAT measures.

The final section of the chapter provides both the logic and evidence for treating measures of implicit and of self-attributed motives as complementary rather than contradictory.

FIFTEEN

The TAT
in Personality
Research Today

I nterest in the TAT seems to appear in waves. The first upsurge followed Morgan and Murray's original work. These studies, published in the 1940s and early 1950s, and described in Chapter 2, were largely descriptive and theoretical in nature, although there were also a number of empirical research studies using the TAT. According to Bellak (1954), in 1941 the TAT had a bibliography of 11 items; by 1953, this number had increased to 780. Much of this work was reviewed by Mayman (1946), and a bibliography of 377 articles on the TAT was assembled by Holt and Thompson (1950). Another wave appeared in the early 1960s, with increased attention being given to research. Much of this work has been summarized in Kagan and Lesser (1961), Murstein (1963a), and Zubin, Eron, and Schumer (1965).

It was at this time, also, that the "new wave" of research with the TAT gained momentum, originating with the work of McClelland and Atkinson and their studies of achievement motivation. The approach they developed for deriving a measure of motivational strength from the TAT has served as the model for a number of younger investigators to study a variety of motives. This new-wave research, which is characterized by experimental rigor and psychometric sophistication, has created renewed enthusiasm for the research potentialities of the TAT in the study of human motivation. Between 1974 and the present, more than 1,000 articles on the TAT have been published.[1] Some of this work has been reviewed in McAdams (1988a), Smith (1992), and Stewart (1982a).

THE "McCLELLAND–ATKINSON TRADITION"[2]

In 1948, Atkinson and McClelland published a paper in the *Journal of Experimental Psychology* in which they demonstrated that the experimental manipulation of hunger influenced the occurrence of themes in TAT stories involving both food deprivation and the removal of the source of the deprivation.[3] The success of this study in demonstrating that the strength of a physiologically based need (hunger) was reflected in the thematic content of subjects' stories provided a strong basis for making the further assumption that the strength of psychological needs, or motives, could also be detected through the analysis of TAT story content.

This idea was tested by McClelland, Clark, Roby, and Atkinson (1949). Choosing the need for achievement (nAch) as the motive to be measured, the experimenters attempted to manipulate the strength of the need by involving groups of male subjects in several short tasks that were designed to be either ego involving, neutral, or relaxed.[4] After the arousal tasks, subjects wrote stories for TAT cards. The assumption was that under ego-involving conditions, the need for achievement would be aroused, and that this arousal should be reflected in story content; in turn, under relaxed or neutral conditions, there should be less evidence of nAch in story content.

In order to assess motivational differences in these groups, the authors established a number of scoring categories designed to reflect different characteristics of nAch, in a manner similar to that used for the scoring of content relevant to hunger motivation. These categories were based on a model of the behavioral sequence that ensues when a motive is aroused or active. The sequence begins when the individual experiences a state of need, or a motive (category N). There may also, at this point in the sequence, be some anticipation of either success or failure regarding the attainment of the goal (category Ga+ or Ga–). The individual may then engage in some activity that is instrumental in attaining the goal (I+) or not attaining it (I–). There may be some obstacle to attaining the goal, due to a block in the outside world (Bw) or to some characteristic in the person him- or herself (Bp). The individual may experience some positive affect (G+) in attaining the goal, or negative affect (G–) if his or her efforts fail. There may be some other individual who is helpful or nurturant (Nup) in aiding the goal-directed behavior. These six categories, plus Thema—a protocol in which the whole story revolves around the motive and there are no other, conflicting or alternate story plots—form the basis for scoring the achievement motive. In subsequent studies of other motives, a similar scheme of scoring categories was adopted.

In the McClelland et al. (1949) study, scores based on these categories were summed to provide an overall score for nAch. The results of this study indicated that, under conditions of ego involvement, scores for nAch were significantly higher than in either the neutral or the relaxed conditions. Further, under conditions of relaxation, nAch scores were lower than in the neutral condition. Additional arousal conditions were studied[5]; the effect of failure arousal conditions was to increase nAch scores, as compared to the other conditions, whereas the effect of success arousal was to produce somewhat lower nAch scores than found under conditions of ego involvement.

This landmark study provided evidence that experimental manipulation of psychological motives would produce predicted and theoretically meaningful changes in TAT scores designed to measure the strength of such motives. Moreover, the use of a detailed, carefully described scoring system made it possible to obtain clear evidence for scoring reliability, which was quite high. Drawing stories at random from the different arousal groups, raters scored the stories for nAch on two separate occasions. The interrater product–moment correlation coefficient for the two sets of nAch scores was .95. The success of this study launched a new approach to the use of the TAT for studying human motivation and was the foundation for the further development of the "McClelland–Atkinson research strategy" (Winter, 1973, p. 37).

Steps in Developing the Scoring System

As described in *The Achievement Motive* (McClelland et al., 1953), this strategy for using the TAT to assess motivation involves several steps (see McAdams, 1982a, 1988a; Winter, 1973). The first step is to identify a group of subjects in whom the motive in question is believed to be strong—often as a result of the experimental arousal of that motive. Next, a sample of TAT stories is obtained from this "strong motive" or "arousal" group. The content or some other quality of these stories is then compared with that of stories obtained from a control group of subjects for whom the motive is not believed to be strong. The differences between the stories obtained from the two groups are assumed to be due to the motive, and are thus taken as a measure of the motive. Underlying this assumption is the belief that the differences in motive strength found between experimentally aroused and nonaroused subjects are similar to the differences in motive strength that reflect personality dispositional differences among people. As a next step, the measure is cross-validated on subsequent groups of aroused and nonaroused subjects; if the measure is successful in differentiating these further groups of subjects for whom the arousal conditions differ, it is considered a valid measure of motive strength. Finally, construct validation is undertaken in which differences in motive scores obtained under neutral conditions are related to other behaviors that have been predicted from theory (McAdams, 1982a, 1988a).

Using this approach, the scoring system for a motive is based on those characteristics of the stories that consistently differentiate between the motive group and the control groups. Often, the selection of these characteristics is guided by theoretical expectations, for example, that certain types of motive-relevant content will be more frequent in the motive group. It is also possible, however, that critically differentiating content or stylistic features will be discovered through empirical examination of the two sets of stories; for example, stories from the low-motive control group may have more of some unpredicted characteristic than is found in the high-motive group. In this way, the discovery of discriminating scoring categories is somewhat similar to the development of criterion-keyed items on self-report personality scales.[6] Also similar is the use of cross-validation procedures; with different subjects, different motive arousal procedures are used, and the results from each arousal group are compared to those from a control group. Only those categories of story content or style that consistently differentiate between motive-aroused subjects and control subjects are included in the final motive scoring scheme.[7]

"Prime Test" and Scoring Subcategories

In addition to establishing story categories that differentiate between the motive and control groups (generally between six and eight such subcategories are developed), the current scoring schemes for several motives (nAchievement, nPower, nAffiliation, and nIntimacy) also require that the story satisfy the requirements of a "prime test" before further scoring of subcategories is undertaken. The prime test looks for more general statements or descriptions of the motive in the TAT story. If the story meets these criteria, further scoring of the motive may be undertaken; if the story does not pass the prime test, no further scoring is allowed.

EXAMPLES OF THIS APPROACH[8]

Achievement Motivation

The refinement of the scoring system to measure need Achievement (nAch) was presented by McClelland et al. (1953). As indicated above, the first task of the scorer is to decide whether the story would pass the prime test. In the case of nAch, this requires that the story contain some reference to an achievement goal, which is defined as "success in competition with some standard of excellence" (McClelland et al., 1953, p. 110). This first criterion is further defined as including stories in which the concern is actually stated, or in which affective concern over goal attainment or instrumental activity to attain a standard of excellence is expressed in the story. Two other criteria that would meet the prime test include descriptions of a unique accomplishment or long-term involvement in achieving a goal. In order to be scored for any of the seven nAch subcategories, the story must meet at least one of these three prime test criteria (see Table 15.1).

The development of this method for assessing nAch from TAT stories was followed by a host of studies relating nAch to performance on

---

TABLE 15.1. Prime Test and Subcategories for Scoring nAch

Prime test criteria

1. Competition with a standard of excellence.
   a. Winning, or doing as well as or better than others is actually stated as a primary concern.
   b. If not actually stated, then affective concern over achievement (vis-à-vis others) is evident.
   c. The competition may be with a self-imposed standard of excellence, rather than with others.
2. Involvement with a unique accomplishment.
3. Involvement in attaining a long-term goal.

Subcategories

1. Need (N): stated desire to reach an achievement goal.
2. Instrumental activity: The person is doing something, including thinking, toward attaining an achievement goal. The outcome of the activity may be successful (I+), unsuccessful (I–) or doubtful (I?).
3. Anticipatory goal states: Someone in the story anticipates goal attainment (Ga+) or frustration/failure in attaining the achievement goal (Ga–).
4. Obstacles or blocks: scored when the progress or goal-directed activity is blocked or hindered in some way. When the obstacle is located in the environment (world), is scored Bw; when it is located in the individual (e.g., lack of confidence), it is scored Bp.
5. Nurturant press (NUP): The character who is engaged in achievement activity is helped or assisted by someone else, in the direction of attaining the achievement goal.
6. Affective states: A positive affective state associated with successful achievement or objective benefits accruing therefrom is scored G+; negative affective states associated with failure to attain an achievement goal, or the objective concomitants thereof, is scored G–.
7. Achievement theme: scored when the entire story is concerned with achievement, and there is no major competing story plot.

Note. Abbreviated from McClelland et al. (1953).

a variety of laboratory tasks (McClelland et al., 1953). Further studies noted the importance of the interaction between nAch and the context for storytelling (including instruction) in determining overt achievement-related action. Many other studies have investigated the relationship between nAch and such behavioral characteristics as risk taking, perceptual sensitivity, and autonomic nervous system reactivity; between nAch and such psychological variables as self-concept and social adjustment; and, of course, between nAch and other psychological motives. Perhaps the most ambitious study involving achievement motivation was that in which evidence of nAch in the published writings of different societies were used to predict the economic growth and decline of various cultures (McClelland, 1961).

Discussion of these studies may be found in Atkinson (1958); Atkinson and Feather (1966); Atkinson and Raynor (1974); Birney (1968); Heckhausen (1968); Koestner and McClelland (1990); McClelland (1961, 1971); Smith (1992); Veroff (1982); Veroff, McClelland, and Ruhlland (1975); and Weiner (1978). A description of the scoring system, and practice, expert-scored stories are available in Smith (1992).

Affiliation Motivation

Following the success of using TAT stories for measuring nAch, and certain observations made in the course of those studies, an attempt was made to measure the need for affiliation (nAff) using a similar procedure. After initial attempts by Roby (1948) and Birney (1950), Shipley and Veroff (1952) devised a more general scoring method based on the procedure of comparing the stories of subjects in whom the affiliation motive had been experimentally aroused with those of control subjects.

The procedure used to arouse the affiliation motive involved having fraternity members complete a series of sociometric tests in which they rated, and were rated by, all the members on a variety of personal attributes, including who they would most like to have as friends. The control group completed a food-preference test. Following this, all the members wrote TAT stories.

A second study was conducted to cross validate the TAT measure derived from this first set of stories. The motive and control groups in the second study were based on subject selection rather than experimental arousal. It was assumed that college freshmen who had indicated their desire to join a fraternity but had been rejected would have stronger affiliation motivation than those men who had been accepted into the fraternity.

Based on the stories from these two studies, TAT imagery that seemed to discriminate between the arousal/motive and control groups was used to form the prime test and scoring subcategories for nAff. As before, the story needed to first pass the prime test before subcategories could be scored. The prime test definition of affiliation imagery was "an objective statement in the story that a person is separated from another and is concerned about it or concerned about possible separation" (Shipley & Veroff, 1952, p. 351). Several further types of imagery that would meet this criterion were given. If the prime test is met, the story may be scored further for six subcategories (see Table 15.2). As with nAch, the development of these categories was based entirely on stories from men.

Although this initial work was successful in differentiating between fraternity members in whom nAff had been aroused and those in whom it had not, the measure was not successful in discriminating between

TABLE 15.2. Prime Test and Subcategories for Scoring nAff

Prime test criteria

1. A concern over establishing, restoring or maintaining a positive affective relationship with another person(s) (Atkinson et al., 1954).
2. Expression of emotional concern over separation or description of an interpersonal relationship which indicates a desire to restore a close relationship.
3. A desire to participate or participation in friendly, convivial activities, such as parties, reunions, or visits.

Subcategories

1. Need (N): stated need for affiliation, as seen in the explicit statement of a desire to affiliate or maintain affiliation with some other person or group or persons.
2. Instrumental activity: The person is doing something, including thinking, toward the attainment of the affiliation goal. This action may be further scored as successful (I+), unsuccessful (I−), or of doubtful success (I?).
3. Anticipatory goal states: Someone in the story thinks of the happiness accompanying an affiliative relationship (Ga+) or thinks of the pain or possibility of separation or rejection (Ga−).
4. Obstacles or Blocks: Some obstacle hinders or blocks the attainment of an affiliative relationship. This obstacle may be due to something in the environment (world) (Bw), or may be due to some personal characteristic or action (Bp).
5. Affective states: emotional states associated with the attainment of affiliation. These may be positive (G+) or negative (G−).
6. Affiliation thema: The whole story is about affiliation and there are no other alternative themas being expressed.

Note. Adapted from Heyns et al. (1958). Copyright 1958 by Van Nostrand Reinhold. Adapted by permission.

aroused and nonaroused subjects in a second study (Atkinson, Heyns, & Veroff, 1954). To help explain these contradictory findings, the authors made use of a two-factor theory of motivation (McClelland, 1951).[9] Briefly, this theory posits two types of motives—those involving approach and those involving avoidance. Thus, in the case of achievement motivation, some individuals hope for success (approach motivation) whereas others fear failure (avoidance motivation). The TAT stories of the former men showed more positive anticipation of the goal (Ga+; see Table 15.1), whereas those who fear failure showed more negative anticipation of the goal (Ga−). In the case of affiliation motivation, it appeared that the initial Shipley and Veroff (1952) study focused more on the avoidance motive (i.e., avoiding or fearing separation or rejection). On the other hand, Atkinson et al. (1954) focused more on the approach tendency—that is, a positive motivation to affiliate, defined as "evidence of concern, in one or more of the characters, over establishing, maintaining, a restoring a positive affective relationship with another person(s)" (Atkinson et al., 1954, p. 406). Based on the results of the Atkinson et al. (1954) study, it was suggested that the definition of affiliation motivation should be expanded to include both the approach and the avoidance tendencies. Thus, in the final scoring system (Heyns, Veroff, & Atkinson, 1958) the prime test categories were expanded to include both the approach definition and the avoidance definition (see Table 15.2). A review of research relating this measure to interpersonal sensitivity, performance on academic and other learning tasks, and the nature of interpersonal relationships is provided by Boyatzis (1973), Jemmott (1987), and Smith (1992). A description of the scoring system, and practice, expert-scored stories are available in Smith (1992).

Intimacy Motivation

Further studies with the measure of nAff yielded inconsistent results, often with curvilinear relationships between nAff and various behavioral and attitudinal variables (see McAdams, 1980). Boyatzis (1973), reviewing research studies with the nAff measure, concluded: "It is difficult to draw any conclusions from the data except that something is not right" (p. 261). He suggested that the confusing findings might stem from the inclusion of both the approach and the avoidance aspects of affiliation motivation in the nAff measure.

From this background, McAdams (1980) took a fresh look at the question of people's motivation to associate with others. He noted that the measure of nAff focuses on the *active striving* to attain a goal—the goal of affiliation—following the model of the nAch measure, in which the focus is on the active striving to attain the goal of achievement. In contrast to this activity and striving of nAff, McAdams proposed a related but different motive in which the focus is on the quality of the interpersonal relationship—a focus on being rather than doing. With this focus on the *quality* of the interpersonal encounter, rather than on the *act* of establishing or maintaining relationships, the issue of approach–avoidance motivation was circumvented (McAdams, 1980; McAdams & Powers, 1981).[10]

McAdams referred to the motive he was investigating as the need for intimacy (nIntimacy), which he described as a recurrent preference or readiness in an individual for "the experiencing of a warm, close, and communicative exchange with another (other) person(s)" (McAdams, 1980, p. 430). To develop the TAT scoring categories, four different arousal experiments were conducted; three of these compared existing groups and one involved a laboratory manipulation. In the first condition, college men and women who were attending fraternity and sorority initiation ceremonies (involving warmth, closeness, and conviviality) were compared with a control group of fraternity and sorority members tested in a classroom under neutral conditions. In the second condition, the arousal group consisted of men and women who were attending a college party and who reported they were having a good time; the control group was the same as in the first experiment. Stories for subjects in the third condition were selected from a previous data set of college heterosexual couples who reported being strongly in love; a control group of college students was matched for age, was not chosen as couples, and generally did not report being in love at the time of testing. In the fourth condition, a within-subjects design was used. Men and women college students were first tested in a neutral setting. This was followed by the arousal procedure: Small groups of subjects participated in games, role playing, and other activities "designed to promote spontaneity, sharing, warmth and occasional frivolity" (McAdams, 1988a, p. 103).

As in the case of nAch and nAff, the scoring system for nIntimacy was based on those aspects of TAT stories that consistently differentiated between subjects in whom the intimacy motive had been aroused and other, nonaroused control subjects. As with the other motives, the identification of differentiating aspects of responses was governed by theoretical predilections, but in order to be included in the scoring system, the category must have successfully differentiated between the aroused and the nonaroused subjects. As was true for nAch and nAff, the scoring system consists of a prime test; for nIntimacy, the prime test is defined as imagery in which a relationship produces such positive affect as love, friendship, or happiness, or a dialogue (verbal or nonverbal exchange of information) that is characterized by reciprocal, noninstrumental communication, by discussion of an interpersonal relationship, or by conversation for the purpose of helping another person in distress (McAdams, 1984). Stories that meet the prime test may then be scored for several subcategories of nIntimacy (see Table 15.3).

Further studies of nAff and nIntimacy showed a moderate correlation between the two measures, and both measures were similarly related to behavioral variables and peer ratings (e.g., McAdams & Powers, 1981). However, when both measures were found to relate to the same variable, the relationship with nIntimacy was generally found to be stronger. Also, when the two measures differ in their relationship with other variables, the intimacy measure "appears to capture a 'being' orientation to interpersonal relations whereas affiliation emphasizes a 'doing' orientation" (McAdams, 1982a, p. 159). A summary of research using the nIntimacy measure appears in McAdams (1988a, pp. 77–83) and Smith (1992). A description of the scoring system, and practice, expert-scored stories are available in Smith (1992).

TABLE 15.3. Prime Test and Subcategories for Scoring nIntimacy

Prime test criteria

1. A relationship produces positive affect (love, friendship, happiness, peace, or tender behavior).
2. Dialogue (verbal or nonverbal) that is characterized by at least one of the following:
   a. Reciprocal, noninstrumental communication
   b. Discussion of an interpersonal relationship
   c. Communication for the purpose of helping another person

Subcategories

1. Psychological growth and coping, as a result of an interpersonal encounter.
2. Commitment or concern, not rooted in guilt or begrudging duty.
3. Time–space: A relationship between (among) people transcends the usual limitations of time and/or space.
4. Union: the physical or figurative coming together of people who have been apart.
5. Harmony: between (among) characters; for example, being "on the same wave length."
6. Surrender: Interpersonal relations are beyond character's own control, and he or she surrenders to that outside control.
7. Escape to intimacy: Characters actively or mentally escape from a particular situation or state to another, in the context of interpersonal relations.
8. Connection with the outside world: an explicit example of a connection between character and the nonhuman outside world (e.g., the feeling of wind rushing past her face).

Note. Adapted from McAdams (1988a). Copyright 1988 by The Guilford Press. Adapted by permission. The complete scoring manual, with examples, practice stories, and expert scored stories, is available in McAdams (1984).

Power Motivation

After the establishment of scoring systems to measure nAch and nAff, Veroff (1957) followed the same model—high-motive versus low-motive groups and a scoring system with a prime test and subcategories—to measure the need for power. Veroff's system was the first of several developed to measure power motivation. His design combined two strategies to construct the arousal group. First, the high-motive subjects were selected: They were candidates running for a student office at the University of Michigan. Second, at the time of testing, the situation was believed to be one of high arousal because the subjects were waiting to learn the outcome of the just-held election, about which they had been asked to estimate their chance of winning. It was believed that this group's concern for power would be especially high at the point that they might, in fact, achieve power. The low-power-motive control group consisted of students in an undergraduate psychology course.

The scoring system was constructed using the same approach as used for nAch and nAff: There was a prime test for power imagery, which had to be passed before further scoring for the subcategories could occur. The designation of the subcategories was taken from the previous scoring systems, including need, instrumental activity, goal anticipation, block or obstacle, affective state, and thema (Veroff, 1957). The definition of each of the scoring categories, as before, was based on the empirical findings of content which differentiated between the high- and low-motive subjects, guided by a general definition of the power motive as "that disposition directing behavior toward satisfactions contingent upon the control of the means of influencing another person(s)" (Veroff, 1957, p. 1). A description of the scoring system, and practice, expert-scored stories are available in Smith (1992). Further, "the means of control can be anything at all that can be used to manipulate another person" (Veroff, 1957, p. 1).

Research with this measure produced unclear or inconsistent results, illustrating, perhaps, the approach–avoidance issue discussed earlier. That is, sometimes the measure predicted power-seeking behavior, whereas other times it was related to avoiding power.[11] Eventually, Veroff and Veroff (1972) decided that this first scoring system stressed the negative side of power motivation, and might better be called fear of weakness. Winter has also noted that the Veroff scoring system seemed to tap the "negative, defensive, and avoidant aspects of the power motive" (Winter, 1973, p. 55).

As a result of some dissatisfaction with Veroff's system, two new approaches were developed (Uleman, 1966, 1972; Winter, 1967, 1973).

Uleman's approach stressed the desire for power or influence for its own sake. His research design differed from the earlier studies in two ways: First, in addition to comparing an aroused and nonaroused group, each subject also served as his own control so that his stories before and after the arousal manipulation could be compared. In one arousal study (Uleman, 1966), subjects were tested before and after observing a convincing demonstration of hypnosis; the assumption was that they would want to be powerful like the hypnotist. In a second arousal study (Uleman, 1972), subjects were tested once before participating in a psychological experiment, and then again when they were about to assume the powerful role of experimenter.

Also different from the earlier studies, Uleman did not have a fixed definition of power to influence the choice of scoring categories, and he did not adopt the standard list of subcategories used in the previous scoring schemes. In contrast to Veroff's scheme, Uleman's approach seemed to reflect a more positive orientation toward power. Perhaps for this reason, scores based on the two different systems did not correlate with each other, nor did either system differentiate the aroused from the nonaroused stories of the other investigator. Eventually, Uleman (1972) considered his measure to reflect the need for influence rather than power.

At about the same time that Uleman was developing his system, Winter (1967) created a separate scoring method. In Winter's (1967) study, the arousal condition consisted of having one group of subjects watch a film of the inaugural address of President John F. Kennedy; the control group watched a film about science demonstration equipment. The scoring system used the traditional model of prime test and subcategories. The latter were not restricted to the standard set used for nAch and nAff; their content was determined empirically through a contrast and cross-validation of stories from aroused and nonaroused subjects.

A comparison of the scores derived from the systems of Veroff (1957), Uleman (1966, 1972), and Winter (1967) indicated that the scores did not intercorrelate very highly, and that the three systems were not very successful in differentiating the aroused and nonaroused groups from the other experimenters. Because there was no clear, rational basis for choosing one of these systems over the other two, Winter decided to try to combine all three, taking his 1967 system as a starting point. In this revised procedure, an effort was made to separate need for power from need for achievement, and to merge Veroff's system with that of Winter.[12] In the final system (Winter, 1973), power is defined in terms of someone having impact. Power imagery in the TAT is scored if, in the story, someone is "concerned about his impact"; that is, about "establishing, maintaining, or restoring his prestige or power" (Winter, 1973, p. 69). Winter's (1973) scoring scheme consisted of a prime test and a number of subcategories, some of which followed the basic framework of nAch and nAff (see Table 15.4).

As with the motives of achievement and affiliation/intimacy, the question of approach–avoidance arose in connection with the power motive. For some subjects, it appeared that the power motive involved getting to (approaching) the positively valued goal (power); for others, the motive was to get away from (avoid) the negatively valued goal (power). One way of distinguishing between these two motives is to assume that a high-motive score indicates approach, or hope for reaching the goal, whereas a low score indicates avoidance, or fear of the goal. This approach was adopted with nAch (McClelland et al., 1953) and with nAff (Hardy, 1957; Byrne, 1962). However, other investigators have taken the position that the hope and fear components of a motive are quite separate.[13] Winter (1973) took the stance that the total motive score obtained through the scoring system described above reflects the overall salience of the motive, which in turn consists of both the positive and

TABLE 15.4. Prime Test and Subcategories for Scoring nPower

Prime test criteria

1. Some person or group of persons in the story is concerned about establishing, maintaining, or restoring power.
2. Some person or group of persons is concerned about impact, control, or influence over another person, group, or the world at large.

Subcategories

1. Prestige: The characters are described in ways that increase or decrease their prestige.
2. Stated need for power: an explicit statement that the character wants to attain a power goal. *Not* inferable from mere instrumental activity.
3. Instrumental act: overt or mental activity by a character indicating that he or she is doing something about attaining a power goal.
4. Block in the world: an explicit obstacle or disruption to the attempt to reach a power goal.
5. Goal anticipation: Some character is thinking about the power goal, with either positive or negative anticipations.
6. Goal states: affective or feeling states associated with attaining or not attaining the power goal.
7. Effect: a distinct response by someone to the power actions of someone else in the story, or an indication of widespread effect on the world at large.

Note. Abbreviated from Winter and Stewart (1978); see also Winter (1973). Copyright 1978 by John Wiley & Sons, Inc. Adapted by permission.

negative (approach and avoidance) aspects of the motive. Thus, "the total nPower score represents the sum of approach and avoidance motives in the area of power" (Winter, 1973, p. 79). However, because the subcategories do not necessarily indicate the valence of the motive, Winter adopted a secondary scoring scheme to classify the stories as hope or fear of power. This scheme was based on the finding that some subjects' TAT stories made frequent use of the word "not," a situation referred to as activity inhibition. McClelland, Davis, Kalin, and Wanner (1972) then developed a set of categories that would differentiate between subjects who were high on nPower and also high on activity inhibition and those who were high on nPower but low on activity inhibition. These categories were applied after the prime test was satisfied and were used as alternatives to the usual subcategories. The new subcategories that characterized the high-power/high-inhibition stories were referred to as socialized power, whereas the high-power/low-inhibition stories were referred to as personalized Power.[14]

Because the activity inhibition score is based on the use of "not"—an indication of approach–avoidance—this seemed to be a possible way to determine the hope–fear aspect of the motive. To do this, Winter (1973) maintained his revised scoring scheme but added at the end a series of criteria, derived from McClelland et al. (1972), to determine whether the story, once scored for nPower in the usual way, should be further classified as hope of power or fear of power. Scoring criteria for hope of power were derived from the personalized power definitions, whereas fear of power criteria were derived from the socialized power categories.

Summaries of the earlier research using this approach to measuring the power motive appear in McClelland et al. (1972), McClelland (1971, 1975), Veroff and Feld (1971), and Winter (1973). More recent work has been discussed by Fodor and Farrow (1979), Jemmott (1987), McAdams (1988a), Smith (1992), and Winter and Stewart (1978). The complete scoring manual, with examples, practice stories, and expert-scored stories, is available in Winter (1973, Appendix 1) and Smith (1992).

A further modification of the interpretation of the power motivation score has been carried out by Winter and Barenbaum (1985). Noting that ideas about power and power getting differ for men and women, the authors developed a TAT measure for "Responsibility," based on the conception that previous gender-based interpretations of the uses of power by males and females may actually have more to do with responsibility than with power per se. The concern in this work was, then, with the possible importance of different ways for expressing power—in a responsible fashion, as compared to a "profligate" fashion—as this might interact with gender.

The method used to develop a responsibility scoring system for the TAT followed the McClelland–Atkinson approach discussed earlier. Using existing data sets, individuals whose background variables included factors likely to promote responsibility (e.g., being the oldest child or being a parent) were compared with a control group lacking these background experiences. The TAT stories of the "responsible" and control groups were compared for mention of several themes or categories that were present more often in the "responsible" group. Eventually, five categories were adopted as the TAT scoring system for responsibility (see Table 15.5).

In studies with both college students and young to middle-aged adults, the importance of the responsibility measure for moderating the relation between nPower and behavior characterized as responsible or profligate was demonstrated. For women who were low in responsibility, profligate behavior was associated with the power motive, but for women who were high in responsibility, the relationship between profligate behavior and nPower was the reverse. The same results were generally found with the male subjects. In other words, for both men and women, profligate behavior was correlated with power motivation if the individuals were also low on the TAT responsibility measure, and differences in the expression of power motivation were thus found to be due not so much to gender as to a responsibility orientation, which in turn seemed to be due to differences in socialization.

These findings support the conclusions of Winter (1988) regarding the role of the power motive in predicting the behavior of men and women. In a review of a large number of published and unpublished

---

TABLE 15.5. Scoring System for Responsibility

1. Moral standard: Actions, people, or things in the story are explicitly described in terms of some abstract standard that involves either morality or legality.
2. Obligation: A character is obliged to act due to some impersonal rule or instruction, or there is an inner feeling of obligation or compulsion to act.
3. Concern for others: One character helps or intends to help, or shows sympathetic concern for another.
4. Concern about consequences: A character is worried or concerned about possible negative consequences of his or her actions; mere concern about success or failure is not scored.
5. Self-judgment: A character critically evaluates his or her character, wisdom, self-control, etc.; the evaluation must refer to the self and not merely to outcomes of an action.

Note. Abbreviated from Winter and Barenbaum (1985). Copyright 1985 by Duke University Press. Adapted by permission.

studies, Winter noted that research results consistently found no differences between men and women in their average level of nPower, nor in the ways in which the power motive is aroused, nor in the relationship between nPower and such responsible power behaviors as the acquisition of social power, prestige, or power-related careers. In all these domains, the power motive functions the same way for both sexes.

However, the finding that the power motive does not predict profligate impulsive behaviors (drinking, drug use, aggression, gambling, and sexual exploitation) for women as it does for men has been striking. Although this initially appeared to be an important sex difference, closer examination of the findings indicated that the socialization experiences of responsibility, attendant upon having younger siblings or children, served as important moderators in the relationship between nPower and profligate behaviors. For women with experiences of younger siblings and children, nPower predicts responsible power-related behaviors; for women without these socialization experiences, nPower does not predict responsible power and does predict the same kind of profligate behaviors usually found among men. A reanalysis of data from men produced a similar finding. Thus, the relationship between nPower and profligate behaviors appears to have more to do with socialization experiences than with gender per se. It is the fact that females are more likely to have socialization experiences involving the responsible caring for others that accounts both for the relationship between nPower and responsible power behaviors found in women and for the absence of a relationship between nPower and profligate behaviors that is found with men who have had the same kind of socialization experiences.

A description of the scoring system, with expert-scored stories, is available in Smith (1992).

OTHER APPROACHES

The McClelland–Atkinson approach to measuring motives demonstrated to many researchers that it was possible to develop reasonably objective, reliable scoring systems for the TAT that were both theoretically meaningful and empirically successful in assessing significant aspects of personality. With this support, the areas of research with the TAT expanded beyond the assessment of motives, and the nature of the scoring systems no longer adhered to the prime test–behavioral sequence subcategories of the earlier model. Whereas the study of motives had been derived from Murray's (1938) theory of personality, more recent research with the TAT has explored concepts derived from psychoanalytic theory.

Emotional Stances in the Process of Adaptation

In *Three Essays on the Theory of Sexuality,* Freud (1905/1962) proposed a theory of psychosexual development, later expanded by Erikson (1950), in which it was hypothesized that individuals normally pass through four important psychosexual stages of development: oral, anal, phallic, and genital. The four stages are age related and cover the period from birth through adolescence; however, the rate of moving from one stage to another will vary across individuals. In certain cases, a person may be fixated at, or regress to, an earlier developmental stage. Based on this theory, Stewart (1973, 1977, 1982b) developed a scoring system, using the TAT stories of male college students, to assess preoccupation with the emotional concomitants of the four psychosexual stages of development. Her first step was to find subjects who best represented a preoccupation with each psychosexual stage. This was accomplished by establishing behaviorally based criteria for each stage. Oral preoccupation was inferred from subjects' reports of oral activity (e.g., eating and smoking). Anal preoccupation was inferred from reports of behavior that was highly ritualized and focused around issues of orderliness and cleanliness. Phallic preoccupation was inferred from reports of extensive high school dating with different girls, characterized by playing the field and a concern for sex and self-image. Genital preoccupation was inferred from having a committed relationship in which time and energy were devoted both to work and to intimate communication (Stewart, 1982b). From a larger sample of 348 men, 6 individuals were chosen to represent each psychosexual stage on the basis of their reporting all the signs of preoccupation with that stage and none of the signs from the other stages. In addition to this group of 24, a second, cross-validation group of 26 was selected on the basis of their showing all the signs from one psychosexual stage and not more than one behavior from another stage. For different purposes, all subjects had previously written stories about five TAT pictures under neutral conditions.

Having identified these criterion groups, the McClelland–Atkinson method of empirical analysis of TAT stories was employed to determine what thematic content would differentiate the stories of individuals with different psychosexual preoccupations. Examination of these stories indicated that four major issues appeared in the stories of all the groups: relationship with authority figures, relationships with other people, inner feelings or affective responses, and orientation to action. However, the approach to these issues differed for individuals from each psychosexual group. Thus, regarding attitude toward authority, individuals in the oral group wrote stories in which authority was portrayed as benevolent, whereas individuals in the anal group characterized authority as critical or reprimanding. Subjects in the phallic group portrayed opposition to authority, while the attitude of those in the genital group was that the power of authority is limited. Similar differences across the four subject groups were found for the other three issues (see Table 15.6).

An inspection of the TAT content that characterized each of the psychosexual groups revealed a meaningful fit with psychoanalytic theory. For example, persons in the oral group, in addition to seeing authority figures as benevolent, also perceived other persons "as sources of immediate gratification of their wishes. Their feelings showed a preoccupation with the issues of loss and abandonment, including confusion and despair, and their orientation to action was entirely passive–receptive" (Stewart, 1982b, p. 1104). This personality description fits very well with the psychoanalytic characterization of the oral character, or of a child in the oral stage of development. Similarly, the TAT concerns of the three other psychosexual groups fit nicely with the theoretical descriptions of those groups in the psychoanalytic literature. In this way, the empirically derived content differences among the TAT stories from the four empirically determined criterion groups provided a meaningful confirmation of psychoanalytic theory.

Because the four thematic fantasy concerns of each psychosexual group did not assess literal preoccupations with erogenous zones, Stewart

TABLE 15.6. Levels of Psychosexual Development (Emotional Stances)

	Attitude toward authority	Relations with others	Feelings	Orientation to action
Oral (receptivity)	Authority is benevolent	Immediate gratification	Loss, despair, confusion	Passivity
Anal (autonomy)	Authority is critical, reprimanding	Lack of gratification	Anxiety about competence	Clearing of disorder
Phallic (assertion)	Opposition to authority	Flight and exploitation	Hostility, anger	Failure, in context of confident attempt
Genital (integration)	Authority is limited	Mutuality, sharing	Ambivalence	Work commitment and involvement

Note. From Stewart (1982b). Copyright 1982 by the American Psychological Association. Adapted by permission.

renamed the fantasy cluster characteristic of each group as representing four different "stances." For the oral group, the fantasy cluster was renamed as reflecting the stance of "receptivity" (taking in, getting, incorporation). The anal group's fantasy concerns were renamed as reflecting the stance of "autonomy" (holding on, maintaining). For the phallic group, the concerns were renamed as reflecting the stance of "assertion" (expanding, reaching out, intruding), and for the genital group, the stance was named "integration" (relating, committing, connecting). It is apparent that this TAT scoring scheme might be considered a measure of Erikson's psychosocial stages of development (see McClelland, 1975). However, Stewart makes it clear that the measure is not intended to represent a developmental sequence but, rather, to represent a process of adaptation which occurs in response to a changed environment.[15]

Application of the scoring system to the cross-validation sample described earlier indicated that scores on each stance (receptivity, autonomy, assertion, and integration) clearly differentiated among the four behavior criterion groups. Further investigation of the psychometric properties of the measure, and of its success in demonstrating the kind of psychological adaptations (e.g., regression to an earlier stance) made by individuals in response to significant environmental changes, has been provided in a number of empirical studies (McClelland, 1975; Stewart & Healy, 1985; Stewart et al., 1982; Stewart et al., 1986). These are discussed in Chapters 11 and 12.

Sexual Concerns

There are two scoring approaches in which the TAT has been used to assess sexual concerns. Both studies established scoring categories on a priori grounds and then used experimental arousal techniques to validate the scoring schemes.

The first approach (Clark, 1952) was prompted by the McClelland et al. (1953) method for the assessment of need achievement. Clark noted that although the expression of nAch may be fairly direct in the TAT, the expression of other motives, such as sex or aggression, may be socially less acceptable. In this latter case, there may be some defensive inhibition that occurs due to anxiety, resulting in a decrease of overt motive expression in TAT stories. (For a discussion of the issue of direct expression vs. the substitutive–defensive position, see Chapter 14.) It was Clark's intent to investigate this issue as it applies to sexual motivation.

In three different experiments, the TAT stories of sexually aroused male subjects were compared with those of a nonaroused, control group. The arousal conditions included (1) exposure to photographic slides of attractive nude females (vs. slides of landscape, architecture, and interior design), (2) using a very attractive female experimenter to administer the TAT (vs. using a male experimenter); and (3) exposure to slides of nude females after 1½ hours of participation in a fraternity beer-drinking party (vs. participation in a beer-drinking party without exposure to any slides). Stories were scored for three categories of sexual imagery and three categories indicating sexual guilt (see Table 15.7).

Significant for the inhibition hypothesis, subjects in the arousal groups of experiments 1 and 2 showed significantly *less* sexual imagery than did their control subjects. However, the beer-drinking arousal subjects in experiment 3 showed more sexual imagery than did their controls. In general, primary sexual imagery[16] was the main contributor to the differences in the scores of subjects in experiments 1 and 3. Moreover, in all three experiments, the subjects who showed the most sexual imagery were also the subjects who had the highest scores for sexual guilt.

Taken together, these findings supported the initial hypothesis. Under normal conditions, the anxiety or guilt attendant on the arousal of the sexual motive led to an inhibition in the expression of this motive in TAT stories, with a resulting lowering of guilt. After drinking, however, the anxiety or guilt over sexual arousal was reduced enough to allow the expression of sexual imagery in TAT stories, resulting in an increase in expressed guilt.

TABLE 15.7. Scoring Categories for Sexual Motivation

Sexual imagery[a]

A. Primary sexual relationships: explicit or implicit evidence for sexual intercourse.
B. Secondary sexual relationships: evidence for the occurrence of such secondary sex activity as kissing, dancing, fondling, etc.
C. Tertiary sexual relationships: characters in the stories perceived as sweethearts, on a date, courting, in love, etc., but not engaged in either primary or secondary sexual activity.

Sexual guilt[b]

A. Someone is ashamed, guilty, sorry, anxiety-ridden, morally concerned, embarrassed, etc., over sexual activity.
B. Someone is punished, criticized, ostracized for sexual activity.
C. Someone punishes himself in some concrete fashion as a result of a sexual activity.

Note. Adapted from Clark (1952). Copyright 1952 by the American Psychological Association. Adapted by permission.
[a]Scored only once for each story; category that is biologically most sexual is given priority.
[b]Guilt is scored only in connection with sexual activity and is scored only once for each story.

The second approach to studying sexual concerns with the TAT attempted to measure castration anxiety (Schwartz, 1955). On the basis of psychoanalytic writings and clinical observations, nine a priori categories were established, describing events that were believed to relate to castration anxiety; a tenth category consisted of nonspecific formal indices of anxiety (see Table 15.8). The experimental design included three groups of male subjects. In the castration-anxiety arousal group, subjects were shown a film explicitly depicting the subincision rites of a Bushman tribe of central Australia. A second arousal group was shown a section of a commercial film in which the severe emotional deprivation of a young boy was portrayed. The control group was shown a section of a Chaplin comedy. Following the films, subjects wrote stories about eight TAT cards.

When the TAT stories were scored according to the castration-anxiety categories, there was a clear difference between the castration-aroused group and the other two groups, with the former having a significantly higher total score and significantly higher scores on a majority of the scoring categories. Also important, the subjects in the other two groups did not differ from each other; thus the effect was specific to the castration-anxiety arousal condition. Interestingly, the typical pattern of the castration-arousal stories is described as beginning with the hero involved in some sexual activity, perhaps with a prostitute. After the sex act, the hero is described as remorseful and/or threatened from external sources and as losing loved ones. The ending of the story was often "bad," including death, debilitation, or some loss of status or possessions.

TABLE 15.8. Scoring Categories for Castration Anxiety

1. Genital injury or loss.
2. Damage to or loss of other parts of the body. Also included are less specific types of damage, such as beating, torture or illness.
3. Damage to or loss of extensions of the body image. This includes prized possessions which may symbolize the self or parts of the self.
4. Sexual inadequacy.
5. Personal inadequacy.
6. General repetitive attempts at mastery.
7. Intrapsychic threat. This includes guilt, remorse, and expectations of punishment.
8. Extrapsychic threat.
9. Loss of cathected objects.
10. Formal characteristics of stories. This includes discontinuities in the stories, "bad" endings, misspellings, etc.

Note. Adapted from Schwartz (1955). Copyright 1955 by Duke University Press. Adapted by permission.

Overall, the description of this pattern is strikingly similar to the pattern described by May (1966; see Chapter 6); enhancement followed by deprivation is the prototypical pattern for representing male sexual identity. That this pattern would be intensified in males whose anxiety about physical sexuality has been increased is understandable and offers support for the validity of May's approach.[17]

Schwartz's measure of castration anxiety has been shown to differentiate between college-age men who experienced loss or absence of their fathers prior to age 6 and those men whose fathers were present (Shill, 1981). The greater castration anxiety among the father-absent men was interpreted as support for the psychoanalytic concept of the Oedipus complex and as a demonstration of the importance of the father's presence in helping the young boy to master castration anxiety.

Self-Definition versus Social Definition

In addition to Westen's approach to using the TAT to assess characteristics of object relations (see Chapter 10), there are two other scoring approaches that also reflect some of the more current concerns of psychoanalytic theory. Stewart and Winter (1974) developed a coding system for the TAT to identify two contrasting patterns used by individuals to organize their experience and to define themselves; Gutman (1964, 1985) developed an approach to assess different styles of ego mastery.

The two patterns identified by Stewart and Winter (1974) are termed "self-definition" and "social definition." The "self-definition" coding categories (scored +1) include causality, defined as the "use of explicit causal language" (p. 1082) and reason–action sequence, in which "the final element of the story is an action or plan for action which follows logically from the preceding elements" (p. 1082). The "social definition" pattern includes four categories (scored −1): "no causality"; "mental state ending," defined as the final element of the story being a character's feeling, expressive behavior, or state of being; "higher power intervention"; and "ineffective actor," defined as the final element of the story being phrased in the passive voice or an impersonal construction, with the explicit statement "that characters are helpless or that action is futile and pointless" (p. 1082) (see Table 15.9).

The coding system was developed from a derivation study in which 49 college women told stories to four TAT-like pictures and responded to a brief questionnaire. On the basis of the questionnaire response, two criterion groups were established: those women who showed a clear career commitment and those who planned marriage and family without a career. The self-definition categories mentioned above were derived from the stories of the women planning a career, whereas the social definition categories were derived from the stories of the women planning a marriage and family.

The scoring system was cross-validated with another sample of women college students who wrote stories about six TAT or TAT-like pictures. On the basis of a questionnaire, the women were grouped into four categories representing career orientation: women who intended (1) lifetime careers in professions considered typically male; (2) lifetime careers in professions typically female; (3) brief jobs, or part time jobs and marriage; and (4) marriage and family, with no mention of jobs or careers. When the stories of these four groups were scored, the highest self-definition (positive) score was found in group (1), followed by group (2). Group (3), and to an even greater extent group (4), had negative scores, indicating social definition. The four groups were statistically different from each other, and there was a strong positive correlation between career orientation and self-definition score. The scores were unrelated to age, college or social class, intelligence, length of stories told, or traditional sex-role measures but were related to a variety of family background and behavioral variables. A description of the scoring system, and practice, expert-scored stories are available in Smith (1992).

TABLE 15.9. Outline of the Scoring System for Self-Definition

Self-definition categories

1. Causality (scored +1). Score any word(s) that explicitly indicate a causal relationship (e.g., because, therefore, thus).
2. Reason–action sequence (scored +1). Score if the final event of the story is an action or purposeful plan for action by any character in the story.

Social definition categories

3. No causality (scored −1). Score if actions or events occur without reason or are merely habitual or routine. Also score if no actions occur or are planned in the story.
4. Mental state ending (scored −1). Score if the story ends with someone's feelings or thoughts, or with a state of being, but not with action or purposeful plan for action.
5. Higher power intervention (scored −1). Score if a "higher power" takes some action that has an effect on the lives of the character(s), without any subsequent action by the character(s).
6. Ineffective actor (scored −1). Score if it is predicted that any action is futile —that is, will have no effect on the situation, or if the resolving (or only) actions of the story are phrased in the passive voice or impersonal construction.

Note. Adapted from Stewart and Winter (1974). Copyright 1974 by Duke University Press. Adapted by permission.

Styles of Ego Mastery

The last TAT scoring system to be discussed in this chapter also relates to psychoanalytic concepts involving ego psychology. Gutmann (1964, 1985) developed a scoring approach to assess different styles of ego mastery. The original system was based on three categories, each delineating a different style of coping with psychic stress (see Table 15.10).[18]

The main categories, "active mastery," "passive mastery," and "magic mastery" were used both for men and for women, but the subcategories differed for each sex, reflecting differences in theme and content of the stories.[19] Men and women of the "active mastery" type were alike in "the formal and structural qualities of their stories. Both sexes impart vigor and conflict to the scene in a framework of logically developed, well-organized, and reasonable stories" (Gutmann, 1964, p. 132). However, for the men, the conflict, or struggle, is with an impersonal environment ("self-asserters") or with passive aspects of themselves ("achievement doubters") that interfere with achievement; for women the conflict is with people ("rebellious daughters"; "moralistic matriarchs").

Both men and women of the "passive mastery" type handle conflict by changing themselves rather than reshaping their environments. For men, this reshaping may be in accord with others' demands ("adaptive conformers") or in terms of disavowing personal motivations and instead

TABLE 15.10. Scoring Scheme for Styles of Ego Mastery

Scoring scheme for men

1. Active mastery
    a. Self-asserters
    b. Achievement doubters
2. Passive mastery
    a. Adaptive conformers
    b. Depersonalized conformers
3. Magical mastery

Scoring scheme for women

1. Active mastery
    a. Rebellious daughters
    b. Moralistic matriarchs
2. Passive mastery
    a. Maternal altruists
    b. Passive aggressors
3. Magical mastery

Note. Adapted from Gutmann (1964).

projecting these onto the world ("depersonalized conformer"). For women, changing the self occurs by way of intropunitive mechanisms. When this is effective, the style involves reaction formation and an identification with their children ("maternal altruists"). When it is not effective, the style is characterized by depression, constriction, and an apathetic conformity to convention ("passive aggressors").

Finally, men and women of the "magical mastery" type show more evidence of distortion of reality in order to create the world as they would like it to be (male) or to justify impulsive or domineering behavior (female). There is evidence of regressive behavior and regressive ego functioning. Studies using these measures of ego mastery are discussed in detail by Gutmann (1987) and are presented in Chapter 12.

SUMMARY

This chapter has described the development of a series of carefully constructed methods for use with the TAT to measure personality characteristics. The pioneering studies of McClelland and Atkinson—their work on the achievement motive and the methodology they created to establish an empirically based scoring system for a psychological disposition, as revealed in TAT stories—are discussed in some detail. It is this approach to developing a scoring system for the TAT that has spawned a host of reliable, valid, and meaningful research studies. It has also has led to the establishment of clearly defined scoring methods for a range of personality variables, including various motives, psychosexual orientation, sexual concerns, self-definition and ego mastery, among others. Detailed descriptions of these scoring methods are provided in the chapter, with references for further follow-up if desired. An understanding of this methodology should make it possible for the researcher to use the TAT to investigate any personality characteristic for which there is an empirical referent.

SIXTEEN

The TAT in Clinical Research Studies: Further Examples

Among psychologists of a psychodynamic persuasion, the TAT is generally considered one of the standard procedures to be included in a psychodiagnostic test battery. At the same time, the question of just how to use the resulting stories, and of whether there are significant markers, or signs, for making differential diagnoses has frequently been a source of puzzlement. In previous chapters, different perspectives for the interpretation of TAT stories from clinical patients have been discussed (see Chapters 8, 9, and 10). In addition to these clinical approaches, there have been a number of research studies relating the TAT to various types of pathology. These latter studies have shown reliable relationships between content and form variables from the TAT with both physical disorders and psychological pathology. In this chapter, aspects of the TAT that relate to physical health and disease, to alcohol and drug use, and to physical and sexual abuse will be discussed, as well as story features that relate to the psychological diagnoses of schizophrenia and other psychotic disorders.[1] A final section discusses the use of the TAT with disturbed children.

PHYSICAL HEALTH AND ILLNESS

There is a substantial body of research demonstrating a relationship between physical health or disease and various motivational dispositions, as measured by the TAT.

Hypertension

One of the first published reports in this area was provided by McClelland (1979), who investigated the relationship between high blood pressure and TAT motive scores. In this investigation, three different groups of men were studied. The first group consisted of 127 German men, 77 of whom were diagnosed with essential hypertension; the other 50 were normal with respect to blood pressure. The second sample consisted of 235 male college freshmen for whom measures of blood pressure were available. Stories about six TAT-like pictures were obtained concurrently from both of the samples. The third sample comprised 78 men whose blood pressure had first been recorded during their junior year of college (about 1940) and had subsequently been recorded about every 5 years thereafter until 1972–1974. During 1950–1952, this last group gave stories about five TAT pictures.

The stories from each sample were scored for nAchievement, nPower, and nAffiliation motivation and for "activity inhibition."[2] From these data, scores on the "inhibited power motive syndrome" were derived. In all three samples, subjects who showed the inhibited power motive syndrome also had higher blood pressure than did subjects with other motive pattern combinations. In the third, longitudinal study, the inhibited power motive syndrome, as measured when these men were in their early 30s, was a significant predictor of elevated blood pressure and hypertensive pathology which appeared 20 years later.[3]

This report clearly demonstrated the relationship between TAT motivational measures and one significant health problem. In recent years, the study of the relationship between TAT measures of social motives and physical illness has been greatly expanded to include a variety of physical problems. Investigators have used TAT stories to investigate possible personality differences associated with health problems such as arthritis, diabetes, and cancer.

Arthritis

For example, one study (Koestner, Ramey, Kelner, Meenan, & McClelland, 1989) found that adults suffering from arthritis, as compared to normal control subjects, had lower TAT scores for achievement and power motivation. Those arthritics with poor health status had especially low levels of achievement motivation. These findings were in contrast to the consciously stated desires of the arthritic subjects and suggested to the authors that the subjects had "an implicit motivational deficit" of which they were unaware.

A second study of adults with three different types of arthritis (Vollhardt, Ackerman, & Shindledecker, 1985) looked for evidence of alexithymia[4] in their TAT stories. Contrary to the hypotheses of the authors, the three groups did not differ in the overall assessment of alexithymic characteristics; unfortunately, there was no nonarthritic control group with which to compare their responses. Further, within the arthritic patients, TAT-based alexithymic scores were significantly correlated with lower socioeconomic class.

Diabetes

The TAT has also been used to detect the presence of alexithymia in adult and adolescent insulin-dependent diabetics. In a study by Abramson, McClelland, Brown, and Kelner (1991), diabetic subjects used fewer emotion words in their TAT stories as compared to controls; in turn, this was found to be associated with poorer metabolic control. It was concluded that the lack of awareness of emotions contributed to the diabetics' difficulty in managing their illness and in regulating glucose levels.

Similar findings were obtained from a study of adolescents who had poor control over their diabetes (Koski, Holmberg, & Torvinen, 1988). As compared to a control group of similar age and sex distribution, the TAT stories of the diabetic adolescents indicated less capacity to express emotions. In addition, their stories demonstrated the use of lower-level defense mechanisms and indicated they were in the earlier stages of the second individuation process characteristic of adolescence (Blos, 1967). Interestingly, the evidence for alexithymia was strongest in those adolescents for whom the onset of diabetes occurred prior to age 6, next strongest in those with an onset between 6 and 11 years, and absent in those with onset after age 12.

Other Health Problems

Two further investigations have used the TAT with patients suffering from physical disorders in an attempt to assess the presence of alexithymic characteristics. A study in Finland (Keltikangas-Jarvinen, 1985) compared the TAT stories of patients with duodenal ulcer, ulcerative colitis, and irritable colon syndrome (disorders believed to have a psychological component) with those of patients with gallstone disease, inguinal hernia, and varicose veins (the control group). The author concluded that the former group showed greater evidence of alexithymia, as evidenced by deficiencies in verbalizing emotions. However, inspection of the results shows that the lower level of reference to emotions in that group is due to the fact that it includes relatively more men, as compared to the control group.[5] In general, men expressed fewer emotions than women; this was true in both groups. In fact, the mean scores of the men in the two groups are identical, as are the mean scores of the women in the two groups.

A second study, carried out in India, used the TAT to assess alexithymia in 30 patients with psychogenic pain disorder who were matched with 30 normal individuals for background variables (Sriram, Chaturvedi, Gopinath, & Shanmugam, 1987). There was some indication that the pain patients used fewer and a narrower range of words than the normals, but the differences were not statistically significant.

The TAT was used to study motivational differences between cancer patients and controls in another study (Cella & Tress, 1986). Sixty men who were diagnosed as either in the early or late stages of Hodgkin's disease were studied; half of each group had recently finished multimodal treatment (surgery, radiation, and chemotherapy),[6] and half had concluded treatment in the more distant past.[7] The TAT stories from both the cancer patients and age- and sex-matched physically healthy controls[8] were scored for intimacy motivation by a single, reliable rater who was blind to diagnosis. The results indicated that all patient groups had lower nIntimacy scores than did the controls. The authors suggest that the experience of cancer may increase the patients' sense of alienation, as well as their refusal to accept a dependent role, resulting in lower nIntimacy scores. Although the four patient groups did not differ statistically, those patients in the early stages of the disease tended to have lower scores than those in the late stages.

Another investigation looked at differences in the TAT stories of women with eating disorders (Williams & Manaster, 1990). Restricter anorexics, bulimic anorexics, and bulimics were contrasted with 30 comparison subjects. The three eating disordered groups had higher scores than the controls on TAT-rated passivity, external locus of control, and negative affect. Avoidance was rated higher in the two bulimic groups than the control group, while detaching from others was greater in the two anorexic groups than in the controls. Both the bulimic and restricter anorexic groups scored lower on maternal empathy than did the controls; the restricter group also scored lower than the controls on achieving as a priority. Measures of maternal malevolence and frustration of autonomy did not show differences between the eating disordered subjects and the controls, and there were very few mentions of food in the stories of the clinical subjects.

MOTIVES AND THE SUPPRESSION OF IMMUNE FUNCTIONS: A THEORY

Stemming from these and other studies, investigators have begun to identify the mediating links between TAT-assessed motives and physical health. Work by McClelland (1989) and Jemmott (1987) has provided a theory about the relationship between social motives and disease suscep-tibility and has marshalled a large body of supporting evidence for the theory. On the behavioral level, the theory holds that if a person with a strong need for power finds that power motivation inhibited, challenged, or blocked, susceptibility to disease will be increased. This means that a person who is above average in nPower and high in self-control (i.e., the inhibited power motive syndrome) is more vulnerable to disease than other people. Also, a person who is above average in nPower, if exposed to high power-related stress ("stressed power motivation"), should be more vulnerable to disease. Thus, the person most vulnerable to disease would be above average on three dimensions: nPower, inhibited power motivation, and life stress. On the other hand, affiliation motivation is seen as having healthy effects on the individual. Thus, a person who is above average in "relaxed affiliation" (defined as having a high nAffilia-tion score, which is greater than nPower, with low activity inhibition) and above average in "unstressed affiliation" (defined as high nAffiliation, which is greater than nPower, with a low degree of life stress) should be the least vulnerable to disease.

Supporting this theory are the results of a study by McClelland and Jemmott (1980). Male and female college students wrote TAT stories and subsequently completed a self-report inventory on life events and illnesses during the preceding 6 months. Stories were scored for nPower, nAffili-ation, and activity inhibition; in addition, number of power and affiliative life stresses were determined. While neither nPower nor nAffiliation alone was related to severity of physical illness, those individuals who were high in nPower,[9] high in activity inhibition, and high in power stress showed overwhelmingly the greatest severity of physical illness. Although the presence of all three of these variables determined which subjects showed the most illness, those who were high on nPower and on just one of the other two variables (activity inhibition or power stress) were also significantly more likely to report severe illness than were other subjects. Also, for subjects who were high on nPower and activity inhibition, high affiliative stress produced the same results as high power stress. This was not true for subjects low in activity inhibition. In general, however, it appeared that stress related to the dominant motive disposition was more likely to be associated with physical illness.

In this study, McClelland and Jemmott (1980) hypothesized about the possible biological explanation for the relationship observed between physical illness, motive dispositions, and life stresses. They noted that events of the power stress type have been found to increase the activation of the sympathetic nervous system. This activation may be an important mediating mechanism for explaining increases in illness because chronic sympathetic activation may suppress immune functions. Jemmott (1987) went on to provide a further explanation for how social motives may be linked to disease susceptibility by citing studies that show that individuals who are high in power motivation are lower in certain parameters of immunological competence, and that for these individuals, immunological competence is further decreased when they are exposed to life stress events. McClelland (1989) concluded that "the explanation for these findings appeared to be that stressed power motivation leads to sympathetic [nervous system] activation, which, if chronic, could raise blood pressure and could lead to more infectious illness through releasing stress hormones that weaken immune defenses against illness" (p. 676).

One of the immunological parameters that has been tested in several studies is secretory immunoglobulin (S-IgA), which is an aspect of humoral immunity. S-IgA is found in serum and secretory fluids (e.g., saliva), which cover mucosal surfaces through which most infective agents enter the body. The S-IgA antibodies present at these surfaces provide an important defense against infection. Thus, an individual who is low in S-IgA antibodies is more susceptible to disease. The fact that individuals who are high in nPower tend to have lower concentrations of S-IgA antibodies explains the physiological link between the social motive of nPower and the higher incidence of physical illness in these individuals.

Jemmott (1987) also cites some evidence that high affiliation motivation is related to better immunological functioning, as well as to lower reports of severe illnesses. Several investigations found that subjects who were high in nAffiliation, or who had affiliation motivation aroused experimentally, had stronger immune functions (S-IgA); this appears to be especially true during high-stress periods. According to McClelland, a particular aspect of nAffiliation is involved in this phenomenon, which he terms "affiliative trust," defined as an orientation toward cooperative, affiliative relationships in contrast to cynical, mistrustful relationships.

This assumption was supported by experimental investigations. In a study by McClelland and Krishnit (1988), the arousal of two different motives had a differential effect on immunocompetence. The experimental arousal of Affiliation motivation (via a film viewing) was followed by an increase in S-IgA if the subjects continued to dwell on affiliation; on the other hand, the experimental arousal of power motivation was followed by a reduction in S-IgA levels among those subjects who had the inhibited power motive syndrome. A similar result was obtained by McKay (1991), who demonstrated a relationship between experimentally aroused affiliation motivation and immune function (S-IgA) concentration. Subjects watched a film designed to arouse feelings about relationships and then provided stories about TAT-like pictures. Persons who told stories in which relationships were described as benevolent (affiliative trust) showed an increase in S-IgA level, whereas subjects who subsequently described malevolent relationships (affiliative mistrust) had a decrease in S-IgA concentration. A second study confirmed that high mistrust scores were associated with poorer immune function and more frequent illnesses.

In a further study, McClelland (1989) was able to demonstrate that the motive–immunological association does not simply reflect differences in motivational factors that occur as a *response* to illness. In a study carried out in a community health center, patients with varying physical complaints were assigned to behavioral medicine treatment groups designed to reduce the effects of stress and increase the sense of personal power or control over their lives. The subjects were tested immediately before treatment, at the end of treatment (6 weeks), and 6 months later. At the end of the treatment period, all patients showed fewer symptoms and fewer visits to the clinic. However, those patients who were high in affiliative trust showed a greater reduction of symptoms than did those who were low on this dimension. Thus, affiliative trust "enabled the patients to benefit more from the behavioral medicine treatments" (p. 680).

In a further longitudinal study (McClelland, 1989) individuals who scored high in affiliative trust at age 31 had significantly fewer serious illnesses in the subsequent 10 years than did those low in affiliative trust.

Thus motive patterns are not just *responses* to health conditions. Rather, they play a causal role "because they predict illness over a 10 year period and because changes in them produced by therapy precede health improvements" (p. 682). McClelland suggests that "the motive syndrome relationships to health are mediated through the chronic activation of emotional centers in the brain and of the autonomic nervous system, and through the release of various hormones that affect immune defenses or other physiological systems involved in particular diseases" (p. 682). In particular, McClelland (1989) has found evidence for norepinephrine being related to the power motive and dopamine as connected to the affiliative motive.

However, in a study of male prisoners (McClelland, Alexander, & Marks, 1982), the effect of power motivation on severity of illness and on immunological functions was overshadowed by the stresses of prison life. As in other studies, for men who were high in nPower, "high stress was associated with the highest mean of illness-severity scores and the lowest mean concentration of S-IgA. . . . [However,] . . . stress and motive type did not combine significantly" (p. 68). The authors attribute the overriding effect of stress, regardless of motive type, as due to the intensity of tension produced by imprisonment, in contrast to the less intense stress present in earlier studies.

An extensive discussion of these investigations, which have demonstrated the relationship between motives, as measured by the TAT, and physical illness, including in some cases a demonstration of the mediating physiological or hormonal variables, has been provided by McClelland (1989). He contrasts the success of these studies using the TAT to those of others which have attempted to relate illness to self-report inventories. Much of the success with the TAT, McClelland believes, stems from the fact that the measurement of the personality variables (i.e., motives) is not dependent on the self-report of the subject, and that the mediating mechanisms (behavioral or physiological) are identified and measured.

ALCOHOL USE

A number of studies have been carried out in which the TAT was used to investigate personality variables and thought processes associated with the use of alcohol. Several of these studies are discussed in this section.

In one of the most complete studies of the personality correlates associated with alcohol use in men, McClelland et al. (1972) found a clear relationship between TAT motive scores and excessive drinking. Those men who were high in nPower but had low inhibition scores were most likely to be heavy drinkers. Further, it was found that a particular type of power imagery was likely to be associated with heavy drinking—namely, "personalized power"—defined as an orientation to the world in which a man must seek to win out over opponents, and where interactions with others are as in a competitive jungle.[10] Men who are heavy drinkers are likely to have a high need for personal power before they start a drinking episode, and the strength of this motivation increases after drinking. Thus drinking is seen as a means to increase their "desire to dominate others who could oppose them" (p. 161).

A concern with "socialized power," defined as thoughts about exerting influence over others, but including doubts about the worth of power, was also related to drinking.[11] Socialized power was found to increase with drinking, especially with moderate amounts of drinking. However, socialized power scores declined in relative importance as drinking progressed. Overall, the problem drinker was best identified from TAT stories in which the standard score for personalized power was higher than the standard score for socialized power. McClelland et al. (1972) summarized their findings: "The heavy drinker's interest in personalized power is always greater both before and after drinking than his interest in socialized power, whereas the reverse is true of light drinkers" (p. 161).

In an earlier study (Kalin, McClelland, & Kahn, 1965), several clear relationships were found between the *amount* of alcohol consumed and changes in TAT stories. A large sample of college males freely consumed alcoholic drinks at their own pace during typical social occasions and wrote TAT stories at three points: on arrival, after about 25 minutes of drinking, and after another 25 minutes of drinking. The amount of alcohol consumed by each man was monitored. A control group[12] followed the same story-writing procedures but consumed only nonalcoholic drinks. Whereas the protocols of the control subjects showed little change over the three testings, those of the drinking subjects changed significantly. Verbal expression of physical aggression increased to a maximum after three or four drinks[13] and then decreased for a time, being replaced by an increasing expression of physical sex thoughts from six drinks on. Inhibitory thoughts—such as restraints on aggression, fear, anxiety and time concern—decreased after 6 drinks. After 10 drinks, expression of physical aggression in the stories again increased. Interestingly, the prealcohol scores for sex and aggression, less the scores on the inhibitory categories which decreased, actually predicted the amount of alcohol that would subsequently be consumed.

In a further study, the effects of alcohol on the presence of violent and aggressive fantasy in TAT stories were tested, after being primed with violent content (Gustafson, 1987). Male undergraduate subjects watched a violent video movie for 1 hour and 41 minutes, after half of them had consumed orange juice spiked with alcohol, and half drank only orange juice. After the movie, subjects told stories about three TAT cards[14]; stories were then scored for aggression and violence by two independent judges, with differences reconciled. Although the results were not statistically significant, the alcohol group did show somewhat greater aggressive and violent fantasy. This finding is difficult to interpret because no prealcohol measure was taken.

A relationship between TAT motive scores and drinking behavior was also found in Veroff's (1982) large-scale 1976 national study (see Chapter 12). In that sample, a high score on either the "fear of weakness" or the "hope for power" component of nPower was correlated, for men, with having a drinking problem that caused family troubles. For women, "hope for power" was related to problem drinking.

The relationship between alcohol consumption and motive scores in women has also been investigated. Wilsnack (1974) used an experimental design similar to that of Kalin et al. (1965), in which women participated in typical social occasions that were either "wet" (alcohol served) or "dry" (soft drinks served). TAT stories were written at the beginning of the parties and again after 70 minutes of party interaction. In order to explore two different theories regarding the motivation for drinking—the dependency theory and the power theory—stories were scored for the presence of dependency imagery[15] and for power motivation according to the system used by McClelland et al. (1972) in their study of male drinking (reported earlier).

The effects of drinking were determined by comparing the wet group with the dry group for changes on these TAT variables after beverage consumption. The results indicated there were no differences between the two groups in changes on dependency measures. However, contrary to the finding with men, subjects in the wet group showed a *de*crease in power scores as compared to the dry group, which showed an increase. Comparisons were also made between those women who consumed more than two drinks (i.e., more than 3 ounces of 86 proof alcohol; "heavy" drinkers) and those who consumed two drinks or less ("light drinkers"). The heavy drinkers were found to have higher power motivation scores at the beginning of the parties, and a tendency to write more stories of the masculine enhancement/deprivation (E/D) type.[16] "Heavy" versus "light" drinking was not associated with scores on dependency imagery.

Overall, the results did not provide support for either the dependency or the power theory of drinking. However, although consuming alcohol did not enhance power, those women with strong power motivation did consume more alcohol. With regard to the "enhancing womanliness" theory, the results suggested that the effect of alcohol on women may be not so much to increase feelings of womanliness as to decrease the salience of masculine concerns.

In a subsequent study of drinking in college women (Schnur & MacDonald, 1988), an interesting relationship between problem drinking and May's TAT D/E measure of sexual identity (see Chapter 6) was observed. As discussed in Chapter 6, women in the freshman year of college show a dramatic change in their D/E score, from strongly feminine (positive) to slightly masculine (negative); by senior year, their D/E scores are again strongly feminine. However, in this sample of 75 college women, those who were in the early years of college (freshmen and sophomores) *and* were identified as being problem drinkers deviated from the expected D/E pattern; the problem drinkers had significantly more positive D/E scores than did the nonproblem drinkers. Similarly, the older problem drinkers (juniors and seniors) deviated from the expected pattern: Those who were problem drinkers had significantly more negative D/E scores than did the nonproblem drinkers of this age group. The authors interpreted these findings to mean that college women with drinking problems lagged behind in their development of sexual identity; they "had not yet entered into the age-appropriate developmental stages of dedifferentiation and identity integration, respectively" (p. 363).

In one study of men and women drinking together (Gustafson, 1988), real-life couples were assessed under conditions in which neither member of the couple drank, or in which only the man or only the woman drank alcohol. Power motivation fantasies, as measured by the TAT, decreased for both men and women only when women were the drinkers.

DRUG USE

The effects of drug use, especially the use of marijuana, also have been studied with the TAT. Here, the interest has been in the change in language use and thought content after marijuana injestion. To compare the TAT stories written by young adult males before and after drug administration, the *Regressive Imagery Dictionary*[17] was employed to index the language used (West, Martindale, Hines, & Roth, 1983). As compared to those of a control placebo group, the stories written under the influence of marijuana showed an increase in the presence of primary process thought.

Data from the same study were reported by Roth, Rosenbloom, Darley, Tinkleberg, and Kopell (1975) to study thought content. In this report, the TAT stories were rated by two independent raters for "stoned thinking" and for hostile and sexual content, with moderate interrater reliability. The results indicated that although the placebo subjects did not differ from time 1 to time 2 on any scale, marijuana ingestion resulted in significant shifts toward the "stoned" end of several scales as a result of drug ingestion. None of the hostility or sexuality scales showed any drug effect.[18]

Another study of marijuana effects, with both male and female young adults, had subjects tell stories to 10 TAT pictures administered on two occasions, 1 week apart (Crockett, Klonoff, & Clark, 1976). Subjects were assigned to one of seven experimental groups, representing different combinations of test occasion (1 or 2) and drug dosage (placebo, low-dose marijuana, or high-dose marijuana). All stories were scored on 13 rating scales by two independent judges; interrater reliability was good. The results indicated significant drug effects for three of the four Thought Process scales: Integration/organization and abstraction were both lower as a function of drug use, while multiplicity of meaning was higher. Also, two of the three Emotional Tone scales showed significant drug effects; "negative emotion" and "anxiety" were lower in the drug condition. As in Roth et al. (1975), there were no drug-related effects for any of the Aggression or Sexual Content scales.

The TAT has also been used to study the personality of opiate-addicted individuals (Wilson, Passik, Faude, Abrams, & Gordon, 1989). Based on a theory of failure in self-regulation, the authors devised a scoring scheme for the TAT to measure three factors reflecting aspects of self-regulation: the capacity to anticipate and plan, the capacity for impulse control, and the presence–absence of themes involving anaclitic depression, hopelessness, and abandonment. The subjects were 50 young adult men and women; half were receiving treatment in a methadone maintenance program and half were controls, screened for psychiatric disorder. All were of normal intelligence and without gross organic factors. Stories were scored for the Scale for Failures of Self-Regulation (SFSR)[19] to yield the three factors described above. The results indicated that the opiate-addicted subjects scored significantly higher than did the control subjects on all three factors reflecting failures in self-regulation. Interestingly, the SFSR scores were not correlated with self-reports of depression on the well-known Beck Depression Inventory,[20] suggesting that the failures in self-regulation are not readily accessible to conscious report.

In an anecdotal paper, Patalano (1986) suggested that TAT Card 3BM may be especially useful with drug abusers, who often describe the single figure in the picture as a drug addict and tend to misperceive the gun on the floor as a hypodermic needle. It is suggested that the story told to this card may be helpful in determining the coping resources of the addicted individual, as well as attitude toward drug taking.

One finding from the Roth et al. (1975) study reported earlier should be considered seriously for any research undertaken in the study of drug effects on TAT stories. In their investigation, an independent rater without knowledge of the drug–placebo condition, was able to classify 54% of the marijuana stories accurately, notably better than the 25% that would be expected by chance.[21] This finding suggests the possibility of an unwitting bias factor in this and other drug studies. For example, although raters in the Roth et al. (1975) study were blind as to the condition of storytelling, their ratings could have been affected by a general impression that the story was written under the influence of the drug. Clearly, some control is needed for this possible source of bias.

ABUSE

The TAT has also been used to study the personality of children who have been victims of abuse and of adults who have been abusive. In a study by Stovall and Craig (1990), 60 girls between the ages of 7 and 12 were selected to represent one of three groups: sexually abused, physically abused, and nonabused but living in a "distressed home environment" and seeking psychotherapy. Their TAT stories were rated on eight Object Relations subscales by two raters, with good interrater reliability. The results indicated that the two groups of abused girls scored significantly lower (more poorly developed object relations) than the nonabused group, on seven of the eight subscales. On the remaining subscale (Self–Other Differentiation), the sexually abused girls scored significantly lower than either of the other groups, which did not differ. Also, the abused girls were more likely to portray positive conscious images of self and others, but their unconscious perceptions revealed quite disturbed, negative perceptions of self and others; this discrepancy was not found in the nonabused girls.

In another study of the object relations of sexually abused girls (Henderson, 1990), the TAT stories of 56 abused girls were compared with those of 56 nonabused girls. The representations of mother figures in the abused group were characterized by more hostility, rivalry, and resistance, whereas the relationships portrayed between father and daughter were more ambivalent, affectionate, and sexualized. Self-representations in the TAT stories of the abused group reflected more felt inadequacy and helplessness.

Two studies compared the TAT stories of sexually abused girls (ages 6 to 16) with those of nonabused girls of similar age, IQ, and race who had been referred for psychological evaluation. One investigation found that the stories of the abused girls contained significantly more themes indicating sexual preoccupation and, secondarily, guilt (Pistole & Ornduff, 1994). The other study used Westen's SCORS approach (see Chapter 10) to determine the level of object relations present in the TAT stories of the two groups (Ornduff, Freedenfeld, Kelsey, & Critelli, 1994). The results indicated that girls in the abused group had a greater number of stories indicating primitive (level 1) object relations on all four of the SCORS scales.

A minimal amount of information about the TAT responses of abusive *parents* is given in a study by Hamilton, Stiles, Melowsky and Beal (1987). Ten abusive parents, sex unspecified, were given 10 TAT cards; there were no control subjects. The TAT protocols were scored for "succorance" themes using Murray's (1943) guidelines. The results indicated that there were 3.7 succorance themes per TAT card, as compared to 10 such themes in Murray's normative group of college students. According to the authors, these findings were contrary to the hypothesis and findings of other studies (see Evans, 1981; Melnick & Hurley, 1969), which suggested that abusive parents have unusually high needs for nurturance. Given the numerous problems with the design of this study, it is difficult to interpret the results.

Melnick and Hurley (1969) studied 10 primarily African-American mothers who were believed to be the abusers of their children, who were under age 3. These women were matched on a variety of background variables with 10 control mothers of nonabused children of similar ages. Their TAT stories were scored according to two systems: the Pathogenic Index, which focuses on the inability to empathize with others or to feel basic trust in the environment, and a series of motivational variables, including nAffiliation, nDependence, nDominance, nIndependence, nNurturance, and nAggression. Indications of the frustration of the first four needs were also scored. The results of the study indicated that the mothers suspected of being abusive had lower scores for the need to give nurturance than did the control mothers. Their scores also showed higher frustration of the need for dependence, and they were higher on the Pathogenic Index. The authors interpreted the results to suggest that the mothers with abused children had experienced prior frustration of their own emotional needs, and that they were deficient in the capacity to empathize with and provide for their children's needs.

In a carefully conducted study (Evans, 1981), 40 mothers who were receiving Aid for Dependent Children told stories about 14 TAT cards. Twenty of the mothers were known to have been moderately abusive; the other 20, from the same socioeconomic class, were not abusive. Other background variables were treated as covariates and were found not to influence the TAT scores. Analysis of the TAT scores indicated that the abusive mothers scored higher on rated aggression (seen in themes of murder, death, and demons) and lower on frustrated independence. For both groups of mothers, the measure of aggression correlated positively with frustrated nurturance, seen in themes of desertion, quarreling, and nonnurturance of others, although the correlation was stronger for the abusive mothers. For the abusive mothers only, aggression correlated with frustrated dominance and frustrated independence. The author concluded that aggression in the nonabusive mothers was more related to attitudes around punishment and objective characteristics of the family, whereas aggression in abusive mothers was more related to psychopathology and unsatisfactory interpersonal relationships.

The personality of adult males who had been abusive to their spouses was found to differ on TAT measures from that of men who were in conflicted, but nonabusive marriages and from that of satisfactorily married men (Dutton & Strachan, 1987). Using as stimulus cards pictures that depicted ambiguous male–female relationships, the spouse abusers had higher nPower scores than did the satisfactorily married men and lower spouse-specific assertiveness scores than did either of the other two groups. These two TAT scores, when entered into a discriminant analysis, correctly identified the abusive and the nonabusive men with 90% accuracy. The authors concluded that the abusive men had a high need to exert power but lacked the verbal resources to do so.

PSYCHOSES

In addition to the early work of Rapaport et al. (1946; see Chapter 10), other approaches have been used to identify or describe patients with serious pathology. Many of these approaches have focused on schizophrenia, but some have included other psychotic disorders.

Communication Deviance

One of the most interesting approaches to using the TAT for the study of psychopathology is that developed by Singer and Wynne (1966; see also Wynne & Singer, 1964). Their assessment approach, referred to as communication deviance, is designed to assess communication defects and deviance in the TAT. The general rationale for Singer and Wynne's (1966) approach is based on the observation that certain individuals, when telling stories, fail to establish and to maintain a shared focus of attention with the listener. This failure appeared to be especially characteristic of the parents of young adult schizophrenics. The resulting deviance in communication is seen in closure problems, disruptions, and peculiar language and logic.[22] Aspects of *closure problems* include the failure to create a story; the use of fragments of words, phrases, or ideas that are dropped into the story and left incomplete; the expression of passages that are unintelligible, inconsistent, contradictory, or that the listener is expected to interpret; omissions or confusions about central aspects of the picture; and, finally, the failure to complete the story. Aspects of *disruptive behavior* include interruptions either of the examiner while giving instructions or of the storyteller him- or herself while telling the story, as well as disruptions of the set to tell a story and instead embarking on some different task. *Peculiar perceptions and verbalizations* include significant misperceptions of the card, the assignment of idiosyncratic meaning to details of the picture, referring to the picture as representing a dream, the use of odd phrases or words, slips of the tongue, peculiar reasoning, and the undue repetition of words, phrases, or ideas. Each of these categories may be scored for each story to yield a total communication deviance (CD) score for the individual.[23]

A number of studies have been conducted with the parents of schizophrenic and other psychiatric patients, using their TAT stories to investigate the occurrence of CD. For example, Jones (1977) studied the TAT stories of the parents of 20 young adult patients with varying psychiatric diagnoses. These diagnoses were ordered on a scale of 1 to 6, with 1 indicating "normal," 3 indicating hospitalized neurotics and personality disorders, and 6 indicating unremitting or chronic schizophrenics. The parents' TAT stories were scored using the Singer–Wynne

CD manual (Singer & Wynne, 1966). Although the correlation between diagnosis and deviance scores was low and nonsignificant, when the factor scores for CD were transformed to standard scores, mothers and couples (mother plus father) who had at least one factor score that was 1 standard deviation above the mean were more likely to have children who had more serious pathology. Thus, although a single score did not identify the parents of schizophrenics, substyles of CD, as revealed in factor scores, were related to schizophrenic pathology.

In particular, there were two substyles, or factors, that discriminated the parents of hospitalized schizophrenics from all other parents. One of these factors involved misperceptions of the content of the picture, and the other involved an omission of some important part of the picture, with a failure to bring the story to a close. The use of these styles by the parents resulted in the listener's wondering if he or she were attending to the same reality as the storyteller.

Sass, Gunderson, Singer, and Wynne (1984) attempted to demonstrate a more specific correspondence between the amount and type of CD in the parents and the degree of formal thought disorder found in their schizophrenic offspring.[24] The offspring were all male, natural children of the parents, between the ages of 15 and 30, with no organic impairment; the parents were under the age of 67. TAT stories were scored for several types of CD. The results indicated that CD characterized by disorganization and impaired focus occurred more frequently in the parents whose schizophrenic offspring had high and moderate degrees of thought disorder than in either the parents of patients with low degrees of thought disorder or the parents of nonschizophrenic patients.

Communication deviance, as revealed in TAT stories, was also used to compare the parents of schizophrenic and manic patients (Miklewitz, Velligan, Goldstein, & Neuchterlein, 1991). Although the total level of CD did not differentiate between the two parent groups, more instances of odd word usage were found among the parents of patients with a diagnosis of bipolar manic disorder. These findings suggest that high levels of parent CD are not unique to schizophrenia.

In another study of communication deviance, Rund (1986) studied 100 Norwegian fathers and mothers who were the parents of schizophrenic patients, nonpsychotic psychiatric patients, or normal offspring. The parent groups were matched on a number of background variables. Verbatim transcriptions of the parents' TAT stories were scored for communication deviance.[25] Reasonable interrater reliability was obtained. Although the results indicated that the three parent groups did not differ on total CD score, when only extreme scores were considered (scores 1 standard deviation above the mean), the three groups showed clear differences. Among the parents of schizophrenics, 19% of the parent couples had high CD scores, as compared to 0% of the parents of nonpsychotic psychiatric patients and 5% of the parents of normal offspring. Also, a stepwise discriminant analysis, using the TAT categories as predictors, significantly categorized the parents into the schizophrenic group and normal group, and within the schizophrenic group, into the parents of paranoid and nonparanoid patients. Prediction was improved when the scores from both mothers and fathers were included. Certain categories were especially successful in differentiating between the schizophrenic and normal parent groups. The common factor of these categories appeared to be a certain reluctance to take responsibility for what was communicated in the story, as seen in an attribution of intention to the cards (rather than to the storyteller), or in describing elements of the story in terms of what they are *not*, or by presenting incomplete words or ideas in the story. Further, a significant correlation was found between the TAT CD measure and a behaviorally based measure of communication deviance.

The assessment of CD in the parents of schizophrenics was studied in yet another language culture by Doane et al. (1989). Sixty-four parents of schizophrenic patients (32 Mexican-Americans and 32 Anglo-Americans), matched for a number of background variables, told stories about seven TAT cards. The stories were transcribed and coded according to Jones and Doane's (1979) system. A native Spanish speaker coded the Mexican-American stories and a native American speaker coded the Anglo-American stories.[26] A comparison of the TAT stories from the mothers and fathers of the two ethnic groups indicated no differences attributable to language or cultural differences. From this, the authors conclude that the rates of CD in parents of schizophrenics "is not a culture-bound phenomenon but is rather a marker of an underlying process" (Doane et al., 1989, p. 489), a conclusion supported by the results of Rund (1986) discussed earlier.[27]

In a further study of parents of children (ages 7 to 14 years) with psychiatric disorders (Tomson, Asarnow, Goldstein, & Miklowitz, 1990), it was found that the TAT stories of parents whose children were diagnosed as schizophrenic spectrum disorders contained higher rates of CD than did the stories of parents of depressed children. This difference was not apparent in a family interaction task.

The occurrence of CD in patients themselves was investigated in a longitudinal study (Doane & Mintz, 1987) using TAT stories obtained from male and female adolescents with behavior disorders who were tested again 15 years later. The results provided only modest support for the hypothesis that CD is an enduring stylistic attribute. Overall, CD increased with age for both males and females. For females only, there was a moderate correlation between adolescent and adult CD type. For the total group, only the "peculiar language" factor correlated across time. Perhaps most significant, those subjects with the highest CD scores in adulthood were more likely to have a DSM-III diagnosis of mental illness and/or personality disorder.

Other Approaches to Schizophrenia

Bellak (1975), although skeptical about the use of the TAT for the differential diagnosis of schizophrenia, does discuss some diagnostic indicators. These include bizarre content, blatant symbolic expressions, and examples of thought disorder not apparent in interviews, along with certain suggestive "signs."

In another approach, Alkire, Brunse, and Houlihan (1974) rated TAT stories from 65 successive patient admissions to a Veterans Administration hospital for the degree of family relationship or closeness of kinship. The ratings ranged from "nuclear family member" to "extended family member" (e.g., aunt or cousin) to "friend" to "total avoidance of character." The results indicated that patients diagnosed as schizophrenic had significantly lower scores (indicating less close relationships) than did nonschizophrenics; within the schizophrenic group, the nonparanoid patients had significantly lower scores than did the paranoids. At the same time, IQ, age, and severity of disorder were generally unrelated to kinship scores. The authors concluded that the avoidance of nuclear family relationships, as revealed on the TAT, is a relevant diagnostic indicator in schizophrenia.

The TAT was also used to study change in a small group of chronic schizophrenics, some of whom were participating in intensive group psychotherapy and some not (Revere, Rodeffer, & Dawson, 1989). All patients were tested five times across a period of 24 months. The results indicated that patients in the therapy group, as compared to the controls, showed an increase in "reality perception" as assessed by the TAT; this difference was not found for a comparable Rorschach measure. The TAT results were consistent with positive changes in the ward behavior of the therapy group.

Other Disorders

The TAT has been used to discriminate among other diagnostic categories of patients, including both psychotic and severe neurotic or character disorders. For example, in a study of depressive and psychotic (primarily schizophrenic) patients, Sharkey and Ritzler (1985) found that hospitalized depressives scored higher on activity level in their TAT stories than did outpatient depressives, whereas normals scored higher on TAT passivity than did depressives or psychotics.[28] Hospitalized depressives also showed more perceptual distortions than did outpatient depressives.

The TAT has also been used to assess defense mechanisms in hospitalized psychotic and severe neurotic and character-disorder patients (Cramer et al., 1988). For this population, the use of the lower-level defenses of denial and projection was related to independent ratings of degree of psychopathology and poor interpersonal relationships, whereas the opposite was found for patients using the higher-level defense of identification. Moreover, in a follow-up study, a decrease in the use of defense mechanisms was associated with a reduction in psychiatric symptoms (Cramer & Blatt, 1990). This work has been discussed in Chapter 7.

A computer-based content analysis of TAT stories has been successful in differentiating among four diagnostic groups (paranoia, depression, somatization disorder, and cancer) (Rosenberg et al., 1990).

Finally, the TAT has been used to detect aspects of cognitive impairment in patients with Alzheimer's disease (Johnson, 1994). A group of 20 hospitalized Alzheimer patients (mean age = 74) was compared with a group of 20 hospitalized psychiatric patients (mean age = 54) without central nervous system impairment. Both groups told stories about the same set of eight TAT cards. Due to the age differences between the two patient groups, age was controlled for in the analysis of the results. The findings showed that the Alzheimer patients used fewer words in their stories. They also were more likely to lose the instructional set to tell a story and were more likely to describe the picture rather than tell a story. Card rejection or refusal was not different in the two groups.

PSYCHOPATHOLOGY
IN CHILDREN AND ADOLESCENTS

Clinicians have also found the TAT to be useful in the clinical assessment of children and adolescents. Numerous examples of TAT stories from children and adolescents with varying levels of psychological disturbance have been provided by Schwartz and Eagle (1986) and by Eagle and Schwartz (1994) (see Chapter 11). In the remainder of this chapter, the use of the TAT to study psychopathology in this age range—including psychosis, emotional disturbance, "at risk" children, borderline personality disorder, schizophrenia, and attention deficit disorder—is discussed.

In an early study with psychotic children ages 5 to 17, Leitch and Schafer (1947) noted that the TAT, among a battery of other tests, was crucial for differentiating between psychotic and nonpsychotic degrees of maladjustment. In particular, they indicated that the analysis of formal characteristics of the TAT stories was very useful for the purpose of diagnosis rather than simply focusing on the ideational content. Diagnostic indicators for psychosis included stories characterized by incoherence, contradictions, queer ideas and verbalizations, repetition of a phrase, neologisms and nonsense rhyming, introduction of the examiner into the story, manneristic speaking, overgeneralizations and symbolic interpretations, autistic logic, and themes unrelated to the picture. In addition, several disturbances in the perceptual sphere differentiated the stories of psychotic from nonpsychotic children. These included the omission of important details in the picture, uncommon misrecognitions or distortions, and the expression of perceptual uncertainties that were not resolved.

In a systematic review of 13 earlier studies, McGrew and Teglasi (1990) noted that the TAT stories of disturbed children and adolescents could be characterized by the following formal elements: more bizarre ideas, more incoherences or loose associations, more perceptual distortions or omissions, more perseverations, more aggression to unaggressive cards, and more magical thinking but fewer complete stories, fewer positive responses or outcomes, and shorter or more verbally constricted stories.

This approach, with a focus on the formal aspects of the stories, was used by McGrew and Teglasi (1990) in a very well-conducted study of 80 white boys, ages 6 to 12 years, from middle and upper-middle SES families. Half the boys were well adjusted and half were emotionally disturbed; the groups were matched for IQ, which ranged from low average to superior. Stories were told about 9 TAT cards and were transcribed and scored for 12 different categories by three independent raters, with adequate interrater reliability. The categories, which are clearly defined and illustrated by the authors, include two dealing with the adequacy of the story (perceptual organization and internal logic), three with characteristics of verbalization (perceptual personalization, expression of inadequacy, and inappropriate or bizarre comments or actions), three with adequacy of judgment (positive action, negative action, and outcome), and four with the modulation of content in terms of the stimulus properties and social conventionality (including hostility, hostility to the less aggressive cards, positive feelings, and negative feelings). When these 12 categories were entered into a discriminant function analysis, 95% of the comparison group and 85% of the disturbed group were correctly identified. Furthermore, *all* the categories except negative feelings significantly differentiated between the two groups.

In a different approach, the TAT stories of a group of 24 disturbed adolescents and their parents were studied by Goldstein, Gould, Alkire, Rodnick, and Judd (1970) for two formal variables: the degree of kinship represented by characters in the stories and the quality of interpersonal involvements. The adolescents' disturbance was categorized on the basis of its locus of expression (inside or outside of the home) and its activity level (active or passive).[29] The results of this study provided a number of interesting findings regarding the parents of the adolescents but relatively few for the disturbed adolescents themselves. For the *parents*, an analysis of the stories for kinship patterns revealed the greatest differences for those parents whose adolescents had difficulties outside the home. Within this group, the parents of the active adolescents had the *lowest* kinship scores, whereas parents of the passive adolescents had the *highest* scores. Parents of the other two (inside) groups were similar, with scores falling between the "outside" groups. An analysis of the quality of interpersonal involvements indicated that for positive involvement, there was a significant interaction between activity level and locus of difficulty. Very few positive involvements were mentioned by parents of "active-outside" or "passive-inside" adolescents; parents of the other two groups referred to twice as many positive involvements. An analysis of negative interpersonal involvements yielded a significant interaction between activity level and parent (mother or father). Fathers of the active adolescents perceived *fewer* negative involvements than did their wives, whereas fathers of the passive adolescents perceived *more* negative involvements. These findings indicate that it is possible to use the TAT to characterize some differences in the structure of family relationships for different categories of disturbed adolescents.

One of the studies reviewed by McGrew and Teglasi (1990) is of special interest due to the clinical groups studied. Shabad, Worland, Lander, and Dietrich (1979) identified a group of 32 children who were "at risk" for developing a psychiatric disturbance on the basis of having one parent who was hospitalized for a psychotic illness. These children, who ranged in age from 7 to 18 years, were evaluated at the time of the parent's hospitalization and were followed up 6 to 10 years later. Three groups of at-risk children were identified: those who were initially evaluated as being seriously disturbed and subsequently had a major disturbance leading to hospitalization (termed the "sick–sick" group; $n = 8$), those who were seriously disturbed at the initial evaluation but were never hospitalized ("sick–well"; $n = 12$), and those initially evaluated as not disturbed and were never hospitalized ("well–well"; $n = 12$). In addition, 12 children with normal parents were included in the study.

Stories about three TAT cards given at the initial evaluation revealed significant differences among the groups as identified 6 to 10 years later.[30] Individuals in the sick–sick group, as compared to all other groups, gave more stories on Card 1 with the hero being outstanding, in combination with magical thinking. On Card 3 (showing a person collapsed over a bed), they gave more blatantly positive outcomes; on Card 7GF, only children in this group mentioned "growing up big" or "getting married." As compared with all other groups, children in this sick–sick group gave fewer stories to Card 7GF in which "her mother" was mentioned, or in which the object in the little girl's arms was mentioned. They also made fewer references to maternal punishment than did the sick–well group, which made *more* references to maternal punishment than did all other groups.

The authors conclude from these TAT results that there appears to be an important difference in the children at risk who do and do not go on to have major psychological disturbances. Those who do eventually become disturbed are noted to be using massive denial and magical thinking, whereas those who do not become seriously disturbed are more likely to openly perceive negative happenings and emotions. These findings are reminiscent of similar results with adult schizophrenics, who also tend to avoid maternal stimuli (see, e.g., Farima & Dunham, 1966; Lefcourt & Steffy, 1967).

The use of the TAT to assess pathology in adolescents with a diagnosis of borderline personality disorder was discussed in Chapter 10 (e.g., Westen, Ludolph, Lerner et al., 1990). Sugarman, Bloom-Feshbach and Bloom-Feshbach (1980) have also used the TAT to diagnose BPD, adopting the same theoretical framework as that of Sugarman (1980; see Chapter 10). These authors discuss several aspects of TAT stories that are especially characteristic of adolescents with BPD. First, there is often evidence of disturbed psychosexual development, as seen in a predominance of oral and oral–aggressive responses, as well as in the avoidance of sexual or heterosexual themes. Also, the lack of establishment of a clear gender identity is seen in overt ruminations about the gender of characters in the TAT pictures. The lack of identity development is also seen in the expression of "negative identity"—expressions of values and roles that are antithetical to those values held by their parents. Disturbances in object relations are seen in the portrayal of characters with minimal elaboration of motives or thought, and through difficulties in establishing relationships with peers, as seen in stories expressing a lack of flexibility when relating to others. Negative self-representations are portrayed in TAT characters who express remorse or guilt about aggressive acts. Difficulties in modulating the expression of emotion are seen in overt expressions of impulse in the stories, or in the expression of disparate emotions that become somewhat fused without the storyteller's becoming aware of it. On the other hand, problems with the verbalization of emotion are also common. Finally, manifestations of a sadistic superego may also appear in content that is punishing or otherwise cruel to the characters in the story.

Another formal variable was used in a study by Strober (1979) of white male adolescent psychiatric patients diagnosed as schizophrenic or nonschizophrenic.[31] It was hypothesized that in schizophrenic disorders, there is a "failure to differentiate between and coordinate separate perspectives of a social event" (p. 310), resulting in lower levels of interpersonal "decentering." TAT stories were rated for level of interpersonal decentering, based on the degree of differentiation between the story figures and the coordination of relationships between them; interrater reliability was adequate. The results indicated that the schizophrenic adolescents had significantly lower decentering scores than did the control patients. Because the two groups did not differ in number of scored interactions, and the scores did not correlate with age or verbal IQ, the findings were not due to a possible spurious confound. Rather, the author suggests that the low-level decentering found in the schizophrenics may be due to the social isolation that is often present in the premorbid development of schizophrenic individuals.

The TAT has also been used in a study of attention deficit disorder by Costantino, Colono-Malgady, Malgady, and Perez (1991). Ninety-five child and adolescent outpatients with a diagnosis of attention-deficit/hyperactivity disorder were compared with 152 normal public school students. Approximately one-third of each group was African-American, one-third Hispanic, and one-third white. Ages ranged from 7 to 15 years, with a mean of 11 years. Stories were told about the 21 cards of the TEMAS test (see Chapter 13). The African-American and Hispanic subjects were given the minority version of the test; the white subjects were given the nonminority version. Tests were given individually, orally, by an examiner of the same ethnicity as the subject. To assess attention deficit (AD), each card was scored for the omission of five kinds of information, regarding the main character, the secondary characters, the event, the setting, and the conflict portrayed. The results indicated that for all five omission categories, there was a significant interaction between group (AD vs. normal) and ethnicity. Within the Hispanic group, the AD subjects had higher omission scores than normals in all categories except conflict. Within the white group, the AD subjects had higher omission scores than normals in all categories except event. Within the African-American group, the AD subjects had higher omission scores than normals for secondary characters, event, and setting.[32] Overall, the results show that AD children and adolescents are more likely to omit stimulus details. This finding was not due to the subjects forgetting the instructions given, for the experimenter used prompts to remind them; such prompting was needed three times more often in the AD than in the normal group.

SUMMARY

As is clear from the material presented in this chapter, the TAT has been used with a variety of clinical groups. The chapter reviews the use of the TAT to study the psychological concomitants of a variety of physical health problems, including high blood pressure, arthritis, cancer, and diabetes. A complex theory has been proposed to explain the connection between physical illness and psychological motives, as assessed by the TAT, based on observed relationships between motives, activation of the sympathetic nervous system, and the suppression of immune functions.

The TAT has also been used in studies of alcohol and drug usage, both to investigate the personality of individuals who typically abuse these substances and to demonstrate changes in personality following on experimental ingestion of the substances. In general, nPower seems to be a significant factor in individuals who abuse alcohol, whereas failures in self-regulation, as assessed from the TAT, have been found to be characteristic of opiate addicts. Experimental introduction of alcohol has been shown to increase both aggressive and sexual ideation in men, while the introduction of marijuana has produced significant changes in thought processes. The personalities of children who have been victims of abuse and of adults who have been abusive have also been studied using the TAT.

A variety of strategies for using the TAT to study psychopathology are discussed in the chapter. The use of the TAT to assess the communication deviance associated with schizophrenia is described. Several empirical studies demonstrating the use of the TAT to differentiate among diagnostic groups are provided. The last section of the chapter focuses on the use of the TAT to study psychopathology in children and adolescents, including emotional disturbance, schizophrenia, and attention deficit disorder.

• SEVENTEEN •

Conclusion

This book began with an apparently simple idea—that the great epic poems of human history are the carriers of the individual's cultural identity, whereas the stories of individual men and women reveal significant aspects of their personal character and life views. Abundant support for the meaningfulness of the individual's story has been provided in every chapter of the book, from the earliest use of the TAT, in which the personal source of stories told was demonstrated, to contemporary studies showing that psychological motives discerned from storytelling can be important predictors of physical and psychological illness. The importance of narrative thought as a way to discover "meaning" has been illustrated and issues of reality, truth, and verification with narrative material have been discussed.

In addition, we have seen throughout the book that the stories of clinical patients, as well as of college students, provide a wealth of material illuminating both personality and pathology. For both patients and students, we have applied different interpretive perspectives to the same narrative stories and have related this material to life history information, showing how both inner and outer context will be reflected in stories told. By using this multiperspective interpretive approach, the great richness of narrative stories for illuminating the human psyche is clearly demonstrated.

Yet, the acceptance of the hypothesis that storytelling is a means for accessing significant personal information is not without its complications, and many persons are skeptical that such a procedure may be granted scientific respectability. The various issues and problems attendant on the use of the TAT as a source of reliable information have been presented in this book. Methodological improvements in knowledgeable selection of stimulus pictures, a recognition of an interaction between picture and gender, the possibility of a picture by ethnicity interaction, the importance in any quantitative scoring system of the need to adjust

319

for story length, and the need for relevant approaches to determining the statistical reliability and validity of the results obtained from storytelling have been discussed at length.

Some of these new approaches to the TAT are themselves based on narratives. Locating autobiographical themes in a story is an example of a narrative approach in which the story line comes from the storyteller. May's D/E assessment of gender identity, based on the pattern, or structure of the TAT story, with a concern for intention, emotion, and conflict, is a good example of a narrative approach in which the story line comes from the interpreter and illustrates the way in which an interpreter's narrative may be superimposed on the storyteller's narrative to find new meaning in the story. Other of the approaches—the assessment of defense mechanisms, object relations, and motives—may be considered "partial narratives," or perspectives, used by the interpreter to discern yet other kinds of meaning in the stories.

The "new look" at storytelling with the TAT—what has also been termed the "McClelland–Atkinson tradition"—has led investigators into a large body of fruitful research. Based on empirical studies to derive and then cross-validate coding categories to identify basic human motives, this approach has yielded a large body of reliable information which is not accessible from assessment procedures of the self-report, questionnaire variety. Repeatedly, it has been demonstrated that these empirically based coding systems for the TAT can be learned and applied reliably. It has also been established that measures of motives based on storytelling do a better job of predicting long-term, real-world behavior than do personality trait measures derived from discrete questionnaire items. The range of motives and other psychologically important variables that have been successfully assessed using this new approach to evaluate storytelling is impressive: motives for achievement, affiliation, intimacy, and power, as well as sexual identity, object relations, and defense mechanisms may all be reliably coded, with the results related to real-life behaviors in a way that demonstrates clearly the validity of the measures.

This book has also documented the importance of storytelling for tracing the subtle developmental changes that occur across time and has demonstrated that the interpretive perspectives used with the stories from adults can be equally successful when applied to children's stories. Using narrative material, qualitative changes in the mental operations invoked for approaching the same dilemmas have been clearly tracked in both cross-sectional and longitudinal studies with children, adolescents, and adults. With adults, it has been possible to monitor, in addition, cross-generational differences in personality structure and to relate these differences to important changes in the social environment and culture of the times.

In comparison to the great success of the systematic study of story-telling for revealing important aspects of personality among more or less average children, adolescents, and adults, reports on the use of storytelling as a *diagnostic* tool among individuals suffering from various psychological disturbances have been less positive. On an individual basis, clinicians have demonstrated great skill and sensitivity in extracting from TAT stories important indications of pathology and core conflicts. Yet, the attempts to formulate reliable and valid measures of pathology have not met with the same success as have the research studies of motives and other personality variables. The approach of Westen to assessing the level of object relations represented in TAT stories offers new promise in this domain. Clearly, there is need for good empirical studies to be carried out, to produce diagnostically meaningful coding systems.

In the end, however, the great value of storytelling for understanding personality does not rest on story-derived numerical scores. Rather, it is the storyteller's un-self-conscious presentation of important life thema that provides us, the sensitive listener, with insights into the innermost level of personality. To obtain these insights, we must be ready to find them. This requires a belief in a dynamic, multifaceted, multilayered personality and a belief that the stories people tell have significance. We need an ear attuned to hearing these repeated thema and to detecting modifications and changes as the social context and interpersonal environment changes. To paraphrase a contemporary personologist, unless the observer believes in the existence of an underlying personality, he or she is unlikely to perceive its manifestations in the TAT. "Clinical acumen is essential to discovery" (Vaillant, 1971, p. 115).

Notes

CHAPTER 1

1. The question of just what constitutes a story, as well as the function of a story, has been discussed by McAdams (1988a).

2. In the story by C. S. Lewis, *The Lion, the Witch and the Wardrobe* (1950/1988).

3. Studies of television viewing have repeatedly reported that grade-school children spend between 20 and 30 hours per week watching television. Despite the attempt of the National Association of Broadcasters to screen out excessive violence in children's programs, research studies have demonstrated that this endeavor has been quite ineffective (e.g., Cramer & Mechem, 1982). In February 1992, the American Psychological Association Task Force on Television and Society revealed that a child who watches television between 2 and 4 hours daily will have witnessed 8,000 murders and 100,000 other acts of television violence by the time he or she leaves elementary school.

   There is an extensive literature demonstrating that children who view violent television engage in more violent behavior (e.g., Huesmann, Eron, Berkowitz, & Chafee, 1992; for an earlier report, see Huesmann, Eron, Lefkowitz, & Walder, 1973; see also Comstock & Strasburger, 1990; Turner, Hesse, & Peterson-Lewis, 1986). The large majority of evidence from more than 3,000 studies over two decades indicates that violence portrayed on television influences the attitudes and behavior of children who watch it.

4. The imitation of violent crimes seen on television by children as young as 5 years old has unfortunately become less than a rare occurrence.

5. This issue has been discussed extensively by Spence (1982) and Edelson (1993).

6. A description of these two personality configurations may be found in Blatt and Shichman (1983). They are also discussed in Chapter 9.

7. *PsychLit* records from January 1974 to March 1995 were used for this purpose.

8. For example, the stories collected from George Vaillant's longitudinal study (the Grant study) are available through the Henry A. Murray Research Center, Radcliffe College, 10 Garden Street, Cambridge, MA 02138, as are other sets of stories.

CHAPTER 2

1. "I am going to show you a picture, and I want you to make up a plot or story for which it might be used as an illustration . . . " (Morgan & Murray, 1935, p. 290).

2. An additional 40 subjects wrote stories about the pictures given as a group test. Morgan and Murray (1935) felt this procedure was not as successful as the individual administration of pictures.

3. These pictures are reproduced in *Explorations in Personality* (Murray, 1938, pp. 406, 542, and 543).

4. For a report on the use of the personality assessment approach to select men for the Office of Strategic Services during World War II, see *Assessment of Men* (United States Office of Strategic Services, 1948).

5. For example, the studies of creativity that were carried out at the Institute of Personality Assessment and Research at the University of California, under the direction of Dr. Donald W. MacKinnon (see MacKinnon, 1965).

6. These TAT cards were used by Rapaport et al. (1946) and are reproduced in their book.

7. An extensive discussion of the origin, history, and development of the TAT images is provided by Morgan (1995).

8. Recently, Peterson (1990) has suggested an alternative method for administering the TAT. Based on the principles underlying psychoanalytic and nondirective psychotherapy, it is suggested that the basic instruction given to the storyteller be changed from telling the individual what to do and how to do it to a less directive request, such as, "Tell me a story about what might be happening in this picture." The important issue here is, "Do we tell the patient how to tell the story, or do we listen to and try to explore how the patient tells their story?" (Peterson, 1990, p. 194). It is further suggested that the order in which the TAT pictures are administered might well try to follow a developmental sequence as that sequence is understood by the individual examiner. For example, the first pictures presented might well relate to themes of early symbiosis, differentiation, and separation, whereas later cards might refer to more advanced developmental issues such as the development of the ability to work and to love.

9. There were, however, some differences in usage across the five different types of psychiatric settings queried. The results indicated that the TAT was used most often by psychologists in psychiatric hospitals (88%), community mental health centers (86%), and Veterans Administration medical centers

(76%) but somewhat less in centers for the developmentally disabled and mentally retarded (55%), and least in counseling centers (44%), where the frequency of use of the TAT was tied for last place with several other tests (Lubin et al., 1985).

10. Lubin et al. (1984) may have misjudged faculty attitude. A large-scale study (Wade, Baker, Morton, & Baker, 1978) surveyed every seventh member of the American Psychological Association who was also a member of Division 12 (Clinical Psychology). From the 471 delivered questionnaires, there was a 50% return rate. The respondents were asked for their opinion regarding which psychological tests students of clinical psychology should learn. The highest two ranked tests were the Rorschach and the TAT (mentioned about equally often), which were listed significantly more often than the next two ranked tests (the WAIS and MMPI). This ranking of the TAT and Rorschach was true regardless of whether the clinicians were themselves users of objective or projective tests and regardless of whether they were frequent or infrequent test users. Although clinicians engaged in clinical practice recommended projective tests more often than clinicians not engaged in these activities (i.e., clinicians who were teaching or doing research), the Rorschach and the TAT were still the two tests most frequently recommended by nonpracticing clinicians for students to learn.

These findings were recently replicated by Piotrowski and Zalewski (1993). Directors of doctoral Ph.D. and Psy.D. programs were contacted and asked their opinion about the use of projective tests. One-half of the respondents (with a return rate of 51%) believed that the use of projective assessment in the academic setting will remain the same in the near future. In addition, the TAT was ranked as the second most important projective test with which clinical doctoral candidates should be familiar.

11. See Chapter 13 on this issue.

12. This research was summarized in Bellak (1975).

CHAPTER 3

1. An exception to this statement is found in the work of McAdams (1985, 1988a, 1988b), who does include the concept of narrative in his writings, although the implications of the two modes of thought do not directly inform his work.

2. In fact, this focus on historical *truth* carried a heavy moralistic charge for Freud (see Kohut, 1984).

3. Curiously, the idea of aboriginal reality continues even *within* narrative theory, where a distinction is made between the fabula and the sjuzet, between base and surface structure, between worlds and versions, all of which differentiate between the "true" story and the imperfect manifestations of this truth (see Bruner, 1986, p. 191).

4. A similar construct has been proposed by McAdams (1988a), termed "thematic lines." However, as discussed by McAdams, thematic lines are closely tied to motivational constellations (see McAdams, 1988a, pp. 69–104).

5. See, for example, Cramer (1968) and Neely (1991).

6. In an ongoing discussion (McAdams & Zeldow, 1993; Rosenberg, Schnurr, & Oxman, 1990; Schnurr, Rosenberg, & Oxman, 1992; Schnurr, Rosenberg, & Oxman, 1993; Rosenberg, Blatt, Oxzman, McHugo, & Ford, 1994; Zeldow & McAdams, 1993) regarding the merits, or lack thereof, of TAT techniques based on computerized counts of the occurrence of individual words, McAdams and Zeldow have clarified how such a decontextualized approach to narrative material will ultimately fall short of discovering much about the narrator. They point out that a computerized search for word matches with a list of dictionary terms identifies words or labels that are without any particular psychological meaning or any demonstrated construct validity; such an approach involves "an omnibus word count procedure for sampling a wide ranging gamut of topics and concepts, some of which pertain to personality and some of which do not" (McAdams & Zeldow, 1993, p. 244). For many, or even most of these words, there is no obvious or proven relevance to personality.

Further, the attempt to relate the occurrence of different word types to other psychological variables does not follow from theoretical predictions or psychological significance. Instead, a kind of dust bowl empiricism and expedience seems to inform this computerized approach. McAdams and Zeldow (1993) conclude: "For our taste, well validated measures of carefully articulated constructs are preferable to omnibus systems that promise to cover the universe by presenting a list of theoretically decontextualized terms and topics" (p. 244).

CHAPTER 4

1. For comments on this phenomenon, see Edelson (1993).

2. Other early advocates of the TAT proposed a narrative that focused on the mental steps the interpreter should take, from the first reading of the stories to the final integration of the material (e.g., Shneidman, 1951; Stein, 1955). Some provided general principles of interpretation, usually interwoven with an "interpretive stance" (e.g., Henry, 1956; Bellak, 1954, 1975; Rapaport et al., 1946). Some stressed the importance of a thorough knowledge of the psychodynamics of personality for competent interpretation (Rapaport et al., 1946; Henry, 1956; Holt, 1951, 1978). Each of these approaches is based on the interpreter having adopted a particular narrative.

3. The issue of reliability is discussed in Chapter 14.

4. Rosenwald (1968) has offered an alternative way to conceptualize the process involved in telling a TAT story, based on the level of *interest* and involvement in the task that the storyteller shows, from beginning to end.

Interest level is reflected in the observance of the instructions as they pertain to the completeness of the plot, in the clarity with which the story is told to another person with whom the subject has a (passing) personal relationship, and in the pleasure and naturalness with which he produces individual expressive themes in his stories. The concept of interest . . . is a possible approach to a process theory of storytelling. (p. 182)

5. Using the "story as dream" narrative, Holt (1951) described nine psychological determinants that shape the production of TAT stories. These include the situational context, the directing sets, the perceptual impact of the TAT card, the arousal of needs and affects, defensive circuiting, and associative elaboration, as well as the abilities, personal style, and internal milieu of the storyteller.

6. The skillful examiner for this study was Valerie Aronoff.

7. This is picture number 10 in Rapaport, Gill, and Schafer (1946, Vol. 2, p. 400).

CHAPTER 5

1. Not his real name. All names have been changed to ensure anonymity.

2. This picture is part of a research series (McClelland & Steele, 1972).

3. This picture is also part of the research series (McClelland & Steele, 1972).

4. The strength of nPower did correlate positively with memories involving anger, which was a subcategory of "unpleasant memories."

5. This is the phenomenon of "transference."

CHAPTER 6

1. This theme, referred to as the "Icarus complex," has been discussed by Murray (1955). It is interesting that for both Phaethon and Icarus, the male authority—Zeus for Phaethon and Phoebus for Icarus—intervenes to directly cause the fall. This point is not discussed by May.

2. Note here that "less" means "less than the male"; that is, the male condition is used as the standard of reference.

3. The exception would be in the process of expulsion of the fetus from the womb.

4. A full description of the scoring method is given in May (1980).

5. These research studies have been summarized by May (1980). Research studies with children and adolescents are discussed in Chapter 11.

6. The pictures were a man and a woman doing a trapeze act against a dark background; a young bullfighter walking in the ring; a man and woman

sitting on a stone bench; and a child leaping or running in a field, with a bird flying above.

7. Two raters independently scored each of the 416 stories; their interrater agreement was high (correlations of .77–.79) for three of the stories. The agreement for the couple on the bench was lower, at .42.

8. Gender differences were significant for stories about the pictures of the trapeze artists, bullfighter, and couple on the bench.

9. It should be noted that May did not use the term "narrative" to describe his work. Nevertheless, for the reasons indicated, it seems clearly an example of a narrative approach to the TAT.

10. Females did have more deprivation units in stories told to the bullfighter picture.

11. For a review of gender differences with the Defense Mechanism Inventory, see Cramer (1988).

12. The pictures were trapeze artists, bullfighter, and couple on the bench.

CHAPTER 7

1. Freud (1937/1959), in his later writings, also believed that defense mechanisms were necessary for normal development.

2. This study was mentioned in Chapter 3.

3. In fact, the measure can be applied to any story material, although certain categories of scoring, such as omission (denial, 1), are based on objective descriptions of the standard TAT pictures. However, omission criteria could be established for any additional picture for which a large enough body of stories is available to form a normative comparison group.

4. These findings were especially true of those patients identified as having an anaclitic personality organization.

CHAPTER 8

1. Parenthesis ( ) indicate that some comment, or question (?) was made by the examiner (in this and other chapters in the book).

2. One is reminded here of the use of position responses on the Rorschach.

CHAPTER 9

1. See also Erikson (1950, p. 229).

2. Changes in the Rorschach responses of these four patients after treatment have been discussed in Blatt and Ford (1994, pp. 159–178).

3. For a complete description of the evaluation procedures, see Blatt and Ford (1994).

4. Interestingly, the coldness in the picture is expressed in "ice cubes"—something that might have the potential to provide oral gratification if in another form.

5. Parentheses ( ) indicate that some comment, or question (?), was made by the examiner (in this and other chapters in the book).

6. This story is also discussed in Chapter 10.

7. This story is also discussed in Chapter 10.

8. This story is also discussed in Chapter 10.

9. The enhancement unit is scored under the category "Insight, Realization: . . . recognizing a previously unknown fact or situation, even if it is a negative one."

10. Cards 1, 15, 14, 10, 13MF, and 12M.

CHAPTER 10

1. The description of the TAT pictures are taken from Murray (1943).

2. The majority of the patients quoted in this chapter were diagnosed before the borderline personality disorder became a recognized diagnostic category. At the time these patients were hospitalized, they were diagnosed as severe character pathology. Experienced clinicians familiar with the case material indicate that in terms of the current diagnostic nomenclature, they would be diagnosed as BPD (S. J. Blatt, personal communication, April 16, 1993).

3. See previous note.

4. The picture depicts a young man with his downcast head buried in his arm. Behind him is the figure of a woman lying in bed (Murray, 1943).

5. This patient was diagnosed as psychotic. However, the story provides a good example of the feeling of helplessness that is found in BPD stories as well. Some of the peculiar logic around the location of the graveyard, however, is more typical of psychotic than BPD stories.

6. In keeping with the diagnostic nomenclature of the time of the patient's hospitalization, the diagnosis at admission was schizophrenic character disorder. He would likely be considered a borderline personality disorder today.

7. This patient, at the hospital admission conference, was diagnosed as a schizophrenic character disorder.

8. A detailed scoring manual, with practice stories, is available from Dr. Drew Westen, Department of Psychiatry, Cambridge Hospital, 1493 Cambridge Street, Cambridge, MA 02139.

9. In the 1995 revised version, there are 95 items.

10. In the 1995 revision, two dimensions have only seven items.

11. The number of items to be sorted into each pile is fixed. Pile 1 (not characteristic of stories) consists of 33 items: 1(33). Pile 2 consists of 21 items: 2(21); the remainder of the distribution is as follows: 3(12), 4(6), 5(6), 6(6), 7(5), 8(5), and 9(5).

12. Appreciation is expressed to Dr. Drew Westen, who kindly scored the two stories in this section.

13. The subjects were primarily females.

14. See Emmons (1987) for a full description of this measure.

15. The other two projective tests—Early Memories and the Rorschach—also differentiated significantly among the three subject groups.

CHAPTER 11

1. For this purpose, Bellak developed the CAT-H, a human figure form of the CAT.

2. Similar guidelines are provided for the TAT stories of adolescents (Eagle & Schwartz, 1994).

3. The following abbreviations are used: WH? = What happens? HF? = How is he/she feeling? WF? = What is he/she feeling? HE? = How does it end."

4. The pictures used were: TAT1, TAT17BM, trapeze, and child in field. Interrater reliability for the four pictures varied from .83 to .89, indicating that stories from young children can be scored reliably for D/E.

5. The pictures used were TAT Card 17BM and the trapeze. Interrater reliability was .86 for a subsample of 70 of the stories.

6. The difference did not quite reach statistical significance.

7. However, very little change occurred for either sex on TAT Card 17BM.

8. This study was conducted by Henry Ireys, and is reported in May (1980).

9. This example, and the discussion of it, is taken from Cramer (1991a).

10. This example, and the discussion of it, is taken from Cramer (1991a).

11. This example, and the discussion of it, is taken from Cramer (1991a).

12. These studies are discussed in greater detail in Chapter 7.

13. The subject was not available on the fourth testing occasion.

14. Pearson's r, with Spearman–Brown correction for double coding.

15. The age of the subjects was not given. The TAT cards used were 1, 2, 3BM, 4, 13MF, and 15.

16. Pearson's r, with Spearman–Brown correction for double coding.

17. The differences were not statistically significant.

18. Veroff (1969) stated that pictures about adults may be especially good for assessing achievement motivation.

19. An initial analysis indicated that the correlation between length of story and achievement score was very low (.11), and thus stories were not corrected for length. However, even when story length was used as a covariate, age remained a significant factor, showing that the age effect was not attributable to older children writing longer stories.

CHAPTER 12

1. See Chapter 15.

2. See also *The Gerontological Apperception Test* (Wolk & Wolk, 1971).

3. Six pictures (from Atkinson, 1958, Appendix III) were used for men; six different pictures were chosen for women, making cross-sex comparison inappropriate. Storytellers were asked to respond to four standard questions about the pictures: "Who are these people and what are they doing?" "What has led up to the picture?" "What do the people want and how do they feel?" And, "What will happen—how will it end?"

4. For example, salesmen and skilled workers.

5. For example, semiskilled and unskilled workers.

6. However, in the 1957 sample, fear of weakness increased at middle age (35 to 54 years) for those men who had only a grade-school education (Veroff et al., 1984).

7. In another context, Veroff (1977) suggested that females in U.S. society tend to emphasize the *process* of achieving, whereas males focus on the *impact*, or end results, of the achievement.

8. There was also some evidence that women in cohorts 1 and 3 had higher scores for affiliation motivation in both 1957 and 1976 (Veroff et al., 1984).

9. These data are confounded by the fact that nAchievement declines in old age.

10. Scoring for nPower (hope of power; Winter) was done in 1976 for both the 1957 and 1976 samples of subjects, because Winter's scoring scheme was not available at the earlier date.

11. A similar finding was reported by Tzukerman (cited in Friedman, 1987), based on TAT stories told to Card 4 by Israeli men and women. The presence–absence of children in the family was not a significant factor; nor was kibbutz versus city residence.

12. Statistical tests were not applied to these results.

13. An alternative explanation for the shift in power has been suggested by Rossi (1980), who attributes the shift to hormonal changes and especially to the change in the ratio of androgen to estrogen.

14. An identical set of TAT cards was used on both occasions.

15. No engaged men were included in the study.

16. The scores were transformed to *T* scores.

17. The wife's career level was also related to several background variables. There was a positive relationship with the husband's reported satisfaction with college and the social status of his family of origin and a negative relationship to the husband being a business executive and his having conservative political views.

18. The adolescent stories were corrected for protocol length. For adults, there was no correlation between length and motivational scores; thus no correction was used.

19. The stories were scored as described in Atkinson, 1958. The Veroff method was used to score nPower; in general, only the "imagery" category of the scoring system was used.

20. McClelland (1966) states that the number of significant correlations is significantly greater than chance.

21. Succorance was defined as "desire for support from outside; from people, institutions or supernatural agencies" (Skolnick, 1966a, p. 465).

22. The exact ages of the women as young adults is not given.

23. Similar differences between the two career groups in the relationship of nAchievement to other variables was found during adolescence. For adolescent girls who had career interests, nAchievement was positively related to mother's personality and educational/employment status, as well as to mother–daughter strife. For girls with domestic interests, nAchievement was not related to these qualities of mother. For both groups of girls, nAchievement correlated with a positive image of father. Also, for girls with domestic interests, nAchievement was related to social maturity and stereotyped female attractiveness but not to intellectual accomplishments; for girls with career interests, nAchievement was related to IQ and academic performance (Elder & MacInnis, 1983).

24. It is important to note that these studies were conducted some time ago. There is clearly a need for current follow-up studies to determine whether social change has led to further motivational change.

CHAPTER 13

1. Other sources of TAT norms include Eron (1950), Murstein (1972), and Rosenzweig (1949).

2. The assessments indicated adequate reliability for dependency pattern and locus of control; the reliability for drive expression and defensive pattern was somewhat lower (.65–.76).

3. There were also some differences in card pull as a function of social class. Females with a working-class background wrote more stories with dependency themes to Cards 1 and 12M. They also wrote more stories overall in which the main figure showed an external locus of control or was inactive, whereas the middle-class group had more stories in which the main character demonstrated an internal locus of control Unfortunately, these related findings were not reported in the same article (Ehrenreich, 1990b).

4. In a general way, this finding is consistent with May's D/E theory (see Chapter 6).

5. The following 10 TAT cards elicited the greatest number of different themes (in decreasing order): 4, 6BM, 3BM, 8BM, 10, 18BM, 15, 7BM, 1, and 13B (Cooper, 1981). The results also showed that the number of themes elicited by Card 8BM decreased across ages 11, 14, and 17, whereas the number of themes elicited by Card 20 increased across the three age groups.

6. In the Newmark and Flouranzano (1973) study, Card 18BM was among the top 10 in terms of number of themes elicited. In the Haynes and Peltier study (1985), Card 5 was among the top 10 of the most frequently used cards.

   Orzbut and Boliek (1986) suggest that the cards best suited for children ages 7 to 11 years include Cards 1, 3BM, 7GF, 8BM, 12M, 13B, 14, and 17BM. For adolescents, they suggest that the most productive cards are 1, 2, 5, 7GF, 12M, 15, 17BM, 18BM, and 18GF.

7. The authors of the article described "general concern" as consisting of issues of sexuality, acceptance, and psychological distress.

8. There is some evidence that the sex of examiner—sex of subject pairing may influence responses to projective tests. For example, Milner (1975) found that a male examiner—male subject pairing resulted in a higher frequency of sexual responses.

9. This finding may be understood in terms of the controversy regarding operant (fantasy) versus respondent (self-report) measures. (See Chapter 14, pp. 263–266.)

10. The needs included abasement, achievement, affiliation, aggression, autonomy, counteraction, defendance, deference, dominance, exhibition, harmavoidance, infavoidance, nurturance, order, play, sentience, and sex.

11. Kagan (1959) demonstrated that the stability of motive scores over time (i.e., retest reliability) is dependent on the stimulus properties of the TAT cards; cards that are highly suggestive of the motives elicit stories with greater stability.

12. Other studies in which standardized scores, corrected for story length, have been used include McAdams and Constantian (1983) and McAdams and Vaillant (1982).

13. As classified in *Psychological Abstracts* (1978–1988).

14. On the other hand, it is interesting here to consider Murstein's (1961) conclusion that modifying the test materials to make them highly similar to

the subject "promotes ego-defensiveness and a reduction in the degree of projection" (p. 254).

15. See also Murstein (1961) for a summary of studies using Thompson's cards with African-American and white subjects.

16. The difference was not tested statistically.

17. The difference between the positive ratings to the "matched" cards was 30% or greater. No statistical test was made.

18. See previous note.

19. The difference between the positive rating for the "matched" cards was 20% or less. No statistical test was made.

20. The standard method of scoring these needs was not used. Rather, each need was scored on a 5-point rating scale.

21. In this study, story protocols from 27 public school children were used to determine interrater reliability for each picture scored for personality, structural, and affective variables. The obtained correlation coefficients ranged from .20 to 1.00; the median correlation for each variable (across pictures) ranged from .43 to .96, with the exception of sexual identity (r = .33). Internal consistency reliability (coefficient alpha) for the personality, structural, and affective measures from the 23 TEMAS pictures used with the public school group ranged from .50 to .98. For the nine pictures used with the clinical group, internal consistency was determined only for the structural and affective measures, and ranged from .30 to .90)

22. The effect was greater for girls than for boys.

23. For examples of this, see Entwisle (1972), who suggests that the correlations between TAT achievement motivation scores and school grades may actually be due to a mediating variable of story length.

24. A number of studies have explicitly dealt with this issue; see Cornelius and Lane (1984), Lundy (1985), McAdams and Constantian (1983), McAdams and Vaillant (1982), and Veroff et al. (1984). The general issue has been discussed in Smith (1992, pp. 533–534).

25. All stories with 180 words or more were combined into a single interval.

26. For an example of this approach, see Winter (1982).

27. See also Cramer (1987), Cornelius and Lane (1984), McClelland (1979), and Veroff et al. (1984) for other examples in which TAT-derived scores have been adjusted for story length.

28. The SPSSX REGRESSION program performs this task easily. See Kim and Kohout (1975).

29. Other investigators suggest that the correction should be based on separate correlations for each TAT score with story length, calculated for each story separately (see Smith, 1992, p. 534).

30. For other examples, see Cramer and Gaul (1988) and Winter (1973).

CHAPTER 14

1. Inanimate objects also change over time, although at a much slower rate.

2. Psychologists working in the area of intelligence testing seem to have finally convinced critics that if an IQ score taken at age 2 does not correlate highly with another IQ score obtained at age 18, this is not an indication of unreliability in the IQ measure but rather of change in the nature of intelligence itself.

3. A study by Heckhausen (1963) found a test–retest correlation of .53 with stories to the same six pictures told 5 weeks apart.

4. Although an attempt to replicate this study was unsuccessful (Kraiger et al. 1984), there were several differences in methodology that might account for the different results. In the "replication" study, one of the stimulus pictures was different; the new picture consisted of two men, replacing the original picture of a man and woman. Although the sex composition of the "repli-cation" sample is not given (the original sample was about 50:50), the possibility of this different picture producing a stimulus sex by subject sex interaction cannot be overlooked. Perhaps more important, in the "replica-tion" study, six subjects were eliminated because the experimental manipu-lation was "contaminated" by subject comments during the test. It is not clear from the authors' report whether other subjects were present when this occurred; if so, they too may have been contaminated. If not, this indicates that the size of the subject groups on the second test occasion was quite small (e.g., six), as compared with the groups of the original study (n's = 23, 23, and 24). In addition, in the original study, the same experimenter was used for the first and second test sessions, and oral instruction was given at the beginning of the second test; information on these two factors is not provided in the replication study. Finally, the subjects in the original study were paid volunteers, while the replication subjects participated for course credit.

5. Entwisle (1972) explicitly makes the point that if each item is measuring something unique, it does not make sense to add up item scores to obtain a total score.

6. For further discussion of these issues, see Smith (1992).

7. McClelland (1980) points out that proponents of respondent measures frequently use school grades, another respondent measure, as an external criterion for validity.

8. This could be accomplished in a number of ways, as discussed in Chapter 13. Furthermore, McClelland (1980) pointed out that studies of achievement motivation typically have controlled for story length, a fact overlooked by Entwisle.

9. Thus demonstrating some discriminant validity.

10. McClelland makes it clear that operant measures are not restricted to the

assessment of motives, citing, for example, the approach of Loevinger (1966) for the assessment of levels of ego development.

11. McClelland points out, in a recent paper, that the best prediction of behavior occurs when both implicit and self-attributed motive measures are used. Implicit motives provide an impulse toward certain types of goals, while self-attributed motives define the particular area in which the impulse is expressed (McClelland, Koestner & Weinberger, 1989).

CHAPTER 15

1. According to a search on *PsychLit*.

2. The early work carried out in this tradition has been published in a volume edited by Atkinson (1958).

3. Earlier, Sanford (1936, 1937) had demonstrated the effects that varying degrees of hunger had on imagery and association.

4. In the "achievement-oriented" condition, the intent was to increase the ego involvement of the subjects; they were told that the tests were measures of both intelligence and leadership capacity. In the "neutral" condition, no attempt was made to increase or to decrease the strength of the motive; in the "relaxed" condition, the paper-and-pencil tests were explained as being in the process of development, and their importance was deemphasized. The intent here was to minimize the arousal of achievement motivation.

5. In three further arousal conditions, the same information regarding intelligence and leadership capacity was given; in addition, success and failure were manipulated. In the "success" condition, subjects were given feedback on their performance, with the norms set so low that they were nearly insured to be successful. In the "failure" condition, the norms were set very high, so as to ensure that most subjects would fall below the standard and thus experience feelings of failure. In the "success–failure" condition, subjects experienced success after the initial test but subsequently experienced failure.

6. However, the scoring categories for motives also have some theoretical connection to the motive being scored, which is not necessarily the case for criterion-keyed scale items.

7. For a detailed description of how this was accomplished for nAch, see McClelland et al. (1953); for nPower, see Winter (1973); for nIntimacy, see McAdams (1982a).

8. Extensive discussions of the TAT scoring methods for need achievement, need affiliation, need intimacy, and need power are provided in Smith (1992).

9. Operationally, the difference between the results of the two studies were

attributed to differences in the pictures used and differences in the control conditions.

10. A description of the process whereby nInt evolved out of nAff is discussed by McAdams (1988a, pp. 102–103).

11. This research has been reviewed by Winter (1973). See also Smith (1992).

12. For a description of the development of D. G. Winter's system, see Winter (1972, 1973).

13. This general issue and related studies are discussed by D. G. Winter (1973).

14. The former constellation characterized men who were low drinkers; the latter was associated with high drinking.

15. Nevertheless, Stewart (1982b) provides some empirical evidence for the existence of a developmental sequence in the subjects of the cross-validation sample. Also, her longitudinal studies have shown predicted shifts in level of psychosexual/psychosocial concerns within the same individuals (Stewart et al., 1986).

16. Category A; see Table 15.7.

17. In fact, a similar study was carried out by Bramante (1970), using May's D/E measure. Subjects viewed either a romantic or comedy film and then wrote TAT stories. Exposure to the romantic film intensified the sex-related fantasy pattern: Men had more negative scores and women more positive scores, as compared to the control (comedy film) group.

18. In a later version of the scoring system (Cooper & Gutmann, 1987), four categories of ego mastery were used: active mastery, active bimodal mastery, passive bimodal mastery, and passive mastery. The two bimodal categories were not defined.

19. These categories are also discussed in Chapter 12.

CHAPTER 16

1. The use of the TAT with borderline and narcissistic personality disorders has been discussed in Chapter 10.

2. "Activity inhibition" is defined as the number of times the word "not" appears in the protocol (see Chapter 15). Scores on the "inhibited power motive syndrome" were defined as the subject's standard score (mean = 50, $SD = 10$) for nPower being greater than the standard score for nAffiliation, with a high activity inhibition score.

3. On the other hand, the blood pressure of these men recorded in their college years was not related to their inhibited power motive score assessed in their early 40s. In subsequent studies, there was some evidence that the inhibition variable may be of less importance in demonstrating a relation-

ship between power motivation and illness (McClelland, 1989; McClelland et al., 1982).

4. The term "alexithymia," introduced by Sifneos (1973), refers to difficulties or impoverishment in the expression of affect and fantasy. This condition was hypothesized to be more prevalent in patients with psychosomatic disorders, although more recent studies call this into question.

5. The psychosomatic group consisted of 53 men and 54 women; the control group consisted of 24 men and 63 women.

6. Therapy had been concluded between 6 and 24 months previously.

7. Therapy had been concluded between 30 and 140 months previously.

8. The 20 control subjects were acquaintances of the cancer patients. Mean age of the groups was 31 years.

9. "High" in nPower was defined as the standard score for nPower > 45 and > the standard score for nAffiliation.

10. Operationally, men with high "personalized power" have high nPower and low inhibition scores. For a further discussion of personalized power, see Chapter 15.

11. Operationally, socialized power is defined as high nPower and high inhibition scores.

12. There were 125 men in the drinking group and 62 men in the control group.

13. Each drink consisted of 1.5 ounces of 86 proof liquor.

14. The TAT cards were 2, 14, and 18GF.

15. This scoring system was developed by S. K. Winter (1966). See also S. K. Winter (1969).

16. See Chapter 6 for a discussion of TAT and gender identity. A pattern of enhancement followed by deprivation (E/D) is considered to be masculine.

17. A description of the *Regressive Imagery Dictionary* and its use for content analysis is given in Martindale and Fischer (1977).

18. Subjects in the marijuana group also wrote shorter stories at time 2.

19. The SFSR uses TAT Cards 1, 5, 8BM, 10, 12M, 13MF, 14, 15, and 16. Each story is scored for 11 items relating to self-regulation, with each item rated for degree of intensity.

20. The Beck Depression Inventory did differentiate the opiate-addicted and control subjects, with the addicts scoring significantly higher.

21. There were four sets of stories: marijuana/control and time 1/time 2.

22. These categories of communication deviance are described and illustrated in a manual devised for scoring TAT stories (Singer & Wynne, 1966).

23. Singer and Wynne (1966) scored only Card 1 of the TAT.

24. Four groups were established: schizophrenic offspring with a high degree of thought disorder ($n = 5$ families), schizophrenic offspring with a moderate

degree of thought disorder (n = 7), schizophrenic offspring with a low degree of thought disorder (n = 9), and nonschizophrenic offspring with a diagnosis of obsessive–compulsive or antisocial personality disorder (n = 4). Stories were told about six TAT cards; they were recorded, transcribed, and scored by two independent raters. An adjustment was made for differences in verbal productivity.

25. An unpublished manual, *TAT Communication Deviance Scoring Manual* (Jones & Doane, 1979) was used for scoring. The scoring manual included 29 categories such as "lack of commitment to ideas or percepts, unclear or unintelligible communication of themes or ideas, language anomalies, disruptive speech, and closure problems" (Rund, 1986, p. 136).

26. The two raters had demonstrated interrater reliability on another sample of stories. In the present study, the normative data of Jones (1977) was used to transform each parent's score for each category to a standard z score; the mean of these z scores was calculated to arrive at a composite CD score for each parent.

27. This study did not explore whether there is a difference between the Mexican-American parents of schizophrenics and the Mexican-American parents of normal, nonpatients—results that have been found in both Anglo-American and Norwegian societies.

28. It is not known from the published report whether the hospitalized patients were on antidepressant medication.

29. The four groups were similar in age (range 13 to 19 years; median = 16), IQ, and social status.

30. Nine TAT cards were given as part of the initial evaluation. Responses to Cards 1, 3BM, 7GF, scored by two raters with adequate interrater reliability, produced significant results.

31. The two groups did not differ on IQ (mean = 105, range 85–130) or SES, which was primarily middle class. Stories were told about three TAT cards (2, 6BM, and 7BM).

32. It is important, in considering these findings, to realize that the white subjects were shown different pictures than the African-American and Hispanic subjects.

References

Abramson, L., McClelland, D. C., Brown, D., & Kelner, S. (1991). Alexithymic characteristics and metabolic control in diabetic and healthy adults. *Journal of Nervous and Mental Disease, 179*, 490–494.

Alexander, I. E. (1988). Personality, psychological assessment, and psychobiography. *Journal of Personality, 56*, 265–294.

Alkire, A. A., Brunse, A. J., & Houlihan, J. P. (1974). Avoidance of nuclear family relationships in schizophenia. *Journal of Clinical Psychology, 30*, 398–400.

Alvarado, N. (1994). Empirical validity of the Thematic Apperception Test. *Journal of Personality Assessment, 63*, 59–79.

American Psychiatric Association. (1994). *Diagnostic and Statistical Manual of Mental Disorders* (4th ed.). Washington, DC: Author.

Anastasi, A. (1988). *Psychological testing* (6th ed.). New York: Macmillan.

American Psychological Association. (1978–1988). *Psychological abstracts*. Washington, DC: Author.

Angyal, A. (1951). *Neuroses and treatment: A holistic theory* (E. Hanfmann & R. M. Jones, Eds.). New York: Wiley.

Archer, R. P., Maruish, M., Imhof, E. A., & Piotrowski, C. (1991). Psychological test usage with adolescent clients: 1990 survey findings. *Professional Psychology Research and Practice, 22*, 247–252.

Armstrong, M. (1954). Children's responses to animal and human figures in thematic pictures. *Journal of Consulting Psychology, 18*, 67–70.

Atkinson, J. W. (Ed.). (1958). *Motives in fantasy, action, and society*. New York: Van Nostrand.

Atkinson, J. W. (1982). Motivational determinants of thematic apperception. In A. J. Stewart (Ed.), *Motivation and society* (pp. 3–40). San Francisco: Jossey-Bass.

Atkinson, J. W., & Birch, D. (1970). *A dynamic theory of action*. New York: Wiley.

Atkinson, J. W., & Birch, D. (1978). *Introduction to motivation*. New York: Van Nostrand.

Atkinson, J. W., Bongort, K., & Price, L. H. (1977). Explorations using computer simulation to comprehend thematic apperceptive measurement of motivation. *Motivation and Emotion, 1*, 1–27.

341

Atkinson, J. W., & Feather, N. T. (Eds.). (1966). *A theory of achievement motivation.* New York: Wiley.

Atkinson, J. W., Heyns, R. W., & Veroff, J. (1954). The effect of experimental arousal of the affiliation motive on thematic apperception. *Journal of Abnormal and Social Psychology, 49*, 405–410.

Atkinson, J. W., & McClelland, D. C. (1948). The projective expression of needs: Vol. II. The effects of different intensities of the hunger drive on thematic apperception. *Journal of Experimental Psychology, 38*, 643–658.

Atkinson, J. W., & Raynor, J. O. (Eds.). (1974). *Motivation and achievement.* New York: Wiley.

Avery, R. R. (1985). *The place of self and object representations in personality organization and social behavior.* Unpublished doctoral dissertation, University of Rochester, Rochester, NY.

Bailey, B. E., & Green, J. (1977). Black Thematic Apperception Test stimulus material. *Journal of Personality Assessment, 41*, 25–30.

Bakan, D. (1966). *The duality of human existence: An essay on psychology and religion.* Chicago: Rand McNally.

Barends, A., Westen, D., Leigh, J. Silbert, D., & Byers, S. (1990). Assessing affect-tone of relationship paradigms from TAT and interview data. *Psychological Assessment: A Journal of Consulting and Clinical Psychology, 2*, 329–332.

Bedford, V. H. (1989). A comparison of thematic apperceptions of sibling affiliation, conflict, and separation at two periods of adulthood. *International Journal of Aging and Human Development, 28*, 53–66.

Bellak, L. (1954). *The Thematic Apperception Test and the Children's Apperception Test in clinical use.* New York: Grune & Stratton.

Bellak, L. (1975). *The Thematic Apperception Test: The Children's Apperception Test and the Senior Apperception Technique in clinical use* (3rd ed.). New York: Grune & Stratton.

Benton, C. J., Hernandez, A. C. R., Schmidt, A., Schmitz, M. D., Stone, A. J., & Weiner, B. (1983). Is hostility linked with affiliation among males and with achievement among females? *Journal of Personality and Social Psychology, 45*, 1167–1171.

Biersdorf, K. R., & Marcuse, F. L. (1953). Responses of children to human and animal pictures. *Journal of Projective Techniques, 17*, 455–459.

Birney, R. C. (1950). *The effect of threat on thematic apperception.* Unpublished honors thesis, Wesleyan University, Middletown, CT.

Birney, R. C. (1958). Thematic content and the cue characteristics of pictures. In J. W. Atkinson (Ed.), *Motives in fantasy, action, and society* (pp. 630–643). New York: Van Nostrand.

Birney, R. C. (1968). Research on the achievement motive. In E. Borgatta & W. Lambert (Eds.), *Handbook of personality theory and research* (pp. 857–889). Chicago: Rand McNally.

Blatt, S. J. (1990) Interpersonal relatedness and self-definition: Two personality configurations and their implications for psychopathology and psychotherapy. In J. L. Singer (Ed.), *Repression and dissociation* (pp. 299–335). Chicago: University of Chicago Press.

Blatt, S. J., & Ford, R. Q. (1994). *Therapeutic change: An object relations perspective.* New York: Plenum Press.

Blatt, S. J., & Shichman, S. (1983). Two primary configurations of psychopathology. *Psychoanalysis and Contemporary Thought, 6,* 187–254.

Blos, P. (1967). The second individuation process of adolescence. *Psychoanalytic Study of the Child, 22,* 162–186.

Boyatzis, R. E. (1973). Affiliation motivation. In D. C. McClelland & R. S. Steele (Eds.), *Human motivation: A book of readings* (pp. 252–276). Morristown, NJ: General Learning Press.

Boyd, N., & Mandler, G. (1955). Children's responses to human and animal stories and pictures. *Journal of Consulting Psychology, 19,* 367–371.

Bramante, M. (1970). *Sex differences in fantasy patterns: A replication and elaboration.* Unpublished doctoral dissertation, City University of New York, New York, NY.

Brittain, H. L. (1907). A study in imagination. *The Pedagogical Seminary, 14,* 137–207.

Bruner, J. (1986). *Actual minds, possible worlds.* Cambridge, MA: Harvard University Press.

Budoff, M. (1960). The relative utility of animal and human figures in a picture story test for young children. *Journal of Projective Techniques, 42,* 347–352.

Budoff, M. (1963). Animal vs. human figures in a picture story test for young, mentally backward children. *American Journal of Mental Deficiency, 68,* 245–250.

Byrne, D. (1962). Response to attitude similarity-dissimilarity as a function of affiliation need. *Journal of Personality, 30,* 164–177.

Campus, N. (1976). A measure of needs to assess the stimulus characteristics of TAT cards. *Journal of Personality Assessment, 40,* 248–258.

Carlson, R. (1981). Studies in script theory: I. Adult analogs of a childhood nuclear scene. *Journal of Personality and Social Psychology, 40,* 501–510.

Carlson, R. (1986). After analysis: A study of transference dreams following treatment. *Journal of Consulting and Clinical Psychology, 54,* 246–252.

Castaneda, A., McCandless, B., & Palermo, D. (1956). The children's form of the manifest anxiety scale. *Child Development, 27,* 317–326.

Cella, D. F., & Tress, S. (1986). Psychological adjustment to survival from Hodgkin's disease. *Journal of Consulting and Clinical Psychology, 54,* 616–622.

Chusmir, L. H. (1983). Male-oriented vs. balanced-as-to-sex Thematic Apperception Tests. *Journal of Personality Assessment, 47,* 29–35.

Chusmir, L. H. (1985). Motivation of managers: Is gender a factor? *Psychology of Women Quarterly, 9,* 153–159.

Clark, R. A. (1952). The projective measurement of experimentally induced levels of sexual motivation. *Journal of Experimental Psychology, 44,* 391–399.

Comstock, G., & Strasburger, V. C. (1990). Television violence and aggressive behavior. *Journal of Adolescent Health Care, 11,* 31–44.

Cooper, A. (1981). A basic TAT set for adolescent males. *Journal of Clinical Psychology, 37,* 411–414.

Cooper, K. L., & Gutmann, D. L. (1987). Gender identity and ego mastery style in middle-aged, pre- and post-empty nest women. *The Gerontologist, 27,* 347–352.

Cornelius, E. T., & Lane, F. B. (1984). The power motive and managerial success in a professionally oriented service industry organization. *Journal of Applied Psychology, 69,* 32–29.

Costantino, G., Colon-Malgady, G., Malgady, R. G., & Perez, A. (1991). Assessment of attention deficit disorder using a thematic apperception technique. *Journal of Personality Assessment, 57,* 87–95.

Costantino, G. C., & Malgady, R. G. (1983). Verbal fluency of hispanic, black and white children on TAT and TEMAS, a new Thematic Apperception Test. *Hispanic Journal of Behavioral Sciences, 5,* 199–206.

Costantino, G., Malgady, R. G., Colon-Malgady, G., & Bailey, J. (1992). Clinical utility of the TEMAS with nonminority children. *Journal of Personality Assessment, 59,* 433–438.

Costantino, G. C., Malgady, R. G., & Rogler, L. H. (1988). *Tell-Me-a-Story (TEMAS) Manual.* Los Angeles: Western Psychological Services.

Costantino, G. C., Malgady, R. G., Rogler, L. H., & Tsui, E. C. (1988). Discriminant analysis of clinical outpatients and public school children by TEMAS: A Thematic Apperception Test for Hispanics and blacks. *Journal of Personality Assessment, 52,* 670–678.

Costantino, G. C., Malgady, R. G., & Vazquez, C. (1981). A comparison of the Murray TAT and a new Thematic Apperception Test for urban Hispanic children. *Hispanic Journal of Behavioral Sciences, 3,* 291–300.

Cramer, P. (1968). Mediated priming of polysemous stimuli. *Journal of Experimental Psychology, 78,* 137–144.

Cramer, P. (1975). The development of play and fantasy in boys and girls: Empirical studies. In D. Spence (Ed.), *Psychoanalysis and contemporary science* (Vol. IV, pp. 529–567). New York: International Universities Press.

Cramer, P. (1980). The development of sexual identity. *Journal of Personality Assessment, 44,* 604–612.

Cramer, P. (1987). The development of defense mechanisms. *Journal of Personality, 55,* 597–614.

Cramer, P. (1988). The Defense Mechanism Inventory: A review of research and discussion of the scales. *Journal of Personality Assessment, 52,* 142–164.

Cramer, P. (1991a). *The development of defense mechanisms: Theory, research and assessment.* New York: Springer-Verlag.

Cramer, P. (1991b). Anger and the use of defense mechanisms in college students. *Journal of Personality, 59,* 39–55.

Cramer, P., & Blatt, S. J. (1990). Use of the TAT to measure change in defense mechanisms following intensive psychotherapy. *Journal of Personality Assessment, 54,* 236–251.

Cramer, P., & Blatt, S. J. (1993). Change in defense mechanisms following intensive treatment, as related to personality organization and gender. In U. Hentschel, G. J. W. Smith, W. Ehlers, & J. D. Draguns (Eds.), *The concept of defense mechanisms in contemporary psychology* (pp. 310–320). New York: Springer-Verlag.

Cramer, P., Blatt, S. J., & Ford, R. Q. (1988). Defense mechanisms in the anaclitic and introjective personality configuration. *Journal of Consulting and Clinical Psychology, 56,* 610–616.

Cramer, P., & Bryson, J. (1973). The development of sex-related fantasy patterns. *Developmental Psychology, 8,* 131–134.

Cramer, P., & Carter, T. (1978). The relationship between sexual identification and the use of defense mechanisms. *Journal of Personality Assessment, 42,* 63–73.

Cramer, P., & Gaul, R. (1988). The effects of success and failure on children's use of defense mechanisms. *Journal of Personality, 56,* 729–742.

Cramer, P., & Hogan, K. A. (1975). Sex differences in verbal and play fantasy. *Developmental Psychology, 11,* 145–154.

Cramer, P., & Mechem, M. B. (1982). Violence in children's animated television. *Journal of Applied Developmental Psychology, 3,* 23–39.

Crockett, D., Klonoff, H., & Clark, C. (1976). The effects of marijuana on verbalization and thought processes. *Journal of Personality Assessment, 40,* 582–587.

Dana, R. H. (1986). Personality assessment and Native Americans. *Journal of Personality Assessment, 50,* 480–500.

Demorest, A. P., & Alexander, I. E. (1992). Affective scripts as organizers of personal experience. *Journal of Personality, 60,* 645–663.

Deutsch, H. (1944). *The psychology of women: A psychoanalytic interpretation* (Vols. 1 and 2). New York: Grune & Stratton.

Dlepu, O., & Kimbrough, C. (1982). Feeling-tone and card preferences of black elementary children for the TCB and TAT. *Journal of Non-White Concerns in Personnel and Guidance, 10,* 50–56.

Doane, J. A., Miklowitz, D. J., Oranchak, E., de Apodaca, R. F., Karno, M., Strachan, A. M., & Jenkins, J. H. (1989). Parental communication deviance and schizophrenia: A cross-cultural comparison of Mexican- and Anglo-Americans. *Journal of Abnormal Psychology, 98,* 487–490.

Doane, J. A., & Mintz, J. (1987). Communication deviance in adolescence and adulthood: A longitudinal study. *Psychiatry, 50,* 5–13.

Dollinger, S. J. (1985). Lightning-strike disaster among children. *British Journal of Medical Psychology, 58,* 375–383

Dollinger, S. J., & Cramer, P. (1990). Children's defensive responses and emotional upset following a disaster: A projective assessment. *Journal of Personality Assessment, 54,* 116–127.

Dutton, D. G., & Strachan, C. E. (1987). Motivational needs for power and spouse-specific assertiveness in assaultive and nonassaultive men. *Violence and Victims, 2,* 145–156.

Eagle, C. J., & Schwartz, L. (1994). *Psychological portraits of adolescents.* New York: Lexington Books.

Edelson, M. (1993). Telling and enacting stories in psychoanalysis and psychotherapy: Implications for teaching psychotherapy. *Psychoanalytic Study of the Child, 48,* 293–325.

Ehrenreich, J. H. (1990). Quantitative studies of responses elicited by selected TAT cards. *Psychological Reports, 67,* 15–18.

Elder, G. H., Jr., & MacInnis, D. J. (1983). Achievement imagery in women's lives from adolescence to adulthood. *Journal of Personality and Social Psychology,* *45,* 394–404.

Emmons, R. A. (1987). Narcissism: Theory and measurement. *Journal of Personality and Social Psychology, 52,* 11–17.

Emmons, R. A., & McAdams, D. P. (1991). Personal strivings and motive dispositions: Exploring the links. *Personality and Social Psychology Bulletin, 17,* 648–654.

Entwisle, D. R. (1972). To dispel fantasies about fantasy-based measures of achievement motivation. *Psychological Bulletin, 77,* 377–391.

Erikson, E. H. (1950). *Childhood and society.* New York: Norton.

Erikson, E. H. (1954). The dream specimen of psychoanalysis. *Journal of the American Psychoanalytic Association, 2,* 5–56.

Erikson, E. H. (1968). *Identity: Youth and crisis.* New York: Norton.

Eron, L. D. (1950). A normative study of the Thematic Apperception Test. *Psychological Monographs, 64*(9).

Evans, A. L. (1981). *Personality characteristics and disciplinary attitudes of child-abusing mothers.* Saratoga, CA: Century Twenty-One.

Fakouri, M. E. (1979). Relationship among differences in fantasy pattern, IQ, and sex-role adoption. *Psychological Reports, 44,* 775–781.

Farima, A., & Dunham, R. M. (1966). Measurements of family relationships and their effect. *Archives of General Psychiatry, 9,* 64–73.

Fenichel, O. (1945). *The psychoanalytic theory of neurosis.* New York: Norton.

Fleming, J. (1982). Projective and psychometric approaches to measurement. The case of fear of success. In A. J. Stewart (Ed.), *Motivation and society* (pp. 63–96). San Francisco: Jossey-Bass

Fodor, E. M., & Farrow, D. L. (1979). The power motive as an influence on use of power. *Journal of Personality and Social Psychology, 37,* 2091–2097.

Freud, A. (1936/1946). *The ego and the mechanisms of defense.* New York: International Universities Press.

Freud, S. (1894/1961). The neuro-psychoses of defence. *Standard edition* (Vol. 3, pp. 45–61). London: Hogarth Press.

Freud, S. (1900/1953). The interpretation of dreams. *Standard edition* (Vols. 4 and 5, pp. 1–627). London: Hogarth Press.

Freud, S. (1905/1953). Three essays on the theory of sexuality. *Standard edition* (Vol. 7, pp. 125–243). London: Hogarth Press.

Freud, S. (1908/1959). The poet and day-dreaming. *Collected papers* (Vol. 4, pp. 173–183). New York: Basic Books.

Freud, S. (1909/1955). Analysis of a phobia in a five-year-old boy. *Standard edition* (Vol. 10, pp. 5–149). London: Hogarth Press.

Freud, S. (1911/1959). Psycho-analytic notes upon an autobiographical case of paranoia. *Collected papers* (Vol. 3, pp. 387–470). New York: Basic Books.

Freud, S. (1924/1959). The economic problem in masochism. *Collected papers* (Vol. 2, pp. 255–268). New York: Basic Books.

Freud, S. (1926/1959). Inhibitions, symptoms, and anxiety. *Standard edition* (Vol. 20, pp. 77–86). London: Hogarth Press.

Freud, S. (1930/1961). Civilization and its discontents. *Standard edition* (Vol. 21, pp. 64–145). London: Hogarth Press.

Freud, S. (1933/1964). Femininity. *Standard edition* (Vol. 22, pp. 112–135). London: Hogarth Press.

Freud, S. (1937/1959). Construction in analysis. *Collected papers* (Vol. 5, pp. 358–371). New York: Basic Books.

Friedman, A. (1987). Getting powerful with age: Changes in women over the life cycle. *Israel Social Science Research, 5,* 76–86.

George, B. L., & Waehler, C. A. (1994). The ups and downs of TAT Card 17BM. *Journal of Personality Assessment, 63,* 167–172.

Glasberg, R., & Aboud, F. (1982). Keeping one's distance from sadness: Children's self-reports of emotional experience. *Developmental Psychology, 18,* 287–293.

Gleser, G. C., & Ihilevich, D. (1969). An objective instrument for measuring defense mechanisms. *Journal of Consulting and Clinical Psychology, 33,* 51–60.

Goldstein, M. J., Gould, E., Alkire, A. A., Rodnick, E. H., & Judd, L. L. (1970). Interpersonal themes in the thematic apperception test stories of families of disturbed adolescents. *Journal of Nervous and Mental Disease, 150,* 354–365.

Gurin G., Veroff, J., & Feld, S. C. (1960). *Americans view their mental health.* New York: Basic Books.

Gustafson, R. (1987). Alcohol and aggression: A test of an indirect measure of aggression. *Psychological Reports, 60,* 1241–1242.

Gustafson, R. (1988). The relationship between alcohol intoxication and power in real-life non-alcoholic couples. *Drug and Alcohol Dependence, 22,* 55–62.

Gutmann, D. L. (1964). An exploration of ego configurations in middle and later life. In B. L. Neugarten (Ed.), *Personality in middle and late life* (pp. 114–148). New York: Atherton Press.

Gutmann, D. L. (1985). The parental imperative revisited: Towards a developmental psychology of adulthood and later life. In J. A. Meacham (Ed.), *Family and individual development* (pp. 31–60). New York: Karger.

Gutmann, D. L. (1987). *Reclaimed powers: Toward a new psychology of men and women in later life.* New York: Basic Books.

Haan, N. (1974). The adolescent antecedents of an ego model of coping and defense and comparisons with Q-sorted ideal personalities. *Genetic Psychology Monographs, 89,* 273–306.

Haber, R. N., & Alpert, R. (1958). The role of situation and picture cues in projective measurement of the achievement motive. In J. W. Atkinson (Ed.), *Motives in fantasy, action, and society* (pp. 644–663). New York: Van Nostrand.

Hamilton, A., Stiles, W. B., Melowsky, F., & Beal, D. G. (1987). A multilevel comparison of child abusers with nonabusers. *Journal of Family Violence, 2,* 215–225.

Harder D. W. (1979). The assessment of ambitious–narcissistic character style with three projective tests: The Early Memories, TAT, and Rorschach. *Journal of Personality Assessment, 43,* 23–32.

Hardy, K. R. (1957). Determinants of conformity and attitude change. *Journal of Abnormal and Social Psychology, 54,* 289–294.

Hartman, A. A. (1949). An experimental examination of the thematic apperception technique in clinical diagnosis. *Psychological Monographs, 63*(8, Whole No. 303).

Haynes, J. P., & Peltier, J. (1985). Patterns of practice with the TAT in juvenile forensic settings. *Journal of Personality Assessment, 49,* 26–29.

Healy, J. M. Jr., & Stewart, A. J. (1984). Adaptation to life changes in adolescence. In P. Karoly & J. J. Steffen (Eds.), *Adolescent behavior disorders: Foundations and contemporary concerns* (pp. 39–60). Lexington, MA: Heath.

Heckhausen, H. (1963). *Hoffnung und Furcht in der Leistungsmotivation.* New York: Springer.

Heckhausen, H. (1968). Achievement motive research. In W. J. Arnold (Ed.), *Nebraska symposium on motivation: 1968* (pp. 103–170). Lincoln: University of Nebraska Press.

Henderson, O. (1990). The object relations of sexually abused girls. *Melanie Klein and Object Relations, 8,* 63–76.

Henry, W. F. (1956). *The analysis of fantasy.* New York: Wiley.

Hermans, H. J. M., Kempen, H. J. G., & van Loon, R. J. P. (1992). The dialogical self: Beyond individualism and rationalism. *American Psychologist, 47,* 23–33.

Heyns, R. W., Veroff, J., & Atkinson, J. W. (1958). A scoring manual for the affiliation motive. In J. W. Atkinson (Ed.), *Motives in fantasy, action, and society* (pp. 205–218). New York: Van Nostrand.

Hibbard, S., Farmer, L., Wells, C., Difillipo, E., Barry, W., Korman, R., & Sloan, P. (1994). Validation of Cramer's Defense Mechanism Manual for the TAT. *Journal of Personality Assessment, 63,* 197–210.

Hill, K. T., & Sarason, S. B. (1966). The relation of test anxiety and defensiveness to test and school performance over the elementary-school years. *Monographs of the Society for Research in Child Development, 31*(2), 1–76.

Holt, R. R. (1951). The Thematic Apperception Test. In H. H. Anderson & G. L. Anderson (Eds.), *An introduction to projective techniques* (pp. 181–229). New York: Prentice Hall.

Holt, R. R. (1958). Formal aspects of the TAT—a neglected resource. *Journal of Projective Techniques, 22,* 163–172.

Holt, R. R. (1978). *Methods in clinical psychology.* New York: Plenum Press.

Holt, R. R., & Thompson, C. E. (1950). Bibliography for the TAT. *Journal of Projective Techniques, 14,* 80–1000.

Howard, G. S. (1991). A narrative approach to thinking, cross-cultural psychology, and psychotherapy. *American Psychologist, 46,* 187–197.

Huesmann, L. R., Eron, L. D., Berkowitz, L., & Chafee, S. (1992). The effects of television violence on aggression: A reply to a skeptic. In P. Suedfeld & P. E. Tetlock (Eds.), *Psychology and social policy* (pp. 191–200). New York: Hemisphere.

Huesmann, L. R., Eron, L. D., Lefkowitz, M. M., & Walker, L. O. (1973). Television violence and aggression: The causal effect remains. *American Psychologist, 28,* 617–620.

Ireys, H. T. (1975). *The development of sex differences in play.* Unpublished honors thesis, Williams College, Williamstown, MA.

Jacobs, B. (1958). A method for investigating the cue characteristics of pictures.

In J. W. Atkinson (Ed.), *Motives in fantasy, action, and society* (pp. 617–629). New York: Van Nostrand.

Jemott, J. J. (1987). Social motives and susceptibility to disease: Stalking individual differences in health risks. *Journal of Personality, 55,* 267–298.

Johnson, J. L. (1974). *The measurement of the development of sex differences.* Unpublished honors thesis, Williams College, Williamstown, MA.

Johnson, J. L. (1994). The Thematic Apperception Test and Alzheimer's disease. *Journal of Personality Assessment, 62,* 314–319.

Jones, J. E. (1977). Patterns of transactional style deviance in the TAT's of parents of schizophrenics. *Family Process, 16,* 327–337.

Jones, J. E., & Doane, J. H. (1979). *TAT communication deviance scoring manual.* Unpublished manuscript.

Kagan, J. (1959). The stability of TAT fantasy and stimulus ambiguity. *Journal of Consulting Psychology, 23,* 266–271.

Kagan, J. (1960). Thematic apperceptive techniques with children. In A. I. Rabin & M. R. Haworth (Eds.), *Projective techniques with children* (pp. 105–129). New York: Grune & Stratton.

Kagan, J., & Lesser, G. S. (Eds.). (1961). *Contemporary issues in thematic apperception methods.* Springfield, IL: Charles C Thomas.

Kalin, R., McClelland, D. C., & Kahn, M. (1965). The effects of male social drinking in fantasy. *Journal of Personality and Social Psychology, 1,* 441–452.

Katz, H. E., Russ, S. W., & Overholser, J. C. (1993). Sex differences, sex roles, and projection on the TAT: Matching stimulus to examinee gender. *Journal of Personality Assessment, 60,* 186–191.

Keen, E. (1970). *Three faces of being: Toward an existential clinical psychology.* New York: Appleton-Century-Crofts.

Keiser, R. W., & Prather, E. N. (1990). What is the TAT? A review of ten years of research. *Journal of Personality Assessment, 55,* 800–803.

Keltikangas-Jarvinen, L. (1985). Concept of alexithymia: I. The prevalence of alexithymia in psychosomatic patients. *Psychotherapy and Psychosomatics, 44,* 132–138.

Kernberg, 0. (1967). Borderline personality organization. *Journal of the American Psychoanalytic Association, 15,* 641–685.

Kernberg, O. (1975). *Borderline conditions and pathological narcissism.* Northvale, NJ: Jason Aronson.

Kernberg, O. (1976). *Object-relations theory and clinical psychoanalysis.* Northvale, NJ: Jason Aronson.

Kim, J., & Kohout, F. (1975). Multiple regression analysis. In N. Nie, C. Hull, J. Jenkins, K. Steinbrenner, & D. Bent (Eds.), *Statistical package for the social sciences* (pp. 320–365). New York: McGraw-Hill.

King, L. A. (1995). Wishes, motives, goals and personal memories: Relations of measures of human motivation. *Journal of Personality, 63,* 985–1007.

Klein, R. G. (1986). Questioning the clinical usefulness of projective psychological tests for children. *Developmental and Behavioral Pediatrics, 7,* 378–382.

Koestner, R., & McClelland, D. C. (1990). Perspectives on competence motivation. In L. A. Pervin (Ed.), *Handbook of personality: Theory and research* (pp. 527–548). New York: Guilford Press.

Koestner, R., Ramey, A., Kelner, S., Meenan, R., & McClelland, D. C. (1989). Indirectly expressed motivational deficits among arthritic adults. *Motivation and Emotion*, *13*, 21–29.

Kohut, H. (1979). The two analyses of Mr. Z. *International Journal of Psycho-Analysis*, *60*, 3–27.

Kohut, H. (1984). *How does analysis cure?* (A. Goldberg, Ed.). Chicago: University of Chicago Press.

Koski, M. L., Holmberg, R. L., & Torvinen, V. (1988). Alexithymia in juvenile diabetes: A clinical study based on projective methods (TAT and ORT). *Psychiatria Fennica*, *19*, 21–29.

Kraiger, K., Hakel, M. D., & Cornelius, E. T. III. (1984). Exploring fantasies of TAT reliability. *Journal of Personality Assessment*, *18*, 365–370.

Kwawer, J. S., Lerner, H. D., Lerner, P. M., & Sugarman, A. (Eds.). (1980). *Borderline phenomena and the Rorschach text*. New York: International Universities Press.

Lawton, M. J. (1966). Animal and human CATs with a school sample. *Journal of Projective Techniques and Personality Assessment*, *30*, 243–246.

Lazarus, R. S. (1961). A substitutive–defensive conception of apperceptive fantasy. In J. Kagan & G. S. Lesser (Eds.), *Contemporary issues in thematic apperceptive methods* (pp. 51–71). Springfield, IL: Charles C Thomas.

Lazarus, R. S. (1966). Story telling and the measurement of motivation: the direct versus substitutive controversy. *Journal of Consulting Psychology*, *30*, 483–487.

Lefcourt, M. M., & Steffy, R. A. (1967). Sex-linked censure expectancies in process and reactive schizophrenics as a function of censure, social class and premorbid adjustment. *Journal of Abnormal Psychology*, *72*, 415–420.

Lefkowitz, J., & Fraser, A. W. (1980). Assessment of achievement and power motivation of blacks and whites, using a black and white TAT, with black and white administrators. *Journal of Applied Psychology*, *65*, 685–696.

Leigh, J., Westen, D., Barends, A., & Mendel, M. (1992). Assessing complexity of representations of people from TAT and interview data. *Journal of Personality*, *60*, 809–837.

Leitch, M., & Schafer, S. (1947). A study of the Thematic Apperception Test of psychotic children. *American Journal of Orthopsychiatry*, *17*, 337–342.

Levitt, E. E., & French, J. (1992). Projective testing of children. In C. E. Walker & M. C. Roberts (Eds.), *Handbook of clinical child psychology* (pp. 149–162). New York: Wiley.

Lewis, C. S. (1988). *The lion, the witch and the wardrobe*. New York: Macmillan. (Original work published 1950)

Lezak, M. D. (1987). Norms for growing older. *Developmental Neuropsychology*, *3*, 1–12.

Libby, W. (1908). The imagination of adolescents. *American Journal of Psychology*, *19*, 249–252.

Loevinger, J. (1966). The meaning and measurement of ego development. *American Psychologist*, *21*, 195–206.

Lubin, B., Larsen, R. M., & Matarazzo, J. D. (1984). Patterns of psychological test usage in the United States. *American Psychologist*, *39*, 451–454.

Lubin, B., Larsen, R. M., Matarazzo, J. D., & Seever, M. (1985). Psychological test usage patterns in five professional settings. *American Psychologist, 40*, 857–861.

Lubin, B., Wallis, R., & Paine, C. (1971). Patterns of psychological test use in the United States: 1935–1969. *Professional Psychology, 2*, 70–74.

Luborsky, L. (1984). *Principles of psychoanalytic psychotherapy*. New York: Basic Books.

Lundy, A. (1985). The reliability of the Thematic Apperception Test. *Journal of Personality Assessment, 49*, 141–149.

Lundy, A. (1988). Instructional set and Thematic Apperception Test validity. *Journal of Personality Assessment, 52*, 309–320.

MacKinnon, D. (1965). Personality and the realization of creative potential. *American Psychologist, 20*, 273–281.

Malgady, R. G., Costantino, G., & Rogler, L. H. (1984). Development of a Thematic Apperception Test (TEMAS) for urban Hispanic children. *Journal of Consulting and Clinical Psychology, 52*, 986–996.

Martindale, C., & Fischer, R. (1977). The effect of psilocybin on primary process content in language. *Confinia Psychiatrica, 20*, 195–202.

May, R. R. (1966). Sex differences in fantasy patterns. *Journal of Projective Techniques and Personality Assessment. 30*, 576–586.

May, R. R. (1969). Deprivation–enhancement fantasy patterns in men and women. *Journal of Projective Techniques and Personality Assessment, 33*, 464–469.

May, R. R. (1971). A method for studying the development of gender identity. *Developmental Psychology, 5*, 484–487.

May, R. R. (1975). Further studies on deprivation/enhancement patterns. *Journal of Personality Assessment, 39*, 116–122.

May, R. R. (1980). *Sex and fantasy: Patterns of male and female development*. New York: Norton.

Mayman, M. (1946). Review of the literature on the Thematic Apperception Test. In D. Rapaport, M. M. Gill, & R. Schafer (Eds.), *Diagnostic psychological testing* (Vol. 2, pp. 496–505). Chicago: Mosby–Yearbook.

McAdams, D. P. (1980). A thematic coding system for the intimacy motive. *Journal of Research in Personality, 14*, 413–432.

McAdams, D. P. (1982a). Intimacy motivation. In A. J. Stewart (Ed.), *Motivation and society* (pp. 133–171). San Francisco: Jossey-Bass.

McAdams, D. P. (1982b). Experiences of intimacy and power: Relationships between social motives and autobiographical memories. *Journal of Personality and Social Psychology, 42*, 292–302.

McAdams, D. P. (1984). Scoring manual for the intimacy motive. *Psychological Documents, 14*, 2614.

McAdams, D. P. (1985). The "imago": A key narrative component of identity. In P. Shaver (Ed.), *Self, situations and social behavior* (Vol. 6, pp. 115–141). Beverly Hills, CA: Sage.

McAdams, D. P. (1988a). *Power, intimacy, and the life story*. New York: Guilford Press.

McAdams, D. P. (1988b) Biography, narrative, and lives: An introduction. *Journal of Personality, 56*, 1–18.

McAdams, D. P., & Bryant, F. B. (1987). Intimacy motivation and subjective mental health in a nationwide sample. *Journal of Personality, 55*, 395–413.

McAdams, D. P., & Constantian, C. A. (1983). Intimacy and affiliation motives in daily living: An experience sampling analysis. *Journal of Personality, 45*, 851–861.

McAdams, D. P., Lester, R. M., Brand, P. A., McNamara, W. J., & Lensky, D. B. (1988). Sex and the TAT: Are women more intimate than men? Do men fear intimacy? *Journal of Personality Assessment, 52*, 397–409.

McAdams, D. P., & Powers, J. (1981). Themes of intimacy in behavior and thought. *Journal of Personality and Social Psychology, 40*, 573–587.

McAdams, D. P., & Vaillant, G. E. (1982). Intimacy motivation and psychosocial adjustment: A longitudinal study. *Journal of Personality Assessment, 46*, 586–593.

McAdams, D. P., & Zeldow, P. B. (1993). Construct validity and content analysis. *Journal of Personality Assessment, 61*, 243–245.

McCandless, B. R. (1967). *Children: Behavior and development.* New York: Holt, Rinehart & Winston.

McClelland, D. C. (1951). *Personality.* New York: William Sloan Associates.

McClelland, D. C. (1961). *The achieving society.* New York: Van Nostrand.

McClelland, D. C. (1966). Longitudinal trends in the relation of thought to action. *Journal of Consulting Psychology, 30*, 479–483.

McClelland, D. C. (1971). *Assessing human motivation.* Morristown, NJ: General Learning Press.

McClelland, D. C. (1975). *Power: The inner experience.* New York: Irvington.

McClelland, D. C. (1979). Inhibited power motivation and high blood pressure in men. *Journal of Abnormal Psychology, 88*, 182–190.

McClelland, D. C. (1980). Motive dispositions: The merits of operant and respondent measures. In L. Wheeler (Ed.), *Review of personality and social psychology* (Vol. 1, pp. 10–41). Beverly Hills, CA: Sage.

McClelland, D. C. (1989). Motivational factors in health and disease. *American Psychologist, 44*, 675–683.

McClelland, D. C., Alexander, C., & Marks, E. (1982). The need for power, stress, immune function and illness among male prisoners. *Journal of Abnormal Psychology, 91*, 61–70.

McClelland, D. C., Atkinson, J. W., Clark, R. A., & Lowell, E. L. (1953). *The achievement motive.* New York: Appleton-Century-Crofts.

McClelland, D. C., & Boyatzis, R. E. (1982). Leadership motive pattern and long-term success in management. *Journal of Applied Psychology, 67*, 737–743.

McClelland, D. C., Clark, R. A., Roby, T. B., & Atkinson, J. W. (1949). The projective expression of needs: Vol. IV. The effect of the need for achievement on thematic apperception. *Journal of Experimental Psychology, 18*, 242–251.

McClelland, D. C., Davis, W. N., Kalin, R., & Wanner, E. (1972). *The drinking man.* New York: Free Press.

McClelland, D. C., & Jemott, J. B. III. (1980). Power motivation, stress, and physical illness. *Journal of Human Stress, 6*, 6–15.

McClelland, D. C., Koestner, R., & Weinberger, J. (1989). How do self-attributed and implicit motives differ? *Psychological Review, 96,* 690–702.

McClelland, D. C., & Krishnit, C. (1988). The effect of motivational arousal through films on salivary immunoglobulin. *Psychology and Health, 2,* 31–52.

McClelland, D. C., & Steele, R. S. (1972). *Motivation workshops.* Morristown, NJ: General Learning Press.

McGrew, M. W., & Teglasi, H. (1990). Formal characteristics of Thematic Apperception Test stories as indices of emotional disturbance in children. *Journal of Personality Assessment, 54,* 639–655.

McKay, J. R. (1991). Assessing aspects of object relations associated with immune function: Development of the affiliative trust–mistrust coding system. *Psychological Assessment, 3,* 541–547.

Melnick, B., & Hurley, J. R. (1969). Distinctive personality attributes of child-abusing mothers. *Journal of Consulting and Clinical Psychology, 33,* 746–749.

Menaker, E. (1979). *Masochism and the emergent ego.* New York: Human Sciences Press.

Miklowitz, D. J., Velligan, D. I., Goldstein, M. J., & Neuchterlein, K. H. (1991). Communication deviance in families of schizophrenic and manic patients. *Jouranl of Abnormal Psychology, 100,* 163–173.

Milner, J. S. (1975). Administrator's gender and sexual content in projective test protocols. *Journal of Clinical Psychology, 31,* 540–541.

Morgan, C. D., & Murray, H. (1935). A method for investigating fantasies: The Thematic Apperception Test. *Archives of Neurological Psychiatry, 34,* 289–306.

Morgan, W. G. (1995). Origin and history of the Thematic Apperception Test images. *Journal of Personality Assessment, 65,* 237–254.

Murray, H. A. (1937). Techniques for a systematic investigation of fantasy. *Journal of Psychology, 3,* 115–143.

Murray, H. A. (1938). *Explorations in personality.* New York: Oxford University Press.

Murray, H. A. (1943). *Thematic Apperception Test manual.* Cambridge, MA: Harvard University Press.

Murray, H. A. (1955). American Icarus. In A. Burton & R. Harris (Eds.), *Clinical studies of personality* (pp. 615–641). New York: Harper.

Murstein, B. I. (1961). The role of the stimulus in the manifestation of fantasy. In J. Kagan & G. S. Lesser (Eds.), *Contemporary issues in thematic apperceptive methods* (pp. 229–273). Springfield, IL: Charles C Thomas.

Murstein, B. I. (1963). *Theory and research in projective techniques: Emphasizing the TAT.* New York: Wiley.

Murstein, B. I. (1972). Normative written TAT responses for a college sample. *Journal of Personality Assessment, 36,* 109–147.

Neely, J. H. (1991). Semantic priming effects in visual word recognition: A selective review of current findings and theories. In D. Besner & G. W. Humphreys (Eds.), *Basic processes in reading: Visual word recognition* (pp. 264–336). Hillsdale, NJ: Erlbaum.

Neugarten, B. L. (Ed.). (1964). *Personality in middle and late life.* New York: Atherton Press.

Neugarten, B. L. (Ed.). (1968). *Middle age and aging.* Chicago: University of Chicago Press.

Neugarten, B. L., & Gutmann, D. L. (1968). Age-sex roles and personality in middle age: A Thematic Apperception study. In B. L. Neugarten (Ed.), *Middle age and aging* (pp. 58–71). Chicago: University of Chicago Press.

Newmark, C. S., & Flouranzano, R. (1973). Replication of an empirically derived TAT set with hospitalized psychiatric patients. *Journal of Personality Assessment, 37,* 340–341.

Nunnaly, J. (1968). *Psychometric theory.* New York: Wiley.

Obrzut, J. E., & Boliek, C. A. (1986). Thematic approaches to personality assessment with children and adolescents. In H. M. Knoff (Ed.), *The assessment of child and adult personality* (pp. 173–198). New York: Guilford Press.

Ornduff, S. R., Freedenfeld, R. N., Kelsey, R. M., & Critelli, J. W. (1994). Object relations of sexually abused female subjects: A TAT analysis. *Journal of Personality Assessment, 63,* 223–238.

Pasewark, R. A., Fitzgerald, B. J., Dexter, V., & Cangemi, A. (1976). Responses of adolescent, middle-aged, and aged females on the Gerontological and Thematic Apperception Tests. *Journal of Personality Assessment, 40,* 588–591.

Patalano, F. (1986). Drug abusers and card 3BM of the TAT. *Psychology: A Quarterly Journal of Human Behavior, 23,* 34–36.

Peterson, C. A. (1990). Administration of the Thematic Apperception Test: Contributions of psychoanalytic psychotherapy. *Journal of Contemporary Psychotherapy, 20,* 191–200.

Peterson, C. A., & Schilling, K. M. (1983). Card pull in projective testing. *Journal of Personality Assessment, 47,* 265–275.

Piotrowski, C., & Keller, J. W. (1989). Psychological testing in outpatient mental health facilities: A national study. *Professional Psychology: Research and Practice, 20,* 423–425.

Piotrowski, C., Sherry, D., & Keller, J. W. (1985). Psychodiagnostic test usage: A survey of the Society for Personality Assessment. *Journal of Personality Assessment, 49,* 115–119.

Piotrowski, C., & Zalewski, C. (1993). Training in psychodiagnostic testing in APA-approved PsyD and PhD clinical psychology programs. *Journal of Personality Assessment, 61,* 394–405.

Pistole, D. R., & Ornduff, S. R. (1994). TAT assessment of sexually abused girls: An analysis of manifest content. *Journal of Personality Assessment, 63,* 211–222.

Pollak, S., & Gilligan, C. (1982). Images of violence in Thematic Apperception Test stories. *Journal of Personality and Social Psychology, 42,* 159–167.

Rapaport, D., Gill, M. M., & Schafer, R. (1946). *Diagnostic psychological testing* (Vols. 1 & 2). Chicago: Mosby–Year Book. (Rev. ed., 1968, R. R. Holt, Ed.)

Rapaport, D. (1951). *Organization and pathology of thought.* New York: Columbia University Press.

Reich, W. (1933). *Character analysis.* London: Vision Press.

Reuman, D. A. (1982). Ipsative behavioral variability and the quality of thematic apperceptive measurement of the achievement motive. *Journal of Personality and Social Psychology, 43,* 1098–1110.

Reuman, D. A., Alwin, D. F., & Veroff, J. (1984). Assessing the validity of the achievement motive in the presence of random measurement error. *Journal of Personality and Social Psychology, 47,* 1347–1362.

Revere, V., Rodeffer, C., & Dawson, S. (1989). Changes in long-term institutionalized schizophrenics with psychotherapy. *Journal of Contemporary Psychotherapy, 19,* 203–219.

Richardson, V., & Partridge, S. (1982). Construct validation of imaginative assessment of family orientation and status perception: Theoretical and methodological implications for the Thematic Apperception Test. *Educational and Psychological Measurement, 42,* 1243–1251.

Roby, T. B. (1948). *The effect of need for security on thematic apperception.* Unpublished master's thesis. Wesleyan University, Middletown, CT.

Rosen, B. C., & D'Andrade, R. (1959). The psychological origins of achievement motivation. *Sociometry, 22,* 185–218.

Rosen, J. L., & Neugarten, B. L. (1964). Ego functions in the middle and later years: A thematic apperception study. In B. L. Neugarten (Ed.), *Personality in middle and late life* (pp. 90–101). New York: Atherton Press.

Rosenberg, S. D., Blatt, S. J., Oxman, T. E., McHugo, G. J., & Ford, R. Q. (1994). Assessment of object relatedness through a lexical content analysis of the TAT. *Journal of Personality Assessment, 63,* 345–362.

Rosenberg, S. D., Schnurr, P. P., & Oxman, T. E. (1990). Content analysis: A comparison of manual and computerized systems. *Journal of Personality Assessment, 54,* 298–310.

Rosenwald, G. C. (1968) The Thematic Apperception Test (TAT). In A. I. Rabin (Ed.), *Projective techniques in personality assessment* (pp. 172–221). New York: Springer.

Rosenzweig, S. (1949). Apperceptive norms in the Thematic Apperception Test: I. The problems of norms in projective methods. *Journal of Personality, 17,* 475–482.

Rossi, A. S. (1980). Life span theories and women's lives. *Signs: Journal of Women in Culture and Society, 6,* 4–32.

Roth, W. T., Rosenbloom, M. J., Darley, C. F., Tinkleberg, J. R., & Kopell, B. S. (1975). Marijuana effects on TAT form and content. *Psychopharmacologia, 43,* 261–266.

Rund, B. R. (1986). Communication deviances in parents of schizophrenics. *Family Process, 25,* 133–147.

Sanford, R. N. (1936). The effect of abstinence from food upon imaginal processes: A preliminary experiment. *Journal of Psychology, 2,* 129–136.

Sanford, R. N. (1937). The effect of abstinence from food upon imaginal processes: A further experiment. *Journal of Psychology, 3,* 145–159.

Sarbin, T. R. (1986). *Narrative psychology: The storied nature of human conduct.* New York: Praeger.

Sass, L. A., Gunderson, J. G., Singer, M. T., & Wynne, L. C. (1984). Parental communication deviance and forms of thinking in male schizophrenic offspring. *Journal of Nervous and Mental Disease, 172,* 513–520.

Schafer, R. (1958). How was this story told? *Journal of Projective Techniques, 22,* 181–210.

Schafer, R. (1992). *Retelling a life: Narration and dialogue in psychoanalysis.* New York: Basic Books.

Schatzman, M. (1973). *Soul murder: Persecution in the family.* New York: Random House.

Schnur, R. E., & MacDonald, M. L. (1988). Stages of identity development and problem drinking in college women. *Journal of Youth and Adolescence, 17,* 349–369.

Schnurr, P. P., Rosenberg, S. D., & Oxman, T. E. (1992). Comparison of TAT and free speech techniques for eliciting source material in computerized context analysis. *Journal of Personality Assessment, 58,* 311–325.

Schnurr, P. P., Rosenberg, S. D., & Oxman, T. E. (1993). Issues in the comparison of techniques for eliciting source material in computerized content analysis. *Journal of Personality Assessment, 61,* 237–242.

Schreber, D. P. (1903). *Denkwurdigkeiten eines nervenkranken.* Leipzig: Schloss.

Schwartz, B. J. (1955). The measurement of castration anxiety and anxiety over loss of love. *Journal of Personality, 24,* 204–219.

Schwartz, L. A. (1932). Social situation pictures in the psychiatric interview. *American Journal of Orthopsychiatry, 2,* 124–132.

Schwartz, L., & Eagle, C. J. (1986). *Psychological portraits of children.* Lexington, MA: Lexington Books.

Semrad, E. (1967). The organization of ego defenses and object loss. In D. M. Moriarity (Ed.), *The loss of loved ones* (pp. 126–134). Springfield, IL: Charles C Thomas.

Shabad, P., Worland, J., Lander, H., & Dietrich, D. (1979). A retrospective analysis of the Tats [*sic*] of children at risk who subsequently broke down. *Child Psychiatry and Human Development, 10,* 49–59.

Sharkey, K. J., & Ritzler, B. A. (1985). Comparing diagnostic validity of the TAT and a new picture projective test. *Journal of Personality Assessment, 49,* 406–412.

Sheikh, A. A., & Twerski, M. (1974). Future-time perspective in Negro and white adolescents. *Perceptual and Motor Skills, 39,* 308.

Shill, M. (1981). TAT measures of gender identity (castration anxiety) in father-absent males. *Journal of Personality Assessment, 45,* 136–146.

Shipley, T., & Veroff, J. (1952). A projective measure of need for affiliation. *Journal of Experimental Psychology, 43,* 349–356.

Shneidman, E. S. (1951). *Thematic test analysis.* New York: Grune & Stratton.

Shulman, D. G., & Ferguson, G. R. (1988). Two methods of assessing narcissism: Comparison of the Narcissism–Projective (N-P) and the Narcissistic Personality Inventory. *Journal of Clinical Psychology, 44,* 857–866.

Shulman, D. G., McCarthy, E. C., & Ferguson, G. R. (1988). The projective assessment of narcissism: Development, reliability, and validity of the N-P. *Psychoanalytic Psychology, 5,* 285–297.

Singer, J. L., & Salovey, P. (1991). Organized knowledge structures and personality: Person schemas, self schemas, prototypes, and scripts. In M. J. Horowitz (Ed.), *Person schemas and maladaptive interpersonal patterns* (pp. 33–79). Chicago: University of Chicago Press.

Singer, M. T., & Wynne, L. C. (1966). Principles for scoring communication defects and deviances in parents of schizophrenics: Rorschach and TAT scoring manuals. *Psychiatry, 29,* 260–288.

Skolnick, A. (1966a). Motivational imagery and behavior over twenty years. *Journal of Consulting Psychology, 30,* 463–478.

Skolnick, A. (1966b). Stability and interrelations of motivational imagery over twenty years. *Child Development, 37,* 389–396.

Slaby, R. G., & Frey, K. S. (1975). Development of gender constancy and selective attention to same sex models. *Child Development, 46,* 849–856.

Smith, C. P. (1969). *Achievement-related motives in children.* New York: Russell Sage.

Smith, C. P. (Ed.). (1992). *Motivation and personality: Handbook of thematic content analysis.* New York: Cambridge University Press.

Smith, G. J. W., & Danielsson, A. (1982). *Anxiety and defense strategies in childhood and adolescence.* New York: International Universities Press.

Smith, W. P., & Rossman, B. B. R. (1986). Developmental changes in trait and situational denial under stress during childhood. *Journal of Child Psychiatry, 27,* 227–235.

Spangler, W. D. (1992). Validity of questionnaire and TAT measures of need for achievement. *Psychological Bulletin, 112,* 140–154.

Spence, D. P. (1982). *Narrative truth and historical truth: Meaning and interpretation in psychoanalysis.* New York: Norton.

Sriram, T. G., Chaturvedi, S. K., Gopinath, P. S., & Shanmugam, V. (1987). Controlled study of alexithymic characteristics in patients with psychogenic pain disorder. *Psychotherapy and Psychosomatics, 47,* 11–17.

Stang, D. J., Campus, N., & Wallach, C. (1975). Exposure duration as a confounding methodological factor in projective testing. *Journal of Personality Assessment, 39,* 583–586.

Steele, R. S. (1986). Deconstructing histories: Toward a systematic criticim of psychological narratives. In T. R. Sarbin (Ed.), *Narrative psychology: The storied narrative of human conduct* (pp. 256–275). New York: Praeger.

Stein, M. I. (1955). *The Thematic Apperception Test, an introductory manual for its clinical use with adults* (Rev. ed.). Cambridge, MA: Addison-Wesley.

Stewart, A. J. (1973). *Scoring system for stages of psychological development.* Unpublished manuscript, Harvard University, Department of Psychology and Social Relations, Cambridge, MA.

Stewart, A. J. (1977). *Scoring manual for stages of psychological adaptation to the environment.* Unpublished manuscript, Boston University, Boston, MA.

Stewart, A. J. (1978). A longitudinal study of coping styles in self-defining and socially defined women. *Journal of Consulting and Clinical Psychology, 46,* 1079–1084.

Stewart, A. J. (1982a). *Motivation and society.* San Francisco: Jossey-Bass.

Stewart, A. J. (1982b). The course of individual adaptation to life changes. *Journal of Personality and Social Psychology, 42,* 1100–1113.

Stewart, A. J., & Chester, N. L. (1982). Sex differences in human social motives: Achievement, affiliation, and power. In A. J. Stewart (Ed.), *Motivation and society* (pp. 172–218). San Francisco: Jossey-Bass.

Stewart, A. J., & Healy, J. M. (1985). Personality and adaptation to change. In R.

Hogan & W. H. Jones (Eds.), *Perspectives in personality* (Vol. 1, pp. 117–144). Greenwich, CT: JAI Press.

Stewart, A. J., Sokol, M., Healy, J. M., & Chester, N. L. (1986). Longitudinal studies of psychological consequences in life changes in children and adults. *Journal of Personality and Social Psychology, 50,* 143–151.

Stewart, A. J., Sokol, M., Healy, J. M., Chester, N. L., & Weinstock-Savoy, D. (1982). Adaptation to life changes in children and adults: Cross-sectional studies. *Journal of Personality and Social Psychology, 43,* 1270–1281.

Stewart, A. J., & Winter, D. (1974). Self-definition and social definition in women. *Journal of Personality, 42,* 238–259.

Stifneos, P. E. (1973). The prevalence of "alexithymic" characteristics in psychosomatic patients. *Psychotherapy and Psychosomatics, 22,* 255–256.

Stovall, G., & Craig, R. J. (1990). Mental representations of physically and sexually abused latency-aged females. *Child Abuse and Neglect, 14,* 233–242.

Strober, M. (1979). The structuring of interpersonal relations in schizophrenic adolescents: A decentering analysis of Thematic Apperception Test stories. *Journal of Abnormal Child Psychology, 7,* 309–316.

Sugarman, A. (1980). The borderline personality organization as manifested on psychological tests. In Kwawer, J. S., Lerner, H. D., Lerner, P. M., & Sugarman, A. (Eds.), *Borderline phenomena and the Rorschach test* (pp. 39–57). New York: International Universities Press.

Sugarman, A., Bloom-Feshbach, S., & Bloom-Feshbach, J. (1980). The psychological dimensions of borderline adolescents. In J. S. Kwawer, H. D. Lerner, P. M. Lerner, & A. Sugarman (Eds.), *Borderline phenomena and the Rorschach test* (pp. 469–494). New York: International Universities Press.

Sullivan, H. S. (1953). *The interpersonal theory of psychiatry.* New York: Norton.

Sundberg, N. (1961). The practice of psychological testing in clinical services in the United States. *American Psychologist, 16,* 79–83.

Thompson, C. E. (1949). The Thompson modification of the Thematic Apperception Test. *Rorschach Research Exchange and Journal of Projective Techniques, 13,* 469–478.

Todd, J., Frindman, S., & Kariuki, P. W. (1990). Women growing stronger with age. *Psychology of Women Quarterly, 14,* 567–577.

Tomkins, S. (1947). *The Thematic Apperception Test.* New York: Grune & Stratton.

Tomkins, S. S. (1978). Script theory: Differential magnification of affects. In *Nebraska symposium on motivation* (Vol. 26, pp. 201–236). Lincoln: University of Nebraska Press.

Tomson, M. C., Asarnow, J. R., Goldstein, M. J., & Miklowitz, D. J. (1990). Thought disorder and communication problems in children with schizophrenia spectrum and depressive disorders and their parents. *Journal of Clinical Child Psychology, 19,* 159–168.

Triplett, S., & Brunson, P. (1982). TCB and TAT response characteristics in black males and females: A replication. *Journal of Non-White Concerns in Personnel and Guidance, 10,* 73–77.

Turner, C. W., Hesse, B. W., & Peterson-Lewis, S. (1986). Naturalistic studies of the long-term effects of television violence. *Journal of Social Issues, 42,* 53–73.

Uleman, J. S. (1966). *The new TAT measure of the need for power.* Unpublished doctoral dissertation, Harvard University, Cambridge, MA.

Uleman, J. S. (1972). The need for influence: development and validation of a measure, and comparison with the need for power. *Genetic Psychology Monographs, 85*, 157–214.

United States Office of Strategic Services. (1948). *Assessment of men.* New York: Rinehart.

Vaillant, G. E. (1971). Theoretical hierarchy of adaptive ego mechanisms. *Archives of General Psychiatry, 24*, 107–118.

Vaillant, G. E. (1977). *Adaptation to life.* Boston: Little, Brown.

Vane, J. R. (1981). The Thematic Apperception Test: A review. *Clinical Psychology Review, 1*, 319–336.

Veroff, J. (1957). Development and validation of a projective measure of power motivation. *Journal of Abnormal and Social Psychology, 54*, 1–8.

Veroff, J. (1961). Thematic apperception in a nationwide survey. In J. Kagan & G. S. Lesser (Eds.), *Contemporary issues in thematic apperceptive methods* (pp. 83–111). Springfield, IL: Charles C. Thomas.

Veroff, J. (1969). Social comparison and the development of achievement motivation. In C. P. Smith (Ed.), *Achievement-related motives in children* (pp. 46–101). New York: Russell Sage.

Veroff, J. (1977). Process vs. impact in men's and women's achievement motivation. *Psychology of Women Quarterly, 1*, 283–293.

Veroff, J. (1982). Assertive motivations: Achievement versus power. In A. J. Stewart (Ed.), *Motivation and society* (pp. 99–132). San Francisco: Jossey-Bass.

Veroff, J., Atkinson, J. W., Feld, S. C., & Gurin, G. (1960). The use of thematic apperception to assess motivation in a nationwide interview study. *Psychological Monographs, 74*(12, Whole No. 499), 1–32.

Veroff, J., Depner, C., Kulka, R., & Douvan, E. (1980). Comparison of American motives: 1957 vs. 1976. *Journal of Personality and Social Psychology, 39*, 1249–1262.

Veroff, J., & Douvan, E., & Kulka, A. (1981). *The inner American.* New York: Basic Books.

Veroff, J., & Feld, S. (1971). *Marriage and work in America: A study of motives and roles.* New York: Van Nostrand.

Veroff, J., McClelland, L., & Ruhland, D. (1975). Varieties of achievement motivation. In M. Mednick, S. Tangri, & L. Hoffman (Eds.), *Women and achievement* (pp. 172–205). Washington, DC: Hemisphere.

Veroff, J., Reuman, D., & Feld, S. (1984). Motives in American men and women across the adult life span. *Developmental Psychology, 20*, 1142–1158.

Veroff, J., & Veroff, J. B. (1972). Reconsideration of a measure of power motivation. *Psychological Bulletin, 78*, 279–291.

Vitz, P. C. (1990). The use of stories in moral development. New psychological reasons for an old education method. *American Psychologist, 45*, 709–720.

Vollhardt, B. R., Ackerman, S. H., & Shindledeckler, R. D. (1986). *Acta Psychiatrica Scandinavica, 74*, 73–79.

Wade, T. C., Baker, T. B., Morton, T. L., & Baker, L. J. (1978). The status of psychological testing in clinical psychology: Relationships between test use and professional activities and orientations. *Journal of Personality Assessment, 42,* 3-10.

Walker, E. L., & Atkinson, J. W. (1958). The expressional of fear-related motivation in thematic apperception as a function of proximity to an atomic explosion. In J. W. Atkinson (Ed.), *Motives in fantasy, action, and society* (pp. 143-159). New York: Van Nostrand.

Weinberger, J., & McClelland, D. C. (1990). Cognitive versus traditional motivational models. In E. T. Higgins & R. M. Sorrentino (Eds.), *Handbook of motivation and cognition* (Vol. 2, pp. 562-597). New York: Guilford Press.

Weiner, B. (1978). Achievement strivings. In H. London & J. E. Exner (Eds.), *Dimensions of personality* (pp. 1-36). New York: Wiley.

Weiner, B., Stone, A. J., Schmitz, M. D., Schmidt, A., Hernandez. A. C. R., & Benton, C. J. (1983). Compounding the errors: A reply to Pollak and Gilligan. *Journal of Personality and Social Psychology, 45,* 1176-1178.

Weisskopf-Joelson, E. A., & Foster, H. D. (1962). An experimental study of stimulus variation upon projection. *Journal of Projective Techniques, 26,* 366-370.

West, A., Martindale, C., Hines, D., & Roth, W. T. (1983). Marijuana-induced primary process content in the TAT. *Journal of Personality Assessment, 47,* 466-467.

Westen, D. (1991a). Social cognition and object relations. *Psychological Bulletin, 109,* 429-455.

Westen, D. (1991b). Clinical assessment of object relations using the TAT. *Journal of Personality Assessment, 56,* 56-74.

Westen, D. (1993). *Social cognition and object relations scale: Q-sort for projective stories (SCORS-Q).* Unpublished manuscript, Department of Psychiatry, Cambridge Hospital and Harvard Medical School, Cambridge, MA.

Westen, D. (1995). *Revision of social cognition and object relations scale: Q-sort for projective stories (SCORS-Q).* Unpublished manuscript, Department of Psychiatry, Cambridge Hospital and Harvard Medical School, Cambridge, MA.

Westen, D., Klepser, J., Ruffins, S. A., Silverman, M., Lifton, N., & Boekamp, J. (1991). Object relations in childhood and adolescence: The development of working representations. *Journal of Consulting and Clinical Psychology, 59,* 400-409.

Westen, D., Lohr, N. E., Silk, K., Gold, L., & Kerber, K. (1990). Object relations and social cognition in borderlines, major depressives, and normals: A thematic apperception test analysis. *Psychological Assessment: A Journal of Consulting and Clinical Psychology, 2,* 355-364.

Westen, D., Lohr, N., Silk, K., & Kerber, D. (1985). *Measuring object relations and social cognition using the TAT: Scoring manual.* Unpublished manuscript, University of Michigan, Ann Arbor, MI.

Westen, D., Ludolph, P., Block, J., Wixom, J., & Wiss, F. C. (1990). Developmental history and object relations in psychiatrically disturbed adolescent girls. *American Journal of Psychiatry, 147,* 1061-1068.

Westen, D., Ludolph, P., Lerner, H., Ruffins, S., & Wiss, C. (1990). Object relations in borderline adolescents. *Journal of the American Academy of Child and Adolescent Psychiatry, 29,* 338-348.

Westen, D., Ludolph, P., Silk, K., Kellam, A., Gold, L. & Lohr, N. (1990). Object relations in borderline adolescents and adults: Developmental differences. *Adolescent Psychiatry, 17,* 360–384.

Williams, E. L., & Manaster, G. J. (1990). Restricter anorexia, bulimic anorexia, and bulimic women's early recollection and the Thematic Apperception Test response. *Individual Psychology, 46,* 93–107.

Wilsnack, S. C. (1974). The effects of social drinking on women's fantasy. *Journal of Personality, 12,* 43–61.

Wilson, A., Passik, S. D., Faude, J., Abrams, J., & Gordon, E. (1989). A hierarchical model of opiate addition: Failures of self-regulation as a central aspect of substance abuse. *Journal of Nervous and Mental Disease, 177,* 390–399.

Winter, D. G. (1967). *Power motivation in thought and action.* Unpublished doctoral dissertation, Harvard University, Cambridge, MA.

Winter, D. G. (1972). The need for power in college men: Action correlates and relationship to drinking. In D. C. McClelland, W. N. Davis, R. Kalin, & E. Wanner (Eds.), *The drinking man* (pp. 99–119). New York: Free Press.

Winter, D. G. (1973). *The power motive.* New York: Free Press.

Winter, D. G. (1982). Motivation and performance in presidential candidates. In A. J. Stewart (Ed.), *Motivation and society* (pp. 244–273). San Francisco: Jossey-Bass.

Winter, D. G. (1988). The power motive in women—and men. *Journal of Personality and Social Psychology, 54,* 510–519.

Winter, D. G., & Barenbaum, N. B. (1985). Responsibility and the power motive in women and men. *Journal of Personality, 53,* 335–355.

Winter, D. G., & Stewart, A. J. (1977). Power motive reliability as a function of retest instructions. *Journal of Consulting and Clinical Psychology, 45,* 436–440.

Winter, D. G., & Stewart, A. J. (1978). The power motive. In H. London & J. E. Exner (Eds.), *Dimensions of personality* (pp. 391–447). New York: Wiley.

Winter, D. G., Stewart, A. J., McClelland, D. C. (1977). Husband's motives and wife's career level. *Journal of Personality and Social Psychology, 35,* 159–166.

Winter, S. K. (1966). *Being orientation in maternal fantasy: A content analysis of the TATs of nursing mothers.* Unpublished doctoral dissertation, Harvard University, Cambridge, MA.

Winter, S. K. (1969). Characteristics of fantasy while nursing. *Journal of Personality, 37,* 58–72.

Wolk, R. L., & Wolk, R. B. (1971). *The Gerontological Apperception Test.* New York: Behavioral Publications.

Wolpe, J., & Rachman, S. (1960). Psychoanalytic "evidence." A critique based on Freud's case of Little Hans. *Journal of Nervous and Mental Disease, 130,* 135–148.

Worchel, F. T., Aaron, L. L., & Yates, D. F. (1990). Gender bias on the Thematic Apperception Test. *Journal of Personality Assessment, 55,* 593–602.

Wyatt, F. (1947). The scoring and analysis of the Thematic Apperception Test. *Journal of Psychology, 24,* 319–330.

Wyatt, F. (1986). The narrative in psychoanalysis: Psychoanalytic notes on storytelling, listening, and interpreting. In T. R. Sarbin (Ed.), *Narrative psychology: The storied nature of human conduct* (pp. 193–210). New York: Praeger.

Wynne, L. C., & Singer, M. T. (1964). Thought disorder and the family relations of schizophrenics. A research strategy. *Archives of General Psychiatry, 9,* 191–198.

Zeldow, P. B., & McAdams, D. P. (1993). On the comparison of TAT and free speech techniques in personality assessment. *Journal of Personality, 60,* 181–185.

Zubin, J., Eron, L. D., Schumer, F. (1965). *An experimental approach to projective techniques.* New York: Wiley.

Index

"Aboriginal world," 23, 24
Abstraction, drug use and, 305
Abuse, 306–308
"Achievement doubter," 218
Achievement motivation
  children, 205, 206, 209
  coding scheme, 31–32
  cue value of picture and, 238
  developmental differences, in
    adults, 210–215
  job satisfaction and, 259
  McClelland–Atkinson research
    strategy and, 271, 273–275
  predictive validity, 259
  TAT measures, longitudinal stud-
    ies, 222–227
Action, landscape of, 33–34
Active mastery, 217, 218, 219, 293
Adaptation, stages, 222
Adaptive conformer style, 218
Adolescents
  achievement motivation, 226
  power motivation, 225
  psychopathology, 313–317, 321
    borderline personality disorder,
      174, 316
    schizophrenia, 317
  TAT stories, identification process
    in, 191–195
Aeneid, 3

Affect-Tone of Relationship Schemas
  scale, 167, 168, 173
Affiliation motivation
  developmental differences, in
    adults, 210–215
  immunosuppression and, 299, 300
  McClelland–Atkinson research
    strategy, 275–277
  TAT measures, longitudinal stud-
    ies, 222–227
African-Americans
  with attention deficit disorder, 317
  cards for, 240–242
  Tell-Me-A-Story study, 242–246
Age
  of children
    defense mechanism usage and,
      195–198
    differences in TAT responses
      and, 180–181
  communication deviance and, 311–
    312
  shift in perceived power of women,
    216–217
Agency, 130
Aggression
  abusive mothers and, 308
  projection, 201
  theme, card pulls for, 234
  toward self, 72

Alcohol use, 302–305
Alexithymia, 297–298
Alzheimer's disease, 313
Ambivalence, 115
Anaclitic personality
    in borderline personality disorder,
        159, 160–161
    clinical examples, 134–140
    defense mechanisms, 149–151
    depression and, 132
    deprivation/enhancement assess-
        ment, 146–147
Anal preoccupation, 286, 287
Anorexia, 298
Anxiety
    castration, 290–291
    denial defense for, 201
    from storytelling situation, 84–85
Arthritis, 296–297
Ascension–decension cycle, 73
Attention deficit disorder, 317
Autobiographical material
    in college student case studies, 51–
        52, 54–56, 59–61, 63–64
        TAT stories of, 52–54, 56–59, 61–
            63
    of hospitalized psychiatric patient,
        103–106, 126
    as narrative theme, 77, 126, 320
    similarities with fantasies, 64–66
Avoidance, 108, 136

B

Beck Depression Inventory, 306
Behaviorism, logicoscientific thought
    and, 21–22
Bhagavadgita, 3
Books, as source for fantasy material,
    10
Borderline personality disorder
    (BPD). See also Narcissistic per-
    sonality disorder
    in adolescents, 316
    anaclitic personality in, 160–161
    boundary disturbances, 158
    defense mechanisms
        projective identification, 163–166
        splitting, 162–163
    diagnostic characteristics, 156–157

differential diagnosis, 173–174
    etiology, 157
    interpretative perspective
        of Sugarman, 158–166
        of Westen, 166–174
    pre-oedipal aggression in, 161
    verbalizations, peculiar, 161–162
Boundary disturbances, in border-
    line personality disorder, 158
BPD. See Borderline personality dis-
    order (BPD)
Bulimia, 298

C

California Psychological Inventory
    (CPI), 225
Cancer, 298
Capacity for Emotional Investment
    in Relationships and Moral
    Standards, 167, 168
Cards
    choice of, 233
    heterogeneity of, 252–253
    number of themes elicited by, 235–
        236
    pictures on, 29
        as context, 41–42, 49
        cue value of, 238–240
        pull of, 42
            cue value of picture and, 238–
                240
        defined, 234
        gender differences in, 236–237
        normative studies, 234–236
    for research studies, 240
    special
        for minority groups, 240–246
        for research, 240
    types of, 13
Castration anxiety, 290–291
CAT (Children's Apperception Test),
    88, 179–180
Children
    achievement motivation, 205
    defense mechanisms
        cross-sectional studies of, 195–
            198
        longitudinal studies of, 198–203
    development of. See Development

emotional stance, 209
gender identity
    cross-sectional studies, 182–185
    deprivation/enhancement measure for, 181–182
    importance of stories for, 4
    media and, 4–5
    object relations, 203–205
    psychopathology in, 313–317, 321
    use of TAT with, 179–180
Children's Apperception Test (CAT), 88, 179–180
Closure problems, 309
Coding schemes, 31–32
Cohort effects, 212–213
College students
    assessment of defense mechanisms, 93, 94–99
    case studies, of life story narrative, 50–64
    educational transition, emotional stance during, 207–208
    gender identity assessment, examples of, 76–80
    TAT stories, narcissism in, 175–176
Communication deviance, 309–312
Communion, 130
Complexity of Representations of People scale, 167, 168, 173
Compulsive defenses, 112
Consciousness, landscape of, 33
Constructions
    narrative, 25, 35
    of reality, 24
    vs. interpretation, 24
Context
    change, interpretation and, 37–39
    clinical, story as comment on, 47–49
    components of, 30
    interpretation and, 29–30
    in motivational narrative, 32
    perspectives, 39–43
    research, story as comment on, 43–47
    TAT pictures as, 41–42
CPI (California Psychological Inventory), 225
Criticism
    defense mechanisms for, 93
    effect on storytelling, 46–47

Cronbach's alpha, 256
Cross-sectional studies
    of children, gender identity in, 182–185
    of children, defense mechanisms in, 195–198
Culture, identity of, 4

D

Daughters, rebellious, 218
Day residue, 43
Defense Mechanism Inventory, 82
Defense mechanisms. See also specific defense mechanisms
    anaclitic personality, 149–151
    assessment, 320
        in college studies, 93, 94–99
        in psychiatric patients, 99–100
    in borderline personality disorder, 157
        projective identification, 163–166
        splitting, 162–163
    of children, 208
        cross-sectional studies of, 195–198
        developmental history of, 189–195
        longitudinal studies of, 198–203
    components of, 190
    definition of, 87
    functioning of, 85
    of hospitalized psychiatric patients, 118–119, 124, 129
    introjective personality, 149–151
    mature, 86
    measure of, 82
    in normal psychological development, 86–87
    personality organizations and, 131
    research studies using TAT, 91–94
    TAT coding system for, 88–91
    TAT stories and, 87–91
Defensive principle, 260–261
Demeter, myth of, 71, 74
Denial
    anaclitic personality and, 135, 137, 150
    interpersonal relatedness and, 131–132

Denial *(cont.)*
  research studies using TAT, 91–94
  usage, 87
    assessment criteria for, 88–91
    in borderline personality disor-
        der, 159
    by children, 86, 190–191, 201–
        202
    by college student, 95–99
    by hospitalized psychiatric pa-
        tient, 118–119
Dependence themes, card pull and,
    235
Depersonalized conformer style,
    218
Depression
  anaclitic. *See* Anaclitic personality
  hospitalization for, 312–313
  introjective, 132
  theme, card pulls for, 234
Deprivation/enhancement (D/E) as-
    sessment
  of anaclitic personality, 146–147
  deprivation followed by enhance-
      ment, 71–72
  enhancement followed by depriva-
      tion, 31, 71, 72
  of gender identity, 42, 148–149,
      320
    in children, 181–182
    cross-sectional studies in chil-
        dren, 182–185
    examples of, 76–80
    longitudinal studies in children,
        186–189
    research studies of, 80–83
  of hospitalized psychiatric patients,
      129
Deprivation units, for TAT scoring,
    74–75
Development
  adult differences, 320
    ego energy, 221
    ego mastery styles, 217–221
    emotional stance, 221–222
    in male/female personality trait
        attribution, 216–217
    in TAT stories, 210–229
  childhood differences
    in achievement motivation, 205,
        206, 209
    in emotional stance, 209

  in object relations level, 208–209
  in TAT responses, 180–181
  in TAT stories, 180–181
  emotional stance, 205–208
  hierarchy, for defense mecha-
      nisms, 195–198
  object relations, 203–205
  TAT study
    of achievement motivation, 205
    of defense mechanisms, 189–203
    of emotional stance, 205–208
    of gender identity, 181–189
    of object relations, 203–205
Diabetes, 297
Dialogue, narrative interpretation
    as, 26–27
Disintegration, 120
Disorganization, 120
Disruptive behavior, 309
Domestic violence, 308
Dominance–independence, abusive
    mothers and, 308
Dominance–submissiveness contin-
    uum, 216
Dreams
  analysis of, 38
  interpretation of, 43
  similarity with stories, 42
Drive, 21–22
Drive expression, card pull and, 235
Drug use, 305–306
Duodenal ulcer, 297
Dynamics-of-action theory, 266–268

E

Eating disorders, 298
Educational transitions, emotional
    stance during, 205–208
Ego mastery
  active, 217, 218, 219, 293
  age-related changes in adults, 217–
      221
  magical, 217, 218, 219, 293, 294
  passive, 217, 218, 219, 293–294
  styles, scoring system for, 293–294
Emotional stance
  in adaptation, 286–288
  developmental differences
    in adults, 221–222
    in children, 205–208, 209

Emotions
  inhibited, in borderline personality
    disorder, 158–159
  as myth focus, 71–72
Empty nest syndrome, 220–221
Enhancement. *See* Deprivation/en-
    hancement assessment
Enhancement units, for TAT scoring,
    74–75
Equivalent forms, reliability and, 256
Escape theme, 199–200, 202
Ethnic groups. *See* Minority subjects;
    specific ethnic groups
Explorations in Personality, Murray,
    11–13

F

Failure experiences, age-appropriate
    defenses for, 92–93
False recognition paradigm, 262–263
Family
  relationships
    in schizophrenia, 312
    theme of, 127–128
    themes, card pulls for, 234
  as source for fantasy material, 10
Fantasy/fantasies
  ascension–decension cycle, 73
  classification, conceptual scheme
    for, 11
  patterns
    deprivation followed by enhance-
      ment, 71–72
    enhancement followed by depri-
      vation, 71, 72
    theoretical bases for, 72–73
  personal, 88–89
  shared by whole culture, 70–71
  sources for, 10
  to study gender identity, 70–72
  violent/aggressive, alcohol use
    and, 303
Feeling tone differences, 242
Females. *See also* Gender differences;
    Gender identity
  achievement motivation, 211–212,
    224–225, 227–228
  active mastery, 218
  affiliation motivation, 211–212,
    224–225, 227

alcohol use, power motivation and,
    303–305
anaclitic personality configuration,
    134–137
deprivation followed by enhance-
    ment pattern, 71–73
ego mastery styles, life-span devel-
    opmental differences in, 220
introjective, 143–145
passive mastery in, 218
perceived power, shift in, 216–217
personality traits, attribution of,
    216–217
self-defined, 227, 228–229
social definition of, 227, 228–229
Feminine masochism, 72–73
Feminine mystique, 213
Food deprivation, TAT story themes
    and, 271–272
Future-time perspective, 241

G

Gender congruence/incongruence,
    145–149
Gender differences
  in achievement motivation, 211
  card pull and, 236–237
  in intimacy, 215
Gender identity
  assessment of, 40–42, 73–75
    examples of, 76–80
    in hospitalized psychiatric pa-
      tient, 119
  in children, 208
    cross-sectional studies, 182–185
    deprivation/enhancement meas-
      ure for, 181–182
  deprivation/enhancement assess-
    ment, 42, 148–149, 181182,
    320
  cross-sectional studies in chil-
    dren, 182–185
  examples of, 76–80
  longitudinal studies in children,
    186–189
  research studies of, 80–83
  fantasy patterns, theoretical bases
    for, 72–73
  of hospitalized psychiatric patients,
    124, 129

Gender identity *(cont.)*
  intensity of pattern, 82
  narrative and, 70–72
  in psychiatric population, 82–83
  TAT measurement, gender congruence/incongruence and, 145–149
  using deprivation/enhancement narrative, research studies of, 80–83
Gender roles, 45
Genital preoccupation, 286, 287
Genotype, 266
Gratification, 126, 128–129, 138–139
Greek mythology, 71–72
Guilt, sexual, 289

H

Health problems, 295–298
Helplessness, 104, 136
Hermeneutics, 25
Hispanics
  with attention deficit disorder, 317
  storytelling procedure for, 242–246
Historical truth, 22–26, 28
Homosexual theme, card pulls for, 234
Hunger motivation, TAT story themes and, 271–272
Hypertension, 296
Hysterical personality disorder, gender identity and, 83

I

Icarus, myth of, 71, 74
Identification
  anaclitic/introjective personality and, 151
  primitive precursor of, 195
  research studies using TAT, 91–94
  secondary, 192–194
  usage
    assessment criteria for, 88–91
    by children, 191–195, 202–203
    by college student, 95–99
    by hospitalized psychiatric patient, 118–119

Identifiers of salience, principle, 67
Identity
  of culture, 4
  individual, 4
  narrative of, 38
Iliad, 3
Imagery, sexual, 288–289
Immune system, suppression, motives and, 298–302
Immunoglobulin, secretory, 300
Implicit motives, vs. self-attributed motives, 265–266
Incorporation, 195
Independence themes, card pull and, 235
Inhibited power motive syndrome, 296, 299
Integration/organization, drug use and, 305
Intentions, 33–34
Internal consistency, 256–258, 262
Internalization, of adult standards, 192
Interpersonal relatedness. *See* Anaclitic personality
Interpretation
  context. *See* Context
  as dialogue, 26–27
  of dreams, 43
  falsification criterion, 26
  good, 34
  as means to future effects, 26
  mechanical, 33
  of narrative truth, 24
  perspectives, 39–41, 49
    choice of, 41
    multiple, 25, 37–39, 49
    for narcissism, 174–176
  subjective, 40–41
  verification of, 25–27, 34
  vs. construction, 24
Interpreter
  intention of, 33–34
  narrative of, 37
    changes in, 38–39, 40
    influence of storyteller narrative on, 32–33
    story lines from, 31
    storyteller narrative and, 30–31
  perspective of, 42, 49
  role of, 37
  story comprehension and, 30
Interrater reliability, 250–252

Intimacy motivation
  in autobiographical material, 65
  developmental differences, in
    adults, 210–215
  gender differences in, 215
  longitudinal study, 228
  McClelland–Atkinson research
    strategy and, 277–279
  themes of, 65–66
Introjection, 135, 138, 147–148
Introjective personality, 151–152
  clinical examples, 141–145
  defense mechanisms, 149–151
  development of, 135
IQ, defense mechanisms and, 86
Irritable colon syndrome, 297
Isolation, interpersonal, 122–123

J

Job performance, 223
Job satisfaction, achievement motiva-
    tion and, 259

L

Landscapes, story, 33
Leadership motive pattern (LMP),
    222, 223
Life experiences, peak, 64–66
Life history
  similarities, in TAT story
    script theory and, 66–69
    unity theme and, 66
  of storyteller, 41
  in TAT stories, 39–40
Life story, narrative as root meta-
    phor for, 36–37
Linguistic context, 29–30
Listening, with narrative sensitivity,
    28, 33
Little Hans, 38
Locus of control, card pull and,
    235
Logicoscientific thought
  behaviorism and, 21–22
  goals of, 22
Longitudinal studies
  achievement motivation, 222–227
  affiliation motivation, 222–227

of children, gender identity in,
    186–189
of children, defense mechanisms
    in, 198–203
power motivation, 222–227

M

McClelland–Atkinson research strat-
    egy, 320
  development of, 271–272
  for emotional stances in adapta-
    tion process, 286–288
  examples of, 273–285
    achievement motivation, 273–275
    affiliation motivation, 275–277
    intimacy motivation, 277–279
    power motivation, 280–285
    responsibility, 283–285
  prime tests, 273, 274, 276, 279, 282
  scoring
    subcategories, 273, 274, 276,
      279, 282
    system development, 272–273
Magical mastery, 217, 218, 219, 293,
    294
Major depressive disorder, vs. border-
    line personality disorder, 173
Male–female relations, 45
Male personality traits, attribution
    of, 216–217
Males. See also Gender differences;
    Gender identity
  abusive, 308
  active mastery, 218
  alcohol use, power motivation and,
    302–303, 305
  anaclitic personality configuration,
    137–140
  enhancement followed by depriva-
    tion pattern, 71, 72
    theoretical bases for, 72–73
  introjective, 141–143
  magical mastery in, 218
  passive mastery in, 218
Marijuana, 305–306
Martyrdom, 72
Masculine sexual identity, 194–195
Masochism
  feminine, 72–73
  moral, 72–73

Maternal altruist style, 218
Matriarchs, moralistic, 218
Meaning
   as constructed, 28
   observer's system of interpretation
      and, 21–22
Means–end sets, 67–68
Media
   children and, 4–5
   as source for fantasy material, 10
Memories
   autobiographical, TAT motive
      strength and, 65–66
   coding of, 65
Men. See Males
Minority subjects, TAT card selec-
   tion and, 233, 240–246, 249. See
   also specific minorities
Moral masochism, 72–73
Motivational narrative, 32
Motivational perspective, 40
Motivational themes, life history of
   storyteller and, 65
Motives
   assessment, 320
   implicit vs. self-attributed, 265–266
   suppression of immune function
      and, 298–302
Movies, as fantasy material source, 4–
   5, 10
Multiple perspectives, 30–33

N

Narcissistic personality disorder,
   174–176
Narratives
   alternative, to explain same data,
      38–39
   as comment on clinical context,
      47–49
   as comment on research context,
      43–47
   concepts of, 36–37
   construction of, 4, 21–25
   defense mechanisms and, 87–91
   developmental differences in
      adults, 210–229
   dialogue nature of, 49
   explanations, 39
   gender identity and, 70–72

gender identity assessment, 83
   research studies of, 80–83
gender-related differences, scoring
   criteria for, 74–75
goals of, 23
identifying scripts in, 40
of identity, 38
importance, for children, 4
interpretation. See Interpretation
of interpreter. See Interpreter, narrative of
length of, 233–234, 246–249
life history in, 39–40
meaning of, 28–29
normative, card pull and, 234–236
of observer/interpreter, 37
patterns in, 31
peak life experiences and, 64–66
in psychoanalysis, 37–39
psychological meaning, interpreter
   narrative and, 40
reality, vs. historical reality, 23–25
role shifts in, 44–45
sensitivity, 28, 33
shifting, in storyteller, 38
similarities with dreams, 43
social science interest in, 6
as storyteller's life story, 50
TAT and, 27–35
themes in, 39–40
true-to-life representation of experience and, 23
as unique, individual expression, 5
unity thema and, 66
Native Americans, cards for, 240
Need, 11
Neuroses, 312–313
Nuclear scene, 68–69

O

Object relations
   in abuse, 306–307
   assessment, 320
   of children, 203–205, 208–209
   disordered, in borderline personal-
      ity disorder, 160
   disturbances in, 157
Obsessional defenses, 112, 141
Obsessive–compulsive disorder, 83,
   112

Odyssey, 3
Operant measures, vs. respondent measures, 263–265
Optimism, 81, 235
Oral preoccupation, 286, 287
Outcome, 11
Overexaggeration, 88
Overstimulation, 120, 160

P

Paradigmatic thought. *See* Logicos-cientific thought
Parent–child themes, card pulls for, 234
Parents
  abusive, 307
  emotional stance development and, 222
  of hospitalized schizophrenics, 310
  of schizophrenics vs. manic patients, 310–311
Passive–aggressive defense, 45
Passive aggressor, 218
Passive mastery, 217, 218, 219, 293–294
Passivity theme
  changes over course of treatment, 112–117
  in hospitalized psychiatric patient, 108–109
Peer variables of status, 260
Perceptions, peculiar, 309
Perfection, wished for, 175
Persephone, myth of, 71, 74
Persecution, 112
Personal experiences, as sources for fantasy material, 10
Personality
  anaclitic. *See* Anaclitic personality
  changes, age-related in adults, 217–221
  development, personality organization and, 131
  disorders. *See specific personality disorders*
  introjective. *See* Introjective personality
  male/female traits, attribution of, 216–217

operant vs. respondent measures of, 264–265
  organization, 130–133
  patterns, as TAT story themes, 39–40
  structure, scenes and, 66
Personality Research Form (PRF), 266
Personalized power, 302
Pessimism, 81, 235
Phaethon, myth of, 71, 74
Phallic preoccupation, 286, 287
Phenotype, 266
Pivotal incident, 74
Plot of a life, 66
Power motivation
  alcohol use and, 302
  in autobiographical material, 65
  developmental differences, in adults, 210–215
  fantasy measures of, 265
  immunosuppression and, 299, 300
  McClelland–Atkinson research strategy and, 280–285
  in narcissistic personality disorder, 175
  TAT measures, longitudinal studies, 222–227
  test–retest reliability, 253–254
  themes of, 65–66
Pre-oedipal aggression, 161
Press, 11
Pride, 71
Projection
  description of, 87
  developmental differences in, 86
  research studies using TAT, 91–94
  usage
    assessment criteria for, 88–91
    by children, 191, 196, 198–199, 201–202
    by college student, 95–99
    by hospitalized psychiatric patient, 118–119
Projective hypothesis, 14–15, 39
Projective tests, 69, 179
Propositional thought. *See* Logicos-cientific thought
Psychiatric patients, hospitalized
  autobiographical material, 103–106
  defense mechanisms of, 99–100, 118–119, 129

Psychiatric patients, hospitalized
  (cont.)
  gender identity assessment, 119
  gender identity of, 119, 129
  initial TAT stories, 106–109, 120–
    124
  treatment course
    TAT stories and, 124–129
    TAT story changes and, 109–119
Psychoanalysis, narrative in, 37–39
Psychoanalytic theory
  dreams and, 42–43
Psychological differentiation, 128
Psychometric approaches. See also
    Thematic Apperception Test
    (TAT)
  contemporary, 263–268
  traditional
    problems with, 262–263
    reliability of, 250–258
Psychopathology. See also specific psy-
    chopathologic disorders
  assessment in TAT stories, 176
  in children/adolescents, 313–317
  diagnosis, 153
Psychoses
  childhood, 313–314
  communication deviance in, 309–
    312
Psychosexual development, 286–288

R

Racial groups. See Minority subjects;
    specific racial groups
Reality. See also Truth
  logicoscientific thought and, 22
  narrative vs. historical, 23–25
  perception, 312
  personal constructions and, 24
Refractory phase, 254–255, 257
Regression analysis, story length,
    248–249
Regression theme, 108–109, 113, 117
Reliability
  defined, 250
  equivalent forms, 251, 256
  internal consistency, 251, 256–258
  interrater, 250–252
  measurement approaches, 252–253
  split-half, 251, 256

test–retest, 251, 253–256
  of traditional psychometric ap-
    proaches, 250–258
  problems with, 262–263
Repression, 132
Research. See also McClelland–Atkin-
    son research strategy
  card pull, 233, 234–240, 249
  clinical
    alcohol use, 302–305
    drug use, 305–306
    motives, suppression of immune
      function and, 298–302
    physical health/illness, 295–298
    psychopathology in chil-
      dren/adolescents, 313–317
    psychoses, 309–313
    sexual abuse, 306–308
  context, story as comment on, 43–
    47
  on defense mechanisms, 91–94
  length of TAT story, 233–234
  minority subject, 233, 240–246, 249
  psychoanalytic theory approaches,
    285–294
  SCORS measure studies, 172–174
  special cards for, 240–246
  story length, 246
    adjustment tables for, 247
    percentage scores, 247
    regression analysis, 248–249
    relative scores, 247–248
Respondent measures, vs. operant
    measures, 263–265
Responsibility
  attribution of, 114
  measurement, McClelland–Atkin-
    son research strategy for, 283–
    285
Reversal, 88
Root fantasies, 252

S

Salience, principles of, 67
Sawtooth effect (refractory phase),
    254–255, 257
Scale for Failures of Self-Regulation
    (SFSR), 306
Schizoaffective disorder, case study
    of, 120–129

Schizophrenia
  in adolescents, 317
  differential diagnosis, 312
Scholastic Aptitude Test (SAT), 257
School transitions, emotional stance
    during, 205–208
Schreber case, 38
Scripts, 40
Script theory, 66–69
Secretory immunoglobulin, 300
Self-attributed motives, vs. implicit
    motives, 265–266
Self-concept, 31
Self-definition
  introjective personality and, 131–
    133, 144–145
  themes, 138
  vs. social definition, 291–292
  of women, 227, 228–229
Self-direction, in borderline personal-
    ity disorder, 159
Self-disclosure, anxiety about, 85
Self-esteem maintenance, defense
    mechanisms and, 92
Self-narrative, changes in, 38
Self-observation, 110
Self-reflection, 110, 115
Self-report questionnaires, 263–264,
    266
Self-revelation, in storytelling, 5
Sensitivity, narrative, 28, 33
Sexual abuse, 306–308
Sexual concerns assessment, 288–
    291
Sexual identity. See Gender identity
Social Cognition and Object Rela-
    tions Scale (SCORS), 203, 307
  assessment example, for border-
    line personality disorder, 170–
    172
  correlation of scales, 169
  description of, 167, 168
  Q-sort procedure, 169–171
  research studies, 172–174
Social definition
  vs. self-definition, 291–292
  of women, 227, 228–229
Social learning theory, 72–73
Sources, for fantasy material, 10
Split-half reliability, 256
Splitting, in borderline personality
    disorder, 157, 162–163

Stimulus cards, TAT, 13
Story/stories. See Narratives
Story interpreter. See Interpreter
Story lines. See also Themes
  multiple, 30–31
  repetition of, 31
  revision of, 33
  self representation and, 27, 40
  in storyteller constructions, 28
Storyteller
  attitude/feelings of, 45
  constructions, story line in, 28–29
  emotionally relevant themes, card
    pull and, 235
  hesitation of, 84–85
  life history of, 41
  life themes, case studies of, 50–64
  narrative, shifting of, 38
  personal context of, 29
  story comprehension and, 30
Storytelling. See also Thematic Apper-
    ception Test (TAT)
  as communication, 36
  to construct meaning, 3–4
  in human history, 3
  in personality determination, 9
  refusal, 5–6
  ridicule/denigration in, 85
  self-revelation in, 5
Stress, physical illness and, 298–302
Stressed power motivation, 299
Strong Vocational Interest Blank
    (SVIB), 226
Substitutive principle, 260–261
Symbolism, 113, 141

T

TAT. See Thematic Apperception
    Test (TAT)
Television, 4–5
Tell Me A Story (TEMAS), 242–246
Test–retest reliability, 253–256
Thematic Apperception Test (TAT),
    6. See also specific aspects of
  administration method, 14
  cards. See Cards
  clinicians' use of previous books
    on, 16–17
  coding system, for defense mecha-
    nisms, 88–91

Thematic Apperception Test (TAT)
    (cont.)
    development of, 9–13
        first version of, 10
        historical aspects, 9–13, 270
    instructional variables, 261–262
    methodological improvements,
        319–320
    number of test items, 257
    previous books on, 15–16
    projective hypothesis, 14–15
    stories. See Narratives
    vs. Children's Apperception Test,
        179–180
Thematic lines, 40
Themes. See also specific themes; Story
    lines
    core, 5
    number elicited by cards, 235–
        236
    personality patterns/life histories
        and, 39
    recurring, 67
Themes Concerning Blacks (TCB),
    241–242
Thought
    modes of, 21–23
    processes, in defense mechanisms,
        87
    qualitative and formal aspects of,
        153–156
Treatment
    context, story as comment on, 47–9
    course, TAT story changes and,
        109–119, 124–129
True-score measurement model, 268,
    269
Truth. See also Reality
    artistic, 26
    historical, 22–26, 28
    narrative, 23–25

U

Ulcerative colitis, 297
Uncertainty, feelings of, 175
Unconscious material, 10–11
Understanding of Social Causality,
    167, 168
Unity thema, 66

V

Validity
    context and, 41
    measurement approaches, 258–
        262, 268–269
    of respondent measures, 264
    of TAT measures, 93
Verbalizations, peculiar
    in borderline personality disorder,
        161–162, 165
    of hospitalized psychiatric patients,
        120–123
    in psychoses, 309
Verification, of interpretation, 25–
    27, 34
Violent imagery, gender differences
    in, 237

W

Weakness, fear of. See Power motiva-
    tion
Wish fulfillment, 43
Women. See Females
Words
    counting of, 33
    linguistic context of, 29–30